Recent Results in Cancer Research

Volume 198

More information about this series at http://www.springer.com/series/392

Michael Baumann · Mechthild Krause
Nils Cordes
Editors

Molecular Radio-Oncology

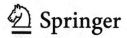 Springer

Editors
Michael Baumann
Department of Radiation Oncology
Faculty of Medicine and University Hospital
  Carl Gustav Carus, Technische
  Universität Dresden
Dresden
Germany

Nils Cordes
Department of Radiation Oncology
Faculty of Medicine and University Hospital
  Carl Gustav Carus, Technische
  Universität Dresden
Dresden
Germany

Mechthild Krause
Department of Radiation Oncology
Faculty of Medicine and University Hospital
  Carl Gustav Carus, Technische
  Universität Dresden
Dresden
Germany

ISSN 0080-0015   ISSN 2197-6767   (electronic)
Recent Results in Cancer Research
ISBN 978-3-662-57020-3   ISBN 978-3-662-49651-0   (eBook)
DOI 10.1007/978-3-662-49651-0

This Springer imprint is published by Springer Nature
The registered company is Springer-Verlag GmbH Berlin Heidelberg

Preface

This textbook on *Molecular Radio-Oncology* is targeting physicians and preclinical researchers with interest in translational radiation oncology.

The first part of the book takes up current knowledge about important molecular radiobiological mechanisms and preclinical investigations on target identification and personalization for combined treatments, DNA repair, and cancer stem cells.

In the second part, potential biomarkers for personalized radiation oncology are described from their preclinical basis to translational and clinical data. The epidermal growth factor receptor (EGFR) and tumor hypoxia are examples of long-identified biomarkers that over time have been used as both prognostic markers and targets for combined treatments. Human papillomavirus infections are increasingly evident in different tumor entities, have been shown to determine prognosis of the patients, and are currently tested as basis for interventions in clinical trials.

The third part of the book refers to the utilization of radiobiological knowledge for the application of molecular imaging techniques in radiation oncology. Fluoro-deoxyglucose (FDG) is the most widely used tracer for positron emission tomography (PET) and indicates not only active tumor tissue with an often higher sensitivity compared to standard sectional imaging techniques, but has also prognostic value for the outcome of radiotherapy. 18F-Misonidazole PET is described as an example of bioimaging of a factor of radioresistance—under the view of utilization as a biomarker for the outcome of radiotherapy as well as of automatic contouring methods for reproducible evaluation.

All chapters are authored by eminent researchers and physicians in the respective fields with a broad experience in preclinical and clinical radiation oncology and long-term teaching experiences who have put a focus on clarity and comprehensiveness of the content of the different chapters.

Michael Baumann
Mechthild Krause
Nils Cordes

Contents

About the Editors

Michael Baumann is a professor of Radiation Oncology and chairman of OncoRay and of the Department of Radiation Oncology at the University Hospital Dresden. His research focus is on preclinical and clinical studies for personalized radiation oncology.

Mechthild Krause is a professor of Translational Radiation Oncology at the German Cancer Consortium (DKTK), Dresden, and the German Cancer Research Center (DKFZ), Heidelberg. Her research focus is on biological individualization of radiotherapy translational and clinical studies.

Nils Cordes is a professor of Molecular Radiobiology at the OncoRay—National Center for Radiation Research in Oncology, Dresden, Germany. His research focus is on interaction of tumor cells with tissue and on preclinical molecular targeting approaches in combination with irradiation.

All three editors are in addition associated with the Helmholtz-Zentrum Dresden-Rossendorf, where radiopharmacy, physics, biology, and clinical research are jointly performed for the improvement of radiooncological patient treatment.

DNA Repair

Kerstin Borgmann, Sabrina Köcher, Malte Kriegs,
Wael Yassin Mansour, Ann Christin Parplys,
Thorsten Rieckmann and Kai Rothkamm

Abstract

Cellular chromosomal DNA is the principal target through which ionising radiation exerts it diverse biological effects. This chapter summarises the relevant DNA damage signalling and repair pathways used by normal and tumour cells in response to irradiation. Strategies for tumour radiosensitisation are reviewed which exploit tumour-specific DNA repair deficiencies or signalling pathway addictions, with a special focus on growth factor signalling, PARP, cancer stem cells, cell cycle checkpoints and DNA replication. This chapter concludes with a discussion of DNA repair-related candidate biomarkers of tumour response which are of crucial importance for implementing precision medicine in radiation oncology.

Keyword

Ionising radiation · DNA damage response · DNA strand breaks · DNA double-strand break repair · Molecular targeting · Biomarkers

K. Borgmann · S. Köcher · M. Kriegs · W.Y. Mansour · A.C. Parplys ·
T. Rieckmann · K. Rothkamm (✉)
Laboratory of Radiobiology and Experimental Radio-Oncology,
University Medical Center Hamburg-Eppendorf, Martinistr. 52,
20246 Hamburg, Germany
e-mail: k.rothkamm@uke.de

T. Rieckmann
Department of Otorhinolaryngology and Head and Neck Surgery,
University Medical Center Hamburg-Eppendorf, Martinistr. 52,
20246 Hamburg, Germany

© Springer-Verlag Berlin Heidelberg 2016
M. Baumann et al. (eds.), *Molecular Radio-Oncology*, Recent Results
in Cancer Research 198, DOI 10.1007/978-3-662-49651-0_1

1   Introduction

DNA is a vitally important biomolecule which stores the genetic information required to create the molecular building blocks for cells, tissues and whole organisms. At the same time, it is surprisingly prone to damage and decay, even in the absence of any exogenous stressors. To counteract endogenous processes such as oxidation and hydrolysis as well as exogenously induced lesions, cells have devised a range of pathways for repairing damaged DNA, without which higher life forms would not have been able to evolve.

Not surprisingly, cellular DNA is also the principal target through which ionising radiation exerts its main biological effects, whether cell killing, neoplastic transformation, mutation induction, growth arrest or cellular ageing (UNSCEAR 2000). Whilst the main aim of radiotherapy is tumour cell inactivation, one needs to consider all of these biological responses to get the full picture of how radiotherapy affects the tumour and the surrounding normal tissue. And in order to understand these cellular responses, it is important to know about the molecular machinery that cells employ to repair DNA that has been damaged by radiation.

Apart from furthering our understanding of the basic mechanisms that govern the cellular radiation response, research into DNA repair also opens up opportunities to (i) learn why some individuals may react more severely to radiotherapy than others, (ii) identify potential markers of individual tumour and patient response to support a move towards personalised treatment and (iii) establish biological targets that can be used for tumour radiosensitisation.

2   Radiation-Induced DNA Damage and Early Cellular Responses

Radiation can damage chromosomal DNA either directly or indirectly via the production of free radical species (such as the hydroxyl radical) in the immediate vicinity of the DNA. The breakage of chemical bonds in the sugar–phosphate backbone of the DNA may result in the formation of strand breaks. Other types of lesions induced by ionising radiation include altered base and sugar moieties as well as cross-links which may form between proteins and DNA. All these modifications are not randomly distributed across the cell nucleus; instead, they form along the track of each ionising particle, as it deposits its energy. The resulting clustered lesions consist of multiple DNA lesions which are closely spaced within a volume of several nanometres, corresponding to up to about 20 base pairs. Occasionally, two strand breaks may be induced on opposite strands within one clustered lesion. These may cause the DNA molecule to break up, if there is insufficient overlap to maintain the DNA double helix via the weak hydrogen bonds between the paired, complementary bases. The resulting DNA double-strand breaks (DSBs) are very deleterious. If left unrepaired, they may cause DNA degradation and loss of chromosomal fragments during the next mitosis. Furthermore, their faithful repair is complicated by the fact that, in contrast to lesions that affect only one of the two DNA strands, there is no template immediately available that could be used to correctly restore the original DNA sequence. For this reason, DSB ends are prone to be misrepaired, causing either small-scale mutations at the break point or chromosomal rearrangements such as translocations if break ends from multiple breaks interact and get misrejoined (Rothkamm and Lobrich 2002). It is for these reasons that DSBs are believed to be the most important DNA lesions induced by ionising radiation. For the same reasons, the remainder of this chapter will focus mainly on the cellular response to DSBs.

Cells respond to ionising irradiation through a highly interactive functional network of partially overlapping DNA damage response pathways (Sulli et al. 2012; Jackson and Bartek 2009). Upon detection of DSBs or extended stretches of single-stranded DNA, molecular DNA damage sensors such as the MRE11-RAD50-Nibrin (MRN) and the KU70-KU86 complexes or RPA, ATRIP and the RAD9-RAD1-HUS1 complex will activate the apical kinases ATM, DNA-PK or ATR, respectively, which belong to the family of phosphatidyl inositol $3'$ kinase-related kinases. These will in turn phosphorylate a plethora of DNA damage mediators and downstream kinases. Examples of mediators—which frequently accumulate at or in the vicinity of DSBs to form microscopically visible DNA damage foci—include MDC1, 53BP1, H2AX, BRCA1 and TOPBP1. Downstream kinases include the checkpoint factors CHK1 and CHK2. Figure 1 exemplifies some of the known and predicted protein interactions for the key DNA damage kinase ATM, according to STRING 10 database (Jensen et al. 2009).

The main outcomes of the DNA damage response include the following:

  (i) Transcriptional activation or repression of DNA damage-responsive genes.
 (ii) Restriction of cell cycle progression at DNA damage-induced checkpoints in order to allow DNA repair to proceed before the cell enters S phase or mitosis. CDC25 and p53 are important effectors to facilitate this outcome.
(iii) Post-translational modification (phosphorylation, acetylation, ubiquitylation, sumoylation, neddylation) of chromatin constituents and associated proteins around the site of the DNA lesion to facilitate repair (Bekker-Jensen and Mailand 2011; Brown and Jackson 2015).
 (iv) Repair of DNA lesions, possibly resulting in mutations and chromosomal aberrations.
  (v) Induction of apoptosis in radiation-damaged cells, which may occur via p53 or in a p53-independent manner.
 (vi) Induction of autophagy, probably via inhibition of mammalian target of rapamycin complex 1 (mTORC1) (Czarny et al. 2015).

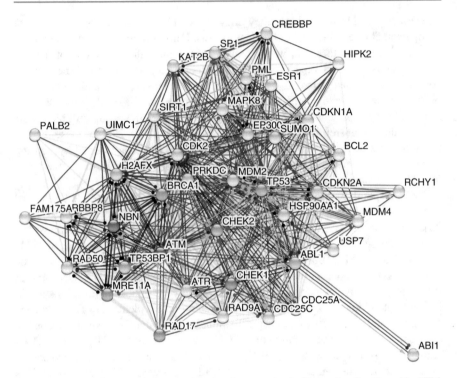

Fig. 1 Network of some of the proteins that interact physically or functionally with ATM, according to STRING 10 database (http://string-db.org; accessed 4 November 2015). *Line colours* indicate the nature of the physical or functional interaction: *green*—activation; *red*—inhibition; *blue*—binding; *turquiose*—phenotype; *purple*—catalysis; *pink*—post-translational modification; *black*—reaction; *yellow*—expression

3 Repair of Single-Stranded DNA Lesions

Several mechanisms for repairing ionising radiation-induced DNA damage exist in human cells which have some overlapping functions and may act as backup pathways for each other to minimise the risk of any damage being left unrepaired. Single-strand breaks and damaged bases such as 7,8-dihydro-8-oxoguanine or thymine glycol are the most common lesions induced by ionising radiation and also form very frequently endogenously, thus requiring efficient repair mechanisms to maintain genome integrity. Thanks to the availability of the complementary sequence on the intact opposite strand which serves as a template for repair, these lesions do not normally give rise to any mutations.

Single-strand breaks caused by damage to the sugar moieties in the DNA are detected by and activate poly(ADP-ribose)polymerase 1 (PARP1) which subsequently modifies itself and other proteins with chains of hundreds of ADP-ribose units. These recruit XRCC1 protein complexes (probably containing DNA polymerase beta, ligase 3 and one of PNKP, APTX or APLF) which process DNA ends. Two alternative options exist for the final two steps, gap filling and DNA ligation, namely short-patch and long-patch repair during which either one or 2–10 nucleotides are incorporated by polymerase beta and/or polymerase delta/epsilon, resulting in the displacement of the damaged strand in the latter case which is then removed by FEN1/PCNA, possibly also with support from PARP1. Repair patches are sealed by the XRCC1/ligase III alpha or PCNA/ligase 1 complexes (Caldecott 2014).

Base lesions are essentially repaired by the same base excision repair (BER) process described above for single-strand break repair, except that this pathway initially employs lesion-specific glycosylases to remove altered bases and then converts the abasic sites into single-strand breaks via an AP endonuclease activity (Brenerman et al. 2014). These breaks are then processed in the same way as those directly induced by radiation.

In global nucleotide excision repair, bulky lesions which distort the helical DNA structure can be recognised by the XPC-hRAD23B-centrin 2 complex which then melts the DNA around the lesion and recruits the TFIIH complex. Subsequently, XPB and XPD unwind the DNA to form a bubble of about 30 nucleotides. XPA then binds the DNA near the 5' end of the bubble, and RPA binds the single-stranded DNA opposite the lesion to protect it from degradation. The first incision is then made by ERCC1-XPF and repair synthesis commences, displacing the damaged strand. Finally, XPG makes the second incision to remove the oligonucleotide contained the lesion, and the newly synthesised DNA patch is sealed by ligase I or ligase III alpha-XRCC1 (Spivak 2015).

In contrast to the above process, which only detects bulky lesions, a transcription-coupled excision repair pathway can repair any DNA lesion located within an actively transcribed gene. In this case, it is the stalling of RNA polymerase II-mediated transcription which detects the lesion and triggers the recruitment of transcription-coupled repair factors. The polymerase is then backtracked or removed to make space for repair which proceeds as described above for global nucleotide excision repair (Spivak 2015).

DNA strand breaks in cellular DNA are commonly measured using alkaline single-cell gel electrophoresis, also called the comet assay (Ostling and Johanson 1984; Olive 2009). In brief, cells are embedded into low-melt agarose and spread onto microscopy slides, lysed, electrophoresed in alkaline running buffer, neutralised and stained with a fluorescent DNA dye, such as ethidium bromide or Sybr Gold, and imaged using a fluorescence microscope. Whilst cells with intact, unirradiated DNA will show round nuclei ('heads') without any DNA leaking out of the nucleus into a tail, cells containing strand breaks will show a comet-like tail of fragmented DNA which migrated out of the nucleus towards the anode during electrophoresis. The percentage of DNA in the tail and the tail length can be measured, and the tail moment be calculated by multiplying the two as a robust indicator of the amount of damage present in the sample. As ionising radiation induces about 30 times more single-strand breaks than DSBs, the initial signal directly after irradiation will be dominated by single-strand breaks. However, the kinetics for repairing single- and DSBs differ considerably, with the former being repaired faster, so that residual damage remaining several hours after irradiation will be greatly enriched for DSBs. In that respect, any signal remaining after many hours in an alkaline comet assay will largely reflect the level of residual DSBs, at least in cells that are BER-competent.

One strategy to measure base lesions utilises glycosylases/AP endonucleases that convert specific base lesions into single-strand breaks (Collins 2014). To this end, lysed cells embedded in agarose slides are incubated with commercially available purified enzymes such as formamidopyrimidine DNA glycosylase or Nth (endonuclease III) to detect oxidised purines or pyrimidines, respectively, prior to electrophoresis. The additional tail moment measured on top of that observed in a parallel sample without glycosylase treatment is then a measure of the amount of base damage. Detailed protocols have been developed in recent years for the application of comet-based assays for various BER and NER substrates in different types of biological material (Azqueta et al. 2013).

4   Pathways for Repairing DNA Double-Strand Breaks

DSBs can be repaired by non-homologous end-joining (NHEJ) processes as well as homology-dependent recombination pathways. Whilst excision repair pathways for single-stranded DNA damage generally use the intact complementary strand as a template, ensuring that repair is mostly error-free, DSB repair is generally more challenging and frequently error-prone. This is especially the case in situations when several DSB ends are sufficiently close to be misaligned and exchanged during repair, giving rise to chromosomal deletions or rearrangements. Promiscuous repair in the presence of multiple DSBs is also responsible for the quadratic increase of deleterious chromosome aberrations with gamma- or X-ray dose, despite a dose-linear increase of DSBs (Barnard et al. 2013). It is therefore important to appreciate that DSB repair efficiency is an important determinant of genome stability and radiosensitivity.

Gel electrophoretic studies of double-stranded DNA fragments following irradiation and immunofluorescence microscopy-based scoring of DNA damage-associated protein 'foci' forming at the sites of DSBs have shown that initial radiation-induced DSB yields do not in general vary very much between genomic loci, organs or individuals. However, some variation has been reported for different tumour cells which cannot be explained by other confounding factors such as DNA content but which may be associated with cellular radiosensitivity (El-Awady et al. 2003; Rube et al. 2008; Rothkamm et al. 2003; Cheng et al. 2015).

X- or gamma-ray-induced DSBs are repaired with biphasic exponential kinetics with half-lives of 5–30 min and several hours, respectively. Repair may reach a plateau of residual, unrepaired and potentially also misrepaired, DSBs (Rothkamm and Lobrich 2003; Dahm-Daphi and Dikomey 1996). Longer half-lives and more residual breaks have been observed in cells exposed to densely ionising particles.

Whilst the time course of DSB repair is generally comparable between tumour cells, lymphocytes or normal fibroblasts, more variability seems to exist between different tumour cell lines. These may reflect bigger differences in the efficiency of DSB processing in tumours, likely caused by deficiencies or upregulation of particular DNA damage response pathways.

Chromatin structure and cell cycle stage also affect both efficiency and kinetics of DSB repair. DSBs in heterochromatic DNA regions are much more difficult to access by repair factors, require additional chromatin relaxation steps mediated by KAP1 and tend to be repaired more slowly (Goodarzi et al. 2008). Repair pathway utilisation depends very much on cell cycle position as it is affected by the avail-ability of a sister chromatid (Rothkamm et al. 2003; Bauerschmidt et al. 2010). Consequently, the radiation response of a normal tissue or a tumour may change during a course of fractionated radiotherapy if cells accumulate in a specific cell cycle phase. One example is the loss of fraction size sensitivity in the basal epidermal layer of irradiated skin which may be explained by the accumulation of cells in the S/G2 phase and consequential increase in the utilisation of homology-dependent repair mechanisms (Somaiah et al. 2012).

Repairing a DSB is of utmost importance for a cell because, if left unrepaired, it would lead to the loss of the affected chromosome fragment and cell death (Helleday et al. 2007). Furthermore, incorrect repair of a DSB may produce dele-tions or chromosome rearrangements which are hallmarks of cancer genomes. For these reasons, efficient DSB repair is of crucial importance for the survival and genomic stability of a cell. Human cells employ two fundamentally different types of DSB repair mechanisms, one relying on the joining of break ends with little or no regard for sequence homology, and the other heavily dependent on the availability of sequence homology. These will be discussed in more detail in the following sections.

4.1 End-Joining Mechanisms

The main DSB repair pathway in mammalian cells is classical non-homologous end-joining (NHEJ). It is active in all phases of the cell cycle (Lieber et al. 2003) except mitosis (Orthwein et al. 2014; Terasawa et al. 2014). NHEJ is initiated by the binding of the Ku70/Ku80 heterodimer to DSB ends, followed by recruitment and activation of the catalytic subunit of the DNA-dependent protein kinase to form the DNA damage kinase DNA-PK. Depending on the nature of the break, the ends may need to be trimmed before they can be ligated, e.g. by nucleolytic resection or by DNA polymerase-mediated fill-in. Then, the ligase complex consisting of ligase IV and its cofactors XRCC4 and XLF binds to the DNA ends and seals the break (Davis and Chen 2013). Intriguingly, whilst the basic NHEJ mechanism has been known for over twenty years, its regulation in human cells is still far from being fully understood.

Cells deficient in NHEJ can repair DSBs via an alternative end-joining mech-anism (Alt-EJ) (Wang et al. 2003; Audebert et al. 2004) which is less efficient than

NHEJ and depends on PARP1 for DSB recognition and on ligase III and its cofactor XRCC1 for the ligation step (Mansour et al. 2010, 2013). It is associated with deletions of DNA at the break site, probably caused by the slower speed of the pathway which prevents nucleolytic degradation less efficiently than classical DNA-PK-dependent NHEJ (Mansour et al. 2013). Whilst Alt-EJ does not strictly require microhomology between overlapping bases at the break ends, it still preferentially uses it if available (Mansour et al. 2010). Interestingly, these features, i.e. deletions and microhomologies at breakpoint junctions, are frequently found in human cancer cells (Welzel et al. 2001; Weinstock et al. 2007; Jager et al. 2000).

4.2 Homology-Dependent Repair Pathways

The main homology-dependent repair pathway, homologous recombination (HR), operates at the replication fork as well as in post-replicative DNA, i.e. during S and G2 phase when the sister chromatid can serve as an intact template to facilitate repair of a DSB by restoring the original sequence. Repair via HR is therefore largely error-free. HR is initiated by a nucleolytic DNA end resection step during which single-stranded overhangs are generated. This is achieved by Mre11-CtIP, followed by Exo1, DNA2 and the BLM helicase (Helleday et al. 2007; Sung and Klein 2006). RPA protects the single-stranded DNA overhangs until RAD51 binds to form a nucleofilament, supported by the RAD51 paralogs RAD51B, RAD51C, RAD51D, XRCC2 and XRCC3 as well as by BRCA2 and RAD52. Following a search for DNA with extensive sequence homology, the RAD51 nucleofilament invades the double helix of, typically, the sister chromatid to form a so-called displacement or D loop. Using the complementary strand as a template, replication polymerases then synthesise DNA until ligase 1 seals the ends. The resulting branched structure of four double-stranded DNA arms joined together, called the Holliday junction, can be resolved either through symmetrical cleavage by GEN1/Yen1, through asymmetrical cleavage (Mus81/Eme1) or through dissolution via the BLM-TopIII-alpha complex to complete the repair process (Andersen et al. 2011; Sarbajna et al. 2014; Wyatt and West 2014).

A different homology-dependent repair mechanism for DSBs does not use a homologous copy such as the sister chromatid but instead utilises homologies between repetitive sequences on the broken chromosome. It is called single-strand annealing (SSA) and is also initiated by a nucleolytic end resection step to produce long single-stranded DNA overhangs to which RPA binds. Subsequently, heptameric rings of RAD52 form at the DNA overhangs and facilitate homology search and annealing of the repeat sequences. Next, the DNA sequences between the repeats are flapped out and cleaved off, most likely be the ERCC1/XPF endonuclease (Shinohara et al. 1998), and an as yet unknown ligase seals the remaining gap. It is clear from the above that SSA is a non-conservative process which results in the deletion of the DNA flanking the breakpoint, including one copy of the repeat sequences used by this mechanism.

4.3   DSB Repair Hierarchy

In normal cells, a functional hierarchy, regulated by an extensive cellular signalling network including cell cycle and DNA damage response factors, determines the use of the DSB repair pathways described above in order to ensure the efficient and faithful processing of DSBs (Mansour et al. 2008). NHEJ usually predominates and suppresses Alt-EJ, HR and SSA pathways. In situations of NHEJ deficiency, most DSBs are repaired by Alt-EJ, although HR and SSA also contribute more strongly to DSB repair (Mansour et al. 2008). Interestingly, DSB repair has been found to be frequently switched to Alt-EJ in tumour cell lines of various origin (Kotter et al. 2014) as well as in primary bladder (Bentley et al. 2004) and head-and-neck tumour cells (Shin et al. 2006). It is tempting to speculate that this switch to a more mutagenic repair mechanism enables tumours to accelerate their genetic diversification in order to overcome further barriers to growth. In any case, this switch to Alt-EJ in tumours offers opportunities for their specific targeting (Kotter et al. 2014).

5   The DNA Damage Response as a Target for Tumour Radiosensitisation

Treatment outcomes could be improved for many tumours treated with radiotherapy if it were possible to selectively enhance tumour cell radiosensitivity without affecting normal tissue responses. Our progress in understanding the cellular radiation response over the past years sets the scene for the development of such strategies, based on targeting signalling and repair pathways that tumours have become addicted to.

5.1   The Epidermal Growth Factor Receptor (EGFR)

The epidermal growth factor receptor (EGFR) is a very important signalling factor in many tumour cells. It is frequently mutated or over-expressed in tumours and can be targeted therapeutically using antibodies such as cetuximab or tyrosine kinase inhibitors such as erlotinib or gefitinib, either as a monotherapy or combined with irradiation (Krause and Van Etten 2005). Combined treatment with cetuximab and radiotherapy has been demonstrated to improve local tumour control in patients with advanced head-and-neck cancer (Bonner et al. 2006). Interestingly, it was especially patients suffering strong cetuximab-associated side effects who benefitted most from the combined treatment. This suggests that there are subgroups of patients with a differential response to this targeted therapy (Bonner et al. 2010).

Cetuximab is thought to radiosensitise tumours at the cellular level (Harari et al. 2007). Although the exact mechanisms are not yet completely understood, DSB repair seems to be involved as it has been shown to be regulated by EGFR and to be suppressed by treatment with cetuximab or tyrosine kinase inhibitors which appear to block both NHEJ and HR (Kriegs et al. 2010; Myllynen et al. 2011). However, the observed repair inhibition was not always associated with enhanced cellular radiosensitivity or improved tumour response (Myllynen et al. 2011; Kriegs et al. 2015; Stegeman et al. 2013). One possible explanation is that these treatments inhibit DSB repair only partially or transiently. Other responses observed following EGFR inhibition in combination with irradiation include the induction of apoptosis (though not confirmed in subsequent studies), semi-permanent cell cycle arrest and premature senescence which correlated with radiosensitisation (Kriegs et al. 2015; Wang et al. 2011). However, recent clinical trials report no improvement of therapy outcome for patients treated with tyrosine kinase inhibitors or cetuximab in combination with radiochemotherapy (Ang et al. 2014; Giralt et al. 2015; Martins et al. 2013; Mesia et al. 2015).

Apart from targeting EGFR function, its sheer abundance in tumours makes it also an ideal target for radioimmunotherapy, in order to selectively irradiate tumour cells (Cai et al. 2008; Saker et al. 2013), thereby allowing tumour control to be achieved with only moderate additional doses given with external beam radiotherapy (Koi et al. 2014). Other cell signalling factors that could be promising targets for DSB repair modulation include MAPK and AKT signalling (Kriegs et al. 2010; Toulany et al. 2006). Furthermore, EGFR-independent targets are being investigated, such as the proto-oncogenes Myc and Ras, and the therapeutic potential of multi-kinase inhibitors such as imatinib, dasatinib or sorafenib is being explored, with promising early results (Laban et al. 2013; Möckelmann et al. 2016). However, it is not at all clear at this stage whether DNA repair plays a significant role in these treatment strategies.

5.2 Poly (ADP-Ribose) Polymerase-1 (PARP1)

PARP1 contributes to a number of cellular tasks, such as DNA repair, replication, transcription and cell cycle regulation. In cancer therapy, it has been identified as an interesting druggable target because of its role in detecting DNA single-strand breaks and facilitating their repair via BER. Following PARP inhibition, single-strand breaks accumulate, resulting in the formation of DSBs especially during replication, which in turn require HR to be efficiently repaired. For this reason, HR-deficient tumours such as those carrying mutations in BRCA1 or BRCA2 have been targeted using PARP inhibitor. The logic behind this 'synthetic lethality' approach is that normal cells will tolerate PARP inhibition because they are HR-proficient, whereas tumour cells which are already compromised in HR, the backup repair pathway for unrepaired single-strand breaks encountered during replication, will struggle to survive upon loss of their main single-strand break repair pathway. PARP inhibition using drugs such as olaparib has been and is being used as a monotherapy in a number of studies which focus mostly on BRCA-deficient tumours (Bryant and Helleday 2004; Benafif and Hall 2015; Mateo et al. 2015). However, the combination of PARP inhibition with DNA-damaging chemo- or radiotherapy is even more promising, due to their synergistic interaction which has been shown in vitro as well as in vivo (Bryant et al. 2005; Fong et al. 2009; Tutt et al. 2010). Given that tumour sensitisation by PARP inhibition is achieved mostly through the formation of DSBs at collapsed replication forks following their collision with unrepaired single-strand breaks, one would expect the best radiosensitising effects of PARP inhibition in tumours with a large S-phase fraction (Noel et al. 2006).

In addition to the 'BRCAness'-dependent effects described above, it is becoming increasingly clear that also tumours that have switched from DNA-PK-dependent NHEJ to PARP-dependent Alt-EJ may also be promising candidates for tumour-specific radiosensitisation by PARP inhibition (Wang et al. 2003; Audebert et al. 2004; Mansour et al. 2010; Kotter et al. 2014).

5.3 Cell Cycle Checkpoint Signalling

Following irradiation, cells arrest at the G1/S and G2/M cell cycle checkpoints to allow time for DNA repair before cells enter the most critical phases of the cell cycle, namely replication and mitosis. In addition, an intra-S-phase checkpoint functions to postpone DNA replication in the presence of DNA damage (Morgan and Lawrence 2015).

DNA damage-induced cell cycle checkpoints are regulated by the kinases ATM and ATR via phosphorylation of the checkpoint kinases Chk2 and Chk1, respectively, which inhibit CDC25 phosphatases and thereby block cyclin-dependent kinase-mediated cell cycle progression. The initiating signals for these signal cascades are either a DSB which activates ATM or an extended stretch of single-stranded DNA coated with RPA (often associated with replication fork stallage and HR intermediates) which activates ATR (Marechal and Zou 2013). Accordingly, the G1/S and G2/M checkpoints are regulated by ATM/Chk2, whilst ATR/Chk1 are essential for the intra-S checkpoint and also contribute to the G2/M arrest. The G1/S checkpoint also requires an intact p53 response and downstream p21/CDKN1A induction and is therefore frequently compromised in tumours. In the absence of a functional G1/S arrest, p53-deficient tumours are very reliant on the ATR/Chk1 pathway to prevent entry into mitosis with too much DNA damage and may therefore be targeted using ATR or Chk1 inhibitors in combination with DNA-damaging agents such as radiotherapy, exploiting the synthetic lethality concept. Indeed, early studies have demonstrated enhanced sensitivity to radio- or chemotherapy of human cell lines derived from various tumour entities (Garrett and Collins 2011; Dillon et al. 2014; Busch et al. 2013).

However, toxicity and lack of specificity of the first generation of inhibitors, such as the Chk1 inhibitor UCN01, has been a serious drawback. More specific and better tolerated inhibitors for the checkpoint kinases, such as SCH 900776/MK-8776 or LY2606368, have been developed more recently and are now being tested in the clinic. Inhibitors for ATR and Wee1—which inhibits CDK1 and thereby delays entry into mitosis—are also being tested in phase I and II trials in combination with chemotherapy. Unfortunately, there are to date only two trials testing inhibitors for the G2/M arrest in combination with radiotherapy (NCT02223923, NCT01922076). As the targeted proteins are also involved in other important aspects of DNA maintenance, such as repair and replication (Sorensen and Syljuasen 2012), their inhibition is also being explored as a monotherapy (McNeely et al. 2014). Furthermore, one could argue that any risk of systemic toxicity of these inhibitors when used in combination with chemotherapy may potentially be avoided or at least reduced when combining them with local radiotherapy treatments.

5.4 Cancer Stem Cells

The concept of cancer stem cells (CSCs) is based on that of normal tissue stem cells. Accordingly, CSC have the potential to self-renew, differentiate and maintain tumour growth and repopulation following radio- or chemotherapy. Two models exist for the organisation of CSC: one that assumes a hierarchically organised system in which only a small proportion of tumour cells actually have any tumourigenic potential whilst most tumour cells are unable to induce tumours (Lapidot et al. 1994; Al-Hajj et al. 2003), and a clonal evolution model in which random changes enable subclones to emerge with new functions and treatment responses within the tumour. In fact, both models may have some merit and could coexist, assuming that clonal evolution may shape the make-up of the small proportion of stem-like cells (Maugeri-Sacca et al. 2014).

Similar to tissue stem cells, CSC are generally thought to be resistant to DNA-damaging agents thanks to upregulated DNA damage response and repair pathways (Maynard et al. 2008; Mandal et al. 2011). Examples include CD133+ glioma stem cells which were shown to have an enhanced Chk1-dependent checkpoint response (Baumann et al. 2008; Bao et al. 2006) and upregulated expression of Nibrin, one component of the MRN complex which is involved in DSB sensing (Cheng et al. 2011). Enhanced DNA damage responses and repair gene expression were also observed in CD133+ CSC in A549 human lung carcinoma cells (Desai et al. 2014), mammary tumour-initiating cells (Zhang et al. 2014), pancreatic putative CSC (Mathews et al. 2011) and patient-derived non-small-cell lung cancer CSC (Bartucci et al. 2012). However, a number of studies showed no difference or even deficient DNA damage responses in CSC (McCord et al. 2009; Ropolo et al. 2009; Lundholm et al. 2013). These conflicting observations suggest that an enhanced DNA damage response may not be a general feature of all CSC and that inter-tumour and possibly even intra-tumour heterogeneity in the DNA damage response functionality may need to be considered (Magee et al. 2012). One important factor that may affect the composition and treatment response of CSC is epithelial–mesenchymal transition (EMT) which has been associated with enhanced radioresistance of mammary CSC. ZEB1, a zinc finger transcription factor which is phosphorylated and stabilised by ATM following DNA damage and then stabilises Chk1, appears to be an important player linking EMT to the DNA damage response (Zhang et al. 2014).

Interestingly, PARP1 inhibition was reported to radiosensitise glioma stem cells (Venere et al. 2014) and Chk1 inhibition reduced the CSC pool in non-small-cell lung cancer cells, suggesting that DNA damage response inhibitors are a promising targeting strategy for CSC (Bartucci et al. 2012). However, as multiple DNA damage response pathways may be simultaneously upregulated in CSC, as shown in glioma stem cells, a multi-targeting approach involving combined inhibition of DNA repair and cell cycle checkpoint mechanisms may be a more promising strategy for overcoming CSC resistance (Signore et al. 2014; Ahmed et al. 2015).

5.5 Replication

One of the most exciting emerging strategies for improving tumour control is the replication-dependent sensitisation of tumours to radiation and chemotherapeutic drugs. It exploits the fact that DNA damage response pathways are of critical importance for replication fork stability, control of origin firing and the resolution of collapsed forks caused by DNA damage (Zeman and Cimprich 2014) (Fig. 2). They serve to counteract replication stress and the formation of secondary DSB induced by cytotoxic cancer therapies (Kotsantis et al. 2015).

The molecular targeting approaches for a range of DNA damage response pathways that are now becoming available for clinical testing provide the opportunity to enhance the toxicity of radio- and chemotherapy during replication (Pearl et al. 2015). Inhibition of the DNA damage response kinases ATR, CHK1 and WEE1 increases the activity of cyclin-dependent kinases, which leads to uncontrolled replication origin firing and depletion of the nucleotide pool, resulting in the

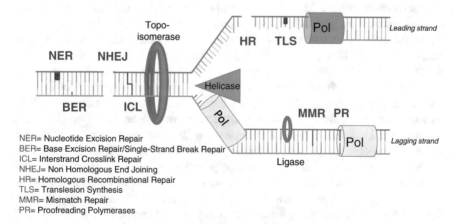

Fig. 2 DNA repair mechanisms active at replication forks to maintain genomic stability. Cells are constantly exposed to insults from endogenous and exogenous agents that can introduce DNA damage and generate genomic instability. Many of these lesions cause structural damage to DNA and can alter or eliminate fundamental cellular processes, such as DNA replication. To counteract harmful effects, cells have developed a higly specialised DNA repair system, which can be subdivided into distinct mechanisms including base excision repair/single-strand break repair, nucleotide excision repair, mismatch repair, interstrand cross-link repair and double-strand break repair, together with the proofreading activity of polymerases and translesion synthesis

accumulation of replication-associated DSBs (Syljuasen et al. 2015). HR proteins which are not only involved in the repair of replication-associated DSBs but also support replication fidelity are also interesting targets (Huang and Mazin 2014). Examples include Rad51-, NUCKS- and RAD51-associated protein 1 whose disruption compromises replication fork progression, increases the firing of replication origins and negatively affects genome stability (Parplys et al. 2014, 2015a, b).

Inhibition of the DNA single-strand break repair factor PARP was first described as a promising strategy for BRCA-deficient mammary cancers, which, due to the associated HR deficiency, cannot efficiently deal with unrepaired DNA damage present during replication. However, PARP1 also senses stalled replication forks and recruits Mre11 which degrades the stalled forks to enable HR-dependent repair and replication fork restart (Ying et al. 2012).

ATR, CHK1 and PARP1 have been shown to be prime targets for radiosensitisation of S-phase cells (Ahmed et al. 2015; Dungey et al. 2008; Pires et al. 2012; Dobbelstein and Sorensen 2015). Furthermore, irradiated cells undergoing replication form secondary DSBs (Groth et al. 2012) and suffer from blocked replication elongation (Parplys et al. 2012). For these reasons, radiation-induced tumour cell killing could potentially be enhanced by enriching the fraction of cells that are in S phase during irradiation, e.g. through the use of replication inhibitors (Dobbelstein and Sorensen 2015).

6 Biomarkers of Treatment Response

Radiotherapy treatment decisions are currently made based on clinical parameters such as tumour size, site and grade. The individual response of patient and tumour, based on their biological make-up, is typically not taken into account, simply because it has not been possible to reliably predict either the tumour or the normal tissue response of a particular patient, except for very rare cases of patients with radiation hypersensitivity syndromes such as ataxia telangiectasia. However, it would be of great benefit if it could be determined prior to the treatment which patients would actually benefit from radiotherapy, what dose should be given and whether the chances of tumour control could be improved using a particular molecular-targeted approach in combination with radiotherapy. Biological markers including mutational or single nucleotide polymorphism (SNP) signatures, gene expression profiles and functional assays for core radiation response mechanisms such as DSB repair capacity are slowly gaining relevance and are starting to pave the way for a precision medicine approach in radiation oncology.

We have reviewed the use of chromosome and DNA damage/repair assays for assessing individual radiation exposures and for predicting normal tissue responses quite extensively in the recent past (Chua and Rothkamm 2013; Pernot et al. 2012; Manning and Rothkamm 2013; Rothkamm et al. 2015) and will therefore focus on biomarkers of tumour response here.

Early attempts to use functional assays for tumour radiosensitivity prediction involved cell suspensions obtained from tumour biopsies which were irradiated in vitro and plated for colony formation to produce survival curves. Cell survival measured in vitro with such an approach was shown to correspond with clinical outcome in cervical cancer (West et al. 1993) and other tumour entities (Bjork-Eriksson et al. 2000), thus demonstrating that therapy outcome can be linked to cellular radiosensitivity. However, due to the amount of effort required for this assay and the long delay before colony counts are available, this method proved unsuitable for routine use in a clinical setting.

A quicker method for assessing the radiation response of tumour cells exploits the fact that cellular radiosensitivity is closely linked to DSB repair capacity. Immunofluorescence microscopic scoring of gamma-H2AX and/or 53BP1 nuclear protein foci, which form at the site of a DSB, is widely used as a surrogate marker of DSBs (Rothkamm et al. 2015) and can be performed in cell lines as well as in frozen or formalin-fixed paraffin-embedded tissue sections (Somaiah et al. 2012; Chua and Rothkamm 2013; Qvarnstrom et al. 2004; Barber et al. 2006; Crosbie et al. 2010; Rothkamm et al. 2012). This method has recently also been applied to determine residual DSBs in xenografts or patient-derived tumour biopsies following in vivo as well as ex vivo irradiation and repair incubation (Menegakis et al. 2015). A recent study demonstrated that residual foci levels obtained with this assay are consistent with the known differences in radioresponsiveness of different tumour types, thus providing proof of concept for this strategy (Menegakis et al. 2015). Additional information about the functionality of DNA damage response pathways in a tumour can be obtained using other biomarkers. For example, Rad51 foci formation following ex vivo treatment can indicate the functionality of the HR pathway and has been used to identify individual breast tumours with HR deficiencies (Naipal et al. 2014). As already mentioned above, patients with such tumours could then benefit from targeted therapy using PARP inhibitor. Biomarkers for other pathways, e.g. for a switch from classical to alternative end-joining, are currently being investigated.

In summary, functional ex vivo assays of biological radiation effects and pathway functions in tumour biopsies are rapid indicators of treatment response which enable treatments to be tailored to the individual characteristics of a tumour. Assaying function, rather than just genetic or expression profiles of a tumour, has the clear advantage of an integrated approach that will register effects, such as epigenetic or post-translational alterations, that may well be missed when using a non-functional method. However, for the assays to be fit for routine use in the clinic, robust, standardised procedures for sample logistics, processing and analysis need to be established and regularly validated.

Aberrant expression of a protein can also indicate whether a particular tumour will respond to a specific treatment strategy. Examples include HPV-positive oropharyngeal cancers which over-express p16/INK4a (Lassen et al. 2009), head-and-neck cancers deficient in the DNA damage response due to downregulated ATM (Mansour et al. 2013), over-expression of EGFR associated with head-and-neck cancer radioresistance (Ang et al. 2002), prostate cancer cells which over-express Bcl2, causing them to use alternative instead of classical end-joining (Catz and Johnson 2003; Wang et al. 2008), or colorectal carcinoma with deregulated HR and over-expression of RAD51 (Tennstedt et al. 2013). Also, over-expression of Ku, but possibly not of other players involved in NHEJ, was found to be associated with radioresistance in head-and-neck cancer (Lee et al. 2005; Moeller et al. 2011).

As gene expression profiling and whole-exome sequencing are becoming more affordable as well as accessible, there is increasing interest in identifying signatures that could be used to predict treatment response and individualise treatment. However, to date, no reliable signatures are available for routine use, although some candidate profiles have been reported (Ahmed et al. 2015; Tinhofer et al. 2015; Spitzner et al. 2010; Pramana et al. 2007).

7 Future Perspectives

Major progress has been made in recent years in the investigation and characterisation of cellular and molecular DNA damage response processes occurring in irradiated tumours and normal tissues. One important driver has been the development of new cellular and molecular methods and techniques. These have facilitated exciting discoveries at the cellular level, especially in the fields of signal transduction, cell cycle regulation and DNA repair. The recent discoveries should not only further our understanding of the cellular response to ionising radiation, but they may also help us develop and refine cancer treatment strategies. For instance, we now understand much better the opportunities—but also the potential caveats— that need to be considered when targeting signalling cascades, such as those involving EGFR, MAP kinase or the mTOR/AKT pathway, to selectively inactivate and/or sensitise tumour cells.

New discoveries have especially been made in the field of DNA repair. They now provide the exciting opportunity to understand the biochemical basis which underpins the large variation of tumour cell radiosensitivity that we have grappled with for so long. Tumour cells frequently suffer from deregulated DNA double-strand break repair, such as a switch from classical to PARP-dependent alternative end-joining or a 'BRCAness' phenotype of HR deficiency, which provides new targets for the selective sensitisation of tumours. The first successful steps in this direction involve the blocking of PARP or the checkpoint factors Chk1 and Chk2.

Gene, miRNA or protein expression profiling as well as functional assays should provide the means to assess the individual radiosensitivity, DNA repair capacity and susceptibility of a tumour to specific targeted therapies. However, overall, one should not underestimate the complexity of the interrelationship between DNA repair, other cellular processes and microenvironmental factors which will necessitate a careful evaluation of any initial findings.

References

Ahmed SU, Carruthers R, Gilmour L, Yildirim S, Watts C, Chalmers AJ (2015) Selective inhibition of parallel DNA damage response pathways optimizes radiosensitization of glioblastoma stem-like cells. Cancer Res

Al-Hajj M, Wicha MS, Benito-Hernandez A, Morrison SJ, Clarke MF (2003) Prospective identification of tumorigenic breast cancer cells. Proc Natl Acad Sci USA 100:3983–3988

Andersen SL, Kuo HK, Savukoski D, Brodsky MH, Sekelsky J (2011) Three structure-selective endonucleases are essential in the absence of BLM helicase in Drosophila. PLoS Genet 7: e1002315

Ang KK, Berkey BA, Tu X, Zhang HZ, Katz R, Hammond EH, Fu KK, Milas L (2002) Impact of epidermal growth factor receptor expression on survival and pattern of relapse in patients with advanced head and neck carcinoma. Cancer Res 62:7350–7356

Ang KK, Zhang Q, Rosenthal DI, Nguyen-Tan PF, Sherman EJ, Weber RS, Galvin JM, Bonner JA, Harris J, El-Naggar AK et al (2014) Randomized phase III trial of concurrent accelerated radiation plus cisplatin with or without cetuximab for stage III to IV head and neck carcinoma: RTOG 0522. J Clin Oncol Official J Am Soc Clin Oncol 32:2940–2950

Audebert M, Salles B, Calsou P (2004) Involvement of poly(ADP-ribose) polymerase-1 and XRCC1/DNA ligase III in an alternative route for DNA double-strand breaks rejoining. J Biol Chem 279:55117–55126

Azqueta A, Langie SA, Slyskova J, Collins AR (2013) Measurement of DNA base and nucleotide excision repair activities in mammalian cells and tissues using the comet assay–a methodological overview. DNA Repair 12:1007–1010

Bao S, Wu Q, McLendon RE, Hao Y, Shi Q, Hjelmeland AB, Dewhirst MW, Bigner DD, Rich JN (2006) Glioma stem cells promote radioresistance by preferential activation of the DNA damage response. Nature 444:756–760

Barber RC, Hickenbotham P, Hatch T, Kelly D, Topchiy N, Almeida GM, Jones GD, Johnson GE, Parry JM, Rothkamm K et al (2006) Radiation-induced transgenerational alterations in genome stability and DNA damage. Oncogene 25:7336–7342

Barnard S, Bouffler S, Rothkamm K (2013) The shape of the radiation dose response for DNA double-strand break induction and repair. Genome Integrity 4:1

Bartucci M, Svensson S, Romania P, Dattilo R, Patrizii M, Signore M, Navarra S, Lotti F, Biffoni M, Pilozzi E et al (2012) Therapeutic targeting of Chk1 in NSCLC stem cells during chemotherapy. Cell Death Differ 19:768–778

Bauerschmidt C, Arrichiello C, Burdak-Rothkamm S, Woodcock M, Hill MA, Stevens DL, Rothkamm K (2010) Cohesin promotes the repair of ionizing radiation-induced DNA double-strand breaks in replicated chromatin. Nucleic Acids Res 38:477–487

Baumann M, Krause M, Hill R (2008) Exploring the role of cancer stem cells in radioresistance. Nat Rev Cancer 8:545–554

Bekker-Jensen S, Mailand N (2011) The ubiquitin- and SUMO-dependent signaling response to DNA double-strand breaks. FEBS Lett 585:2914–2919

Benafif S, Hall M (2015) An update on PARP inhibitors for the treatment of cancer. OncoTargets Ther 8:519–528

Bentley J, Diggle CP, Harnden P, Knowles MA, Kiltie AE (2004) DNA double strand break repair in human bladder cancer is error prone and involves microhomology-associated end-joining. Nucleic Acids Res 32:5249–5259

Bjork-Eriksson T, West C, Karlsson E, Mercke C (2000) Tumor radiosensitivity (SF2) is a prognostic factor for local control in head and neck cancers. Int J Radiat Oncol Biol Phys 46:13–19

Bonner JA, Harari PM, Giralt J, Azarnia N, Shin DM, Cohen RB, Jones CU, Sur R, Raben D, Jassem J et al (2006) Radiotherapy plus cetuximab for squamous-cell carcinoma of the head and neck. N Eng J Med 354:567–578

Bonner JA, Harari PM, Giralt J, Cohen RB, Jones CU, Sur RK, Raben D, Baselga J, Spencer SA, Zhu J et al (2010) Radiotherapy plus cetuximab for locoregionally advanced head and neck cancer: 5-year survival data from a phase 3 randomised trial, and relation between cetuximab-induced rash and survival. Lancet Oncol 11:21–28

Brenerman BM, Illuzzi JL, Wilson DM 3rd (2014) Base excision repair capacity in informing healthspan. Carcinogenesis 35:2643–2652

Brown JS, Jackson SP (2015) Ubiquitylation, neddylation and the DNA damage response. Open Biol 5:150018

Bryant HE, Helleday T (2004) Poly(ADP-ribose) polymerase inhibitors as potential chemotherapeutic agents. Biochem Soc Trans 32:959–961

Bryant HE, Schultz N, Thomas HD, Parker KM, Flower D, Lopez E, Kyle S, Meuth M, Curtin NJ, Helleday T (2005) Specific killing of BRCA2-deficient tumours with inhibitors of poly (ADP-ribose) polymerase. Nature 434:913–917

Busch CJ, Kriegs M, Laban S, Tribius S, Knecht R, Petersen C, Dikomey E, Rieckmann T (2013) HPV-positive HNSCC cell lines but not primary human fibroblasts are radiosensitized by the inhibition of Chk1. Radiother Oncol J Eur Soc Ther Radiol Oncol 108:495–499

Cai Z, Chen Z, Bailey KE, Scollard DA, Reilly RM, Vallis KA (2008) Relationship between induction of phosphorylated H2AX and survival in breast cancer cells exposed to 111In-DTPA-hEGF. J Nucl Med Official Pub Soc Nucl Med 49:1353–1361

Caldecott KW (2014) DNA single-strand break repair. Exp Cell Res 329:2–8

Catz SD, Johnson JL (2003) BCL-2 in prostate cancer: a minireview. Apoptosis Int J Programmed Cell Death 8:29–37

Cheng L, Wu Q, Huang Z, Guryanova OA, Huang Q, Shou W, Rich JN, Bao S (2011) L1CAM regulates DNA damage checkpoint response of glioblastoma stem cells through NBS1. EMBO J 30:800–813

Cheng Y, Li F, Mladenov E, Iliakis G (2015) The yield of DNA double strand breaks determined after exclusion of those forming from heat-labile lesions predicts tumor cell radiosensitivity to killing. Radiother Oncol J Eur Soc Ther Radiol Oncol

Chua ML, Rothkamm K (2013) Biomarkers of radiation exposure: can they predict normal tissue radiosensitivity? Clin Oncol 25:610–616

Collins AR (2014) Measuring oxidative damage to DNA and its repair with the comet assay. Biochim Biophys Acta 1840:794–800

Crosbie JC, Anderson RL, Rothkamm K, Restall CM, Cann L, Ruwanpura S, Meachem S, Yagi N, Svalbe I, Lewis RA et al (2010) Tumor cell response to synchrotron microbeam radiation therapy differs markedly from cells in normal tissues. Int J Radiat Oncol Biol Phys 77:886–894

Czarny P, Pawlowska E, Bialkowska-Warzecha J, Kaarniranta K, Blasiak J (2015) Autophagy in DNA damage response. Int J Mol Sci 16:2641–2662

Dahm-Daphi J, Dikomey E (1996) Rejoining of DNA double-strand breaks in X-irradiated CHO cells studied by constant- and graded-field gel electrophoresis. Int J Radiat Biol 69:615–621

Davis AJ, Chen DJ (2013) DNA double strand break repair via non-homologous end-joining. Transl Cancer Res 2:130–143

Desai A, Webb B, Gerson SL (2014) CD133+ cells contribute to radioresistance via altered regulation of DNA repair genes in human lung cancer cells. Radiother Oncol J Eur Soc Ther Radiol Oncol 110:538–545

Dillon MT, Good JS, Harrington KJ (2014) Selective targeting of the G2/M cell cycle checkpoint to improve the therapeutic index of radiotherapy. Clin Oncol 26:257–265

Dobbelstein M, Sorensen CS (2015) Exploiting replicative stress to treat cancer. Nat Rev Drug Discov 14:405–423

Dungey FA, Loser DA, Chalmers AJ (2008) Replication-dependent radiosensitization of human glioma cells by inhibition of poly(ADP-Ribose) polymerase: mechanisms and therapeutic potential. Int J Radiat Oncol Biol Phys 72:1188–1197

El-Awady RA, Dikomey E, Dahm-Daphi J (2003) Radiosensitivity of human tumour cells is correlated with the induction but not with the repair of DNA double-strand breaks. Br J Cancer 89:593–601

Fong PC, Boss DS, Yap TA, Tutt A, Wu P, Mergui-Roelvink M, Mortimer P, Swaisland H, Lau A, O'Connor MJ et al (2009) Inhibition of poly(ADP-ribose) polymerase in tumors from BRCA mutation carriers. N Eng J Med 361:123–134

Garrett MD, Collins I (2011) Anticancer therapy with checkpoint inhibitors: what, where and when? Trends Pharmacol Sci 32:308–316

Giralt J, Trigo J, Nuyts S, Ozsahin M, Skladowski K, Hatoum G, Daisne JF, Yunes Ancona AC, Cmelak A, Mesia R et al (2015) Panitumumab plus radiotherapy versus chemoradiotherapy in patients with unresected, locally advanced squamous-cell carcinoma of the head and neck (CONCERT-2): a randomised, controlled, open-label phase 2 trial. Lancet Oncol 16:221–232

Goodarzi AA, Noon AT, Deckbar D, Ziv Y, Shiloh Y, Lobrich M, Jeggo PA (2008) ATM signaling facilitates repair of DNA double-strand breaks associated with heterochromatin. Mol Cell 31:167–177

Groth P, Orta ML, Elvers I, Majumder MM, Lagerqvist A, Helleday T (2012) Homologous recombination repairs secondary replication induced DNA double-strand breaks after ionizing radiation. Nucleic Acids Res 40:6585–6594

Harari PM, Allen GW, Bonner JA (2007) Biology of interactions: antiepidermal growth factor receptor agents. J Clin Oncol Official J Am Soc Clin Oncol 25:4057–4065

Helleday T, Lo J, van Gent DC, Engelward BP (2007) DNA double-strand break repair: from mechanistic understanding to cancer treatment. DNA Repair 6:923–935

Huang F, Mazin AV (2014) A small molecule inhibitor of human RAD51 potentiates breast cancer cell killing by therapeutic agents in mouse xenografts. PLoS ONE 9:e100993

Jackson SP, Bartek J (2009) The DNA-damage response in human biology and disease. Nature 461:1071–1078

Jager U, Bocskor S, Le T, Mitterbauer G, Bolz I, Chott A, Kneba M, Mannhalter C, Nadel B (2000) Follicular lymphomas' BCL-2/IgH junctions contain templated nucleotide insertions: novel insights into the mechanism of t(14;18) translocation. Blood 95:3520–3529

Jensen LJ, Kuhn M, Stark M, Chaffron S, Creevey C, Muller J, Doerks T, Julien P, Roth A, Simonovic M et al (2009) STRING 8–a global view on proteins and their functional interactions in 630 organisms. Nucleic Acids Res 37:D412–D416

Koi L, Bergmann R, Bruchner K, Pietzsch J, Pietzsch HJ, Krause M, Steinbach J, Zips D, Baumann M (2014) Radiolabeled anti-EGFR-antibody improves local tumor control after external beam radiotherapy and offers theragnostic potential. Radiother Oncol J Eur Soc Ther Radiol Oncol 110:362–369

Kotsantis P, Jones RM, Higgs MR, Petermann E (2015) Cancer therapy and replication stress: forks on the road to perdition. Adv Clin Chem 69:91–138

Kotter A, Cornils K, Borgmann K, Dahm-Daphi J, Petersen C, Dikomey E, Mansour WY (2014) Inhibition of PARP1-dependent end-joining contributes to Olaparib-mediated radiosensitization in tumor cells. Mol Oncol 8:1616–1625

Krause DS, Van Etten RA (2005) Tyrosine kinases as targets for cancer therapy. N Eng J Med 353:172–187

Kriegs M, Gurtner K, Can Y, Brammer I, Rieckmann T, Oertel R, Wysocki M, Dorniok F, Gal A, Grob TJ et al (2015) Radiosensitization of NSCLC cells by EGFR inhibition is the result of an enhanced p53-dependent G1 arrest. Radiother Oncol J Eur Soc Ther Radiol Oncol 115:120–127

Kriegs M, Kasten-Pisula U, Rieckmann T, Holst K, Saker J, Dahm-Daphi J, Dikomey E (2010) The epidermal growth factor receptor modulates DNA double-strand break repair by regulating non-homologous end-joining. DNA Repair 9:889–897

Laban S, Steinmeister L, Gleißner L, Grob TJ, Grénman R, Petersen C, Gal A, Knecht R, Dikomey E, Kriegs M (2013) Sorafenib sensitizes head and neck squamous cell carcinoma cells to ionizing radiation. Radiother Oncol 109:286–292

Lapidot T, Sirard C, Vormoor J, Murdoch B, Hoang T, Caceres-Cortes J, Minden M, Paterson B, Caligiuri MA, Dick JE (1994) A cell initiating human acute myeloid leukaemia after transplantation into SCID mice. Nature 367:645–648

Lassen P, Eriksen JG, Hamilton-Dutoit S, Tramm T, Alsner J, Overgaard J (2009) Effect of HPV-associated p16INK4A expression on response to radiotherapy and survival in squamous cell carcinoma of the head and neck. J Clin Oncol Official J Am Soc Clin Oncol 27:1992–1998

Lee SW, Cho KJ, Park JH, Kim SY, Nam SY, Lee BJ, Kim SB, Choi SH, Kim JH, Ahn SD et al (2005) Expressions of Ku70 and DNA-PKcs as prognostic indicators of local control in nasopharyngeal carcinoma. Int J Radiat Oncol Biol Phys 62:1451–1457

Lieber MR, Ma Y, Pannicke U, Schwarz K (2003) Mechanism and regulation of human non-homologous DNA end-joining. Nat Rev Mol Cell Biol 4:712–720

Lundholm L, Haag P, Zong D, Juntti T, Mork B, Lewensohn R, Viktorsson K (2013) Resistance to DNA-damaging treatment in non-small cell lung cancer tumor-initiating cells involves reduced DNA-PK/ATM activation and diminished cell cycle arrest. Cell Death Dis 4:e478

Magee JA, Piskounova E, Morrison SJ (2012) Cancer stem cells: impact, heterogeneity, and uncertainty. Cancer Cell 21:283–296

Mandal PK, Blanpain C, Rossi DJ (2011) DNA damage response in adult stem cells: pathways and consequences. Nat Rev Mol Cell Biol 12:198–202

Manning G, Rothkamm K (2013) Deoxyribonucleic acid damage-associated biomarkers of ionising radiation: current status and future relevance for radiology and radiotherapy. Br J Radiol 86:20130173

Mansour WY, Bogdanova NV, Kasten-Pisula U, Rieckmann T, Kocher S, Borgmann K, Baumann M, Krause M, Petersen C, Hu H et al (2013b) Aberrant overexpression of miR-421 downregulates ATM and leads to a pronounced DSB repair defect and clinical hypersensitivity in SKX squamous cell carcinoma. Radiother Oncol J Eur Soc Ther Radiol Oncol 106:147–154

Mansour WY, Borgmann K, Petersen C, Dikomey E, Dahm-Daphi J (2013a) The absence of Ku but not defects in classical non-homologous end-joining is required to trigger PARP1-dependent end-joining. DNA Repair 12:1134–1142

Mansour WY, Rhein T, Dahm-Daphi J (2010) The alternative end-joining pathway for repair of DNA double-strand breaks requires PARP1 but is not dependent upon microhomologies. Nucleic Acids Res 38:6065–6077

Mansour WY, Schumacher S, Rosskopf R, Rhein T, Schmidt-Petersen F, Gatzemeier F, Haag F, Borgmann K, Willers H, Dahm-Daphi J (2008) Hierarchy of nonhomologous end-joining, single-strand annealing and gene conversion at site-directed DNA double-strand breaks. Nucleic Acids Res 36:4088–4098

Marechal A, Zou L (2013) DNA damage sensing by the ATM and ATR kinases. Cold Spring Harbor Perspect Biol 5

Martins RG, Parvathaneni U, Bauman JE, Sharma AK, Raez LE, Papagikos MA, Yunus F, Kurland BF, Eaton KD, Liao JJ et al (2013) Cisplatin and radiotherapy with or without Erlotinib in locally advanced squamous cell carcinoma of the head and neck: a randomized phase ii trial. J Clin Oncol Official J Am Soc Clin Oncol

Mateo J, Carreira S, Sandhu S, Miranda S, Mossop H, Perez-Lopez R, Nava Rodrigues D, Robinson D, Omlin A, Tunariu N et al (2015) DNA-repair defects and olaparib in metastatic prostate cancer. N Eng J Med 373:1697–1708

Mathews LA, Cabarcas SM, Hurt EM, Zhang X, Jaffee EM, Farrar WL (2011) Increased expression of DNA repair genes in invasive human pancreatic cancer cells. Pancreas 40:730–739

Maugeri-Sacca M, Vici P, Di Lauro L, Barba M, Amoreo CA, Gallo E, Mottolese M, De Maria R (2014) Cancer stem cells: are they responsible for treatment failure? Future Oncol 10:2033–2044

Maynard S, Swistowska AM, Lee JW, Liu Y, Liu ST, Da Cruz AB, Rao M, de Souza-Pinto NC, Zeng X, Bohr VA (2008) Human embryonic stem cells have enhanced repair of multiple forms of DNA damage. Stem Cells 26:2266–2274

McCord AM, Jamal M, Williams ES, Camphausen K, Tofilon PJ (2009) CD133+ glioblastoma stem-like cells are radiosensitive with a defective DNA damage response compared with established cell lines. Clin Cancer Res Official J Am Assoc Cancer Res 15:5145–5153

McNeely S, Beckmann R, Bence Lin AK (2014) CHEK again: revisiting the development of CHK1 inhibitors for cancer therapy. Pharmacol Ther 142:1–10

Menegakis A, von Neubeck C, Yaromina A, Thames H, Hering S, Hennenlotter J, Scharpf M, Noell S, Krause M, Zips D et al (2015) gammaH2AX assay in ex vivo irradiated tumour specimens: a novel method to determine tumour radiation sensitivity in patient-derived material. Radiother Oncol J Eur Soc Ther Radiol Oncol

Menegakis A, De Colle C, Yaromina A, Hennenlotter J, Stenzl A, Scharpf M, Fend F, Noell S, Tatagiba M, Brucker S et al (2015) Residual gammaH2AX foci after ex vivo irradiation of patient samples with known tumour-type specific differences in radio-responsiveness. Radiother Oncol J Eur Soc Ther Radiol Oncol

Mesia R, Henke M, Fortin A, Minn H, Yunes Ancona AC, Cmelak A, Markowitz AB, Hotte SJ, Singh S, Chan AT et al (2015) Chemoradiotherapy with or without panitumumab in patients with unresected, locally advanced squamous-cell carcinoma of the head and neck (CONCERT-1): a randomised, controlled, open-label phase 2 trial. Lancet Oncol 16:208–220

Möckelmann N, Rieckmann T, Busch CJ, Becker B, Gleißner L, Hoffer K, Omniczynski M, Steinmeister L, Laban S, Grénman R et al (2016) Effect of sorafenib on cisplatin-based chemoradiation in head and neck cancer cells. Oncotarget doi: 10.18632/oncotarget.8275

Moeller BJ, Yordy JS, Williams MD, Giri U, Raju U, Molkentine DP, Byers LA, Heymach JV, Story MD, Lee JJ et al (2011) DNA repair biomarker profiling of head and neck cancer: Ku80 expression predicts locoregional failure and death following radiotherapy. Clin Cancer Res Official J Am Assoc Cancer Res 17:2035–2043

Morgan MA, Lawrence TS (2015) Molecular pathways: overcoming radiation resistance by targeting DNA damage response pathways. Clin Cancer Res Official J Am Assoc Cancer Res 21:2898–2904

Myllynen L, Rieckmann T, Dahm-Daphi J, Kasten-Pisula U, Petersen C, Dikomey E, Kriegs M (2011) In tumor cells regulation of DNA double strand break repair through EGF receptor involves both NHEJ and HR and is independent of p53 and K-Ras status. Radiother Oncol J Eur Soc Ther Radiol Oncol 101:147–151

Naipal KA, Verkaik NS, Ameziane N, van Deurzen CH, Ter Brugge P, Meijers M, Sieuwerts AM, Martens JW, O'Connor MJ, Vrieling H et al (2014) Functional ex vivo assay to select homologous recombination-deficient breast tumors for PARP inhibitor treatment. Clin Cancer Res Official J Am Assoc Cancer Res 20:4816–4826

Noel G, Godon C, Fernet M, Giocanti N, Megnin-Chanet F, Favaudon V (2006) Radiosensitization by the poly(ADP-ribose) polymerase inhibitor 4-amino-1,8-naphthalimide is specific of the S phase of the cell cycle and involves arrest of DNA synthesis. Mol Cancer Ther 5:564–574

Olive PL (2009) Impact of the comet assay in radiobiology. Mutat Res 681:13–23

Orthwein A, Fradet-Turcotte A, Noordermeer SM, Canny MD, Brun CM, Strecker J, Escribano-Diaz C, Durocher D (2014) Mitosis inhibits DNA double-strand break repair to guard against telomere fusions. Science 344:189–193

Ostling O, Johanson KJ (1984) Microelectrophoretic study of radiation-induced DNA damages in individual mammalian cells. Biochem Biophys Res Commun 123:291–298

Parplys AC, Kratz K, Speed MC, Leung SG, Schild D, Wiese C (2014) RAD51AP1-deficiency in vertebrate cells impairs DNA replication. DNA Repair 24:87–97

Parplys AC, Petermann E, Petersen C, Dikomey E, Borgmann K (2012) DNA damage by X-rays and their impact on replication processes. Radiother Oncol J Eur Soc Ther Radiol Oncol 102:466–471

Parplys AC, Seelbach JI, Becker S, Behr M, Jend C, Mansour WY, Joosse S, Stuerzbecher HW, Pospiech H, Petersen C et al (2015a) High levels of RAD51 perturb DNA replication elongation and cause unscheduled origin firing due to impaired CHK1 activation. Cell Cycle

Parplys AC, Zhao W, Sharma N, Groesser T, Liang F, Maranon DG, Leung SG, Grundt K, Dray E, Idate R et al (2015b) NUCKS1 is a novel RAD51AP1 paralog important for homologous recombination and genome stability. Nucleic Acids Res

Pearl LH, Schierz AC, Ward SE, Al-Lazikani B, Pearl FM (2015) Therapeutic opportunities within the DNA damage response. Nat Rev Cancer 15:166–180

Pernot E, Hall J, Baatout S, Benotmane MA, Blanchardon E, Bouffler S, El Saghire H, Gomolka M, Guertler A, Harms-Ringdahl M et al (2012) Ionizing radiation biomarkers for potential use in epidemiological studies. Mutat Res 751:258–286

Pires IM, Olcina MM, Anbalagan S, Pollard JR, Reaper PM, Charlton PA, McKenna WG, Hammond EM (2012) Targeting radiation-resistant hypoxic tumour cells through ATR inhibition. Br J Cancer 107:291–299

Pramana J, Van den Brekel MW, van Velthuysen ML, Wessels LF, Nuyten DS, Hofland I, Atsma D, Pimentel N, Hoebers FJ, Rasch CR et al (2007) Gene expression profiling to predict outcome after chemoradiation in head and neck cancer. Int J Radiat Oncol Biol Phys 69:1544–1552

Qvarnstrom OF, Simonsson M, Johansson KA, Nyman J, Turesson I (2004) DNA double strand break quantification in skin biopsies. Radiother Oncol J Eur Soc Ther Radiol Oncol 72:311–317

Ropolo M, Daga A, Griffero F, Foresta M, Casartelli G, Zunino A, Poggi A, Cappelli E, Zona G, Spaziante R et al (2009) Comparative analysis of DNA repair in stem and nonstem glioma cell cultures. Mol Cancer Res MCR 7:383–392

Rothkamm K, Barnard S, Moquet J, Ellender M, Rana Z, Burdak-Rothkamm S (2015) DNA damage foci: meaning and significance. Environ Mol Mutagen 56:491–504

Rothkamm K, Crosbie JC, Daley F, Bourne S, Barber PR, Vojnovic B, Cann L, Rogers PA (2012) In situ biological dose mapping estimates the radiation burden delivered to 'spared' tissue between synchrotron X-ray microbeam radiotherapy tracks. PLoS ONE 7:e29853

Rothkamm K, Kruger I, Thompson LH, Lobrich M (2003) Pathways of DNA double-strand break repair during the mammalian cell cycle. Mol Cell Biol 23:5706–5715

Rothkamm K, Lobrich M (2002) Misrepair of radiation-induced DNA double-strand breaks and its relevance for tumorigenesis and cancer treatment (review). Int J Oncol 21:433–440

Rothkamm K, Lobrich M (2003) Evidence for a lack of DNA double-strand break repair in human cells exposed to very low x-ray doses. Proc Natl Acad Sci USA 100:5057–5062

Rube CE, Dong X, Kuhne M, Fricke A, Kaestner L, Lipp P, Rube C (2008) DNA double-strand break rejoining in complex normal tissues. Int J Radiat Oncol Biol Phys 72:1180–1187

Saker J, Kriegs M, Zenker M, Heldt JM, Eke I, Pietzsch HJ, Grenman R, Cordes N, Petersen C, Baumann M et al (2013) Inactivation of HNSCC cells by 90Y-labeled cetuximab strictly depends on the number of induced DNA double-strand breaks. J Nucl Med Official Pub Soc Nucl Med 54:416–423

Sarbajna S, Davies D, West SC (2014) Roles of SLX1-SLX4, MUS81-EME1, and GEN1 in avoiding genome instability and mitotic catastrophe. Genes Dev 28:1124–1136

Shin KH, Kang MK, Kim RH, Kameta A, Baluda MA, Park NH (2006) Abnormal DNA end-joining activity in human head and neck cancer. Int J Mol Med 17:917–924

Shinohara A, Shinohara M, Ohta T, Matsuda S, Ogawa T (1998) Rad52 forms ring structures and co-operates with RPA in single-strand DNA annealing. Genes Cells Devoted Mol Cell Mech 3:145–156

Signore M, Pelacchi F, di Martino S, Runci D, Biffoni M, Giannetti S, Morgante L, De Majo M, Petricoin EF, Stancato L et al (2014) Combined PDK1 and CHK1 inhibition is required to kill glioblastoma stem-like cells in vitro and in vivo. Cell Death Dis 5:e1223

Somaiah N, Yarnold J, Daley F, Pearson A, Gothard L, Rothkamm K, Helleday T (2012) The relationship between homologous recombination repair and the sensitivity of human epidermis to the size of daily doses over a 5-week course of breast radiotherapy. Clinical Cancer Res Official J Am Assoc Cancer Res 18:5479–5488

Sorensen CS, Syljuasen RG (2012) Safeguarding genome integrity: the checkpoint kinases ATR, CHK1 and WEE1 restrain CDK activity during normal DNA replication. Nucleic Acids Res 40:477–486

Spitzner M, Emons G, Kramer F, Gaedcke J, Rave-Frank M, Scharf JG, Burfeind P, Becker H, Beissbarth T, Ghadimi BM et al (2010) A gene expression signature for chemoradiosensitivity of colorectal cancer cells. Int J Radiat Oncol Biol Phys 78:1184–1192

Spivak G (2015) Nucleotide excision repair in humans. DNA repair

Stegeman H, Span PN, Cockx SC, Peters JP, Rijken PF, van der Kogel AJ, Kaanders JH, Bussink J (2013) EGFR-inhibition enhances apoptosis in irradiated human head and neck xenograft tumors independent of effects on DNA repair. Radiat Res 180:414–421

Sulli G, Di Micco R, d'Adda di Fagagna F (2012) Crosstalk between chromatin state and DNA damage response in cellular senescence and cancer. Nat Rev Cancer 12:709–720

Sung P, Klein H (2006) Mechanism of homologous recombination: mediators and helicases take on regulatory functions. Nat Rev Mol Cell Biol 7:739–750

Syljuasen RG, Hasvold G, Hauge S, Helland A (2015) Targeting lung cancer through inhibition of checkpoint kinases. Front Genet 6:70

Tennstedt P, Fresow R, Simon R, Marx A, Terracciano L, Petersen C, Sauter G, Dikomey E, Borgmann K (2013) RAD51 overexpression is a negative prognostic marker for colorectal adenocarcinoma. Int J Cancer 132:2118–2126

Terasawa M, Shinohara A, Shinohara M (2014) Double-strand break repair-adox: restoration of suppressed double-strand break repair during mitosis induces genomic instability. Cancer Sci 105:1519–1525

Tinhofer I, Niehr F, Konschak R, Liebs S, Munz M, Stenzinger A, Weichert W, Keilholz U, Budach V (2015) Next-generation sequencing: hype and hope for development of personalized radiation therapy? Radiat Oncol 10:183

Toulany M, Kasten-Pisula U, Brammer I, Wang S, Chen J, Dittmann K, Baumann M, Dikomey E, Rodemann HP (2006) Blockage of epidermal growth factor receptor-phosphatidylinositol 3-kinase-AKT signaling increases radiosensitivity of K-RAS mutated human tumor cells in vitro by affecting DNA repair. Clin Cancer Res Official J Am Assoc Cancer Res 12:4119–4126

Tutt A, Robson M, Garber JE, Domchek SM, Audeh MW, Weitzel JN, Friedlander M, Arun B, Loman N, Schmutzler RK et al (2010) Oral poly(ADP-ribose) polymerase inhibitor olaparib in patients with BRCA1 or BRCA2 mutations and advanced breast cancer: a proof-of-concept trial. Lancet 376:235–244

UNSCEAR (2000) Sources and Effects of Ionizing Radiation: Annex F: DNA repair and mutagenesis.United Nations scientific committee on the effects of atomic radiation.

Venere M, Hamerlik P, Wu Q, Rasmussen RD, Song LA, Vasanji A, Tenley N, Flavahan WA, Hjelmeland AB, Bartek J et al (2014) Therapeutic targeting of constitutive PARP activation compromises stem cell phenotype and survival of glioblastoma-initiating cells. Cell Death Differ 21:258–269

Wang Q, Gao F, May WS, Zhang Y, Flagg T, Deng X (2008) Bcl2 negatively regulates DNA double-strand-break repair through a nonhomologous end-joining pathway. Mol Cell 29:488–498

Wang M, Morsbach F, Sander D, Gheorghiu L, Nanda A, Benes C, Kriegs M, Krause M, Dikomey E, Baumann M et al (2011) EGF receptor inhibition radiosensitizes NSCLC cells by inducing senescence in cells sustaining DNA double-strand breaks. Cancer Res 71:6261–6269

Wang H, Perrault AR, Takeda Y, Qin W, Wang H, Iliakis G (2003) Biochemical evidence for Ku-independent backup pathways of NHEJ. Nucleic Acids Res 31:5377–5388

Weinstock DM, Brunet E, Jasin M (2007) Formation of NHEJ-derived reciprocal chromosomal translocations does not require Ku70. Nat Cell Biol 9:978–981

Welzel N, Le T, Marculescu R, Mitterbauer G, Chott A, Pott C, Kneba M, Du MQ, Kusec R, Drach J et al (2001) Templated nucleotide addition and immunoglobulin JH-gene utilization in t(11;14) junctions: implications for the mechanism of translocation and the origin of mantle cell lymphoma. Cancer Res 61:1629–1636

West CM, Davidson SE, Roberts SA, Hunter RD (1993) Intrinsic radiosensitivity and prediction of patient response to radiotherapy for carcinoma of the cervix. Br J Cancer 68:819–823

Wyatt HD, West SC (2014) Holliday junction resolvases. Cold Spring Harbor Perspect Biol 6: a023192

Ying S, Hamdy FC, Helleday T (2012) Mre11-dependent degradation of stalled DNA replication forks is prevented by BRCA2 and PARP1. Cancer Res 72:2814–2821

Zeman MK, Cimprich KA (2014) Causes and consequences of replication stress. Nature Cell Biol 16:2–9

Zhang P, Wei Y, Wang L, Debeb BG, Yuan Y, Zhang J, Yuan J, Wang M, Chen D, Sun Y et al (2014) ATM-mediated stabilization of ZEB1 promotes DNA damage response and radioresistance through CHK1. Nature Cell Biol 16:864–875

Cancer Stem Cells

Wendy A. Woodward and Richard P. Hill

Abstract

The cancer stem cell model in solid tumors has evolved significantly from the early paradigm shifting work highlighting parallels between the stem cell hierarchy in hematologic malignancies and solid tumors. Putative stem cells can dedifferentiated, be induced by context, and be the result of accumulated genetic mutations. The simple hypothesis that stem cell therapies will overcome the minority of cells that lead to recurrence has evolved with it. Nevertheless, the body of evidence that this field is clinically relevant in patients and patient care has grown with the complexity of the hypotheses, and numerous clinical strategies to target these cells have been identified. Herein we review this progress and highlight the work still outstanding.

Keywords

Cancer stem cells · Stem cell markers · Stem cell models · Stem cell resistance · Microenvironment

W.A. Woodward (✉)
Department of Radiation Oncology, The University of Texas
MD Anderson Cancer Center, Houston, TX 77030, USA
e-mail: wwoodward@mdanderson.org

R.P. Hill
Princess Margaret Cancer Centre, Ontario Cancer Insitute,
Toronto, ON M5G 2M9, Canada
e-mail: hill@uhnres.utoronto.ca

R.P. Hill
Department of Medical Biophysics, University of Toronto,
Toronto, ON M5G 2M9, Canada

© Springer-Verlag Berlin Heidelberg 2016
M. Baumann et al. (eds.), *Molecular Radio-Oncology*, Recent Results
in Cancer Research 198, DOI 10.1007/978-3-662-49651-0_2

1 Overview of the Evolution of the Cancer Stem Cell Model

Work over the last decade has highlighted the potential importance of stem cell populations in tumors—cancer stem cells (Clarke et al. 2006; O'Brien et al. 2009). Such cells (CSCs) have been argued to represent the critical population for predicting progression and treatment outcome presuming that their number and treatment sensitivity are important for tumor control by radiation and chemotherapy. The prospective demonstration that only small specific populations of cells, derived from a bulk solid tumor population based on expression of specific surface markers, recreated human tumors in outgrowth experiments propelled the subsequent 10 years of cancer stem cell research. The initial concept was that tumors are organized as steep hierarchies from which only a small percentage of cells are capable of self-renewing and recapitulating the tumor heterogeneity. This concept built on normal stem cell data attributing characteristics of normal stem cells—multipotency, unlimited replication potential, and self-renewal—to proposed cancer stem cells. The cancer stem cell hierarchy was initially viewed as a largely rigid top-down progression from the most primitive cancer stem cells at the top to the most differentiated bulk cells at the bottom. It was presumed that individual cancer stem cells reproduced themselves to maintain self-renewal and as needed produced differentiated daughter cells to maintain homeostasis with a small population of cancer stem cells (Fig. 1a). This model presumed the functional and phenotypic differences of stem cells versus differentiated cells were independent of genetic mutation, mediated instead by epigenetics and differentiation commitment. This stood somewhat at odds with the clonal dynamic, driver mutation model of tumor

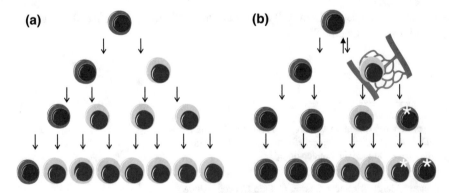

Fig. 1 Increasing complexity in the cancer stem cell model. Drawing from parallels in hematopoietic development, prospective isolation of tumor-initiating cells from solid tumors led to early models of cancer hierarchy similar to the normal state (1A). Primitive, self-renewing cells were presumed to maintain the tumor bulk and the minority population of cancer stem cells. In the last decade has been demonstrated that context and microenvironment can promote tumor initiation, that mutations (*) can confer self-renewing capacity, that some tumors become predominantly composed of self-renewing cells, that markers of self-renewing cells are context dependent, and that functional initiating cells can be both genetically similar or dissimilar (Fig. 1b)

progression and recurrence; the evidence for both was hotly debated. Early on, there were no studies merging genetic analyses with *stemness* studies, and very little consideration was given to the role that context might have in influencing the stem cell population. Over time, however, many new data emerged, challenged the initial paradigm, and were incorporated into this initially simplistic model (Fig. 1b).

After the reports of the first solid tumors to apparently be organized in a cancer stem cell hierarchy (Al-Hajj et al. 2003; Singh et al. 2004), it was demonstrated that the cancer stem cell compartment size and depth of hierarchy depend on tumor type and that self-renewal assays of tumor regrowth in transplants predict for the biology associated with engraftment in animals, which might not faithfully capture the biology of recurrence in situ (Feuring-Buske et al. 2003; Quintana et al. 2008; Notta et al. 2010; Rehe et al. 2013). New markers and strategies to prospectively identify stem cells emerged (Collins et al. 2005; Bao et al. 2006; Dalerba et al. 2007; Ginestier et al. 2007; Hermann et al. 2007; Li et al. 2007; O'Brien et al. 2007; Patrawala et al. 2007; Prince et al. 2007; Ricci-Vitiani et al. 2007; Eramo et al. 2008; Curley et al. 2009; Li et al. 2009a; Piccirillo et al. 2009; Stewart et al. 2011; Wang et al. 2011; Chen et al. 2012; Charafe-Jauffret et al. 2013; Wu et al. 2013; Zhang et al. 2015), and from these, a series of prognostic signatures were derived across tumor types [Table 1 (Gentles et al. 2010; Eppert et al. 2011; Merlos-Suarez et al. 2011; Bartholdy et al. 2014)]. This connection to clinical outcome was reassuring that the cancer stem cell model was relevant. However, the clinical complexity and challenges to incorporation into clinical management were clearly illuminated by findings from patients that the prospectively identified populations that maintain outgrowth potential in tumors may be different in different tumors and patients (Eppert et al. 2011). This further highlighted the need to move to the use of functional demonstrations of stemness rather than the use of markers that are promiscuous, often not linked to function, are potentially transient and depend on context. To this end, the inducible lineage-tracing and re-tracing experiments were developed in genetically engineered mouse models to overcome these issues [reviewed in Roy et al. (2014)], and in some cases, these validated the stem cell model, but they still have some limitations as discussed in more detail below.

Clonal dynamic studies using lineage-tracing approaches in normal tissues demonstrated some common themes across tissues in some cases. In gut and skin, maintaining the frequency of stem cells during homeostasis appeared not as a function of asymmetric division of the primitive stem cell, to create one stem cell and one daughter cell, but rather through maintenance at the population level [reviewed in Blanpain and Simons (2013)]. In other studies, the stem cells identified in lineage-tracing experiments did not align with the prior findings from transplantation experiments, suggesting that transplantation assays may provide circumstances that permit or promote tumor initiation that would not occur in situ. For example, the first lineage-tracing experiments to define cell fate in the developing mammary gland demonstrated that the bipotent differentiation potential of single cells described after transplantation is not identified in situ (Van Keymeulen et al. 2011; van Amerongen 2014). Instead two unipotent basal and luminal stem cells were identified. The same was described in prostate development (Liu et al. 2011;

Table 1 Tumor-initiating cell-related gene signature studies reporting prognostic signatures in independent patient data derived from bulk cells (Glinsky et al. 2005; Phillips et al. 2006; Liu et al. 2007; Shipitsin et al. 2007; Stevenson et al. 2009; Gentles et al. 2010; Eppert et al. 2011; Merlos-Suarez et al. 2011; Becker et al. 2012; Liu et al. 2012; Atkinson et al. 2013; Metzeler et al. 2013; Schwede et al. 2013; Van den Broeck et al. 2013; Peng et al. 2014; Yin et al. 2014; Pfefferle et al. 2015; Yang et al. 2015)

Cancer Type	Signature Source
	Genes identifies in minority stem-like population prognostic in independent tumor samples
Breast, brain, lung prostate	Liu et al. (2007). The prognostic role of a gene signature from tumorigenic breast cancer cells.
Breast	Shipitsin et al. (2007). Molecular definition of breast tumor heterogeneity.
Breast (H2N+)	Liu et al. (2012). Seventeen-gene signature from enriched Her2/Neu mammary tumor-initiating cells predicts clinical outcome for human HER2+: ERalpha- breast cancer.
Breast	Yin et al. (2014). A 41-gene signature derived from breast cancer stem cells as a predictor of survival.
Colon	Merlos-Suarez et al. (2011). The intestinal stem cell signature identifies colorectal cancer stem cells and predicts disease relapse.
Pancreas	Van den Broeck et al. (2013). Human pancreatic cancer contains a side population expressing cancer stem cell-associated and prognostic genes.
Leukemia	Gentles et al. (2010). Association of a leukemic stem cell gene expression signature with clinical outcomes in acute myeloid leukemia.
Leukemia	Eppert et al. (2011). Stem cell gene expression programs influence clinical outcome in human leukemia.
Leukemia	Metzeler et al. (2013). A stem cell-like gene expression signature associates with inferior outcomes and a distinct microRNA expression profile in adults with primary cytogenetically normal AML.
Leukemia	Yang et al. (2015). Systematic computation with functional gene-sets among leukemic and hematopoietic stem cells reveals a favorable prognostic signature for acute myeloid leukemia.
	Genes extracted based on embyonic or developmental correlation prognostic in independent tumor samples
Breast	Pfefferle et al. (2015). Luminal progenitor and fetal mammary stem cell expression features predict breast tumor response to neoadjuvant chemotherapy.

(continued)

Table 1 (continued)

Cancer Type	Signature Source
Prostate, breast, lung, ovarian, bladder, lymphoma, mesothelioma, brain, and leukemia	Glinsky et al. (2005). Microarray analysis identifies a death-from-cancer signature predicting therapy failure in patients with multiple types of cancer.
Lung	Stevenson et al. (2009). Characterizing the clinical relevance of an embryonic stem cell phenotype in lung adenocarcinoma.
Liver	Becker et al. (2012). Genetic signatures shared in embryonic liver development and liver cancer define prognostically relevant subgroups in HCC.
Brain	Phillips et al. (2006). Molecular subclasses of high-grade glioma predict prognosis, delineate a pattern of disease progression, and resemble stages in neurogenesis.
Ovary	Schwede et al. (2013). Stem cell-like gene expression in ovarian cancer predicts type II subtype and prognosis.
Prostate	Peng et al. (2014). An expression signature at diagnosis to estimate prostate cancer patients' overall survival.
	Genes identified in minority stem-like population prognostic in independent normal breast samples from patients with tumor
Breast	Atkinson et al. (2013). Cancer stem cell markers are enriched in normal tissue adjacent to triple negative breast cancer and inversely correlated with DNA repair deficiency.

Wang et al. 2014). Later, Rios et al. highlighting the potential caveats of these approaches identified a single bipotent stem cell in the mammary gland (Rios et al. 2014). Speculation regarding contributors to the dramatic differences in the results of these studies includes differences in promoter specificity and/or transcriptional activity due to approaches used, labeling efficiency in different lineages, and confocal imaging variation across the studies [reviewed in Oakes et al. (2014)]. Alternatively or in addition, it may simply reflect the heterogeneous results of a legitimately complex system revealed through differing studies.

Fate mapping was carried out in tumors including benign papilloma and squamous cell carcinoma, glioma, and intestinal adenomas (Chen et al. 2010; Driessens et al. 2012; Schepers et al. 2012). Progression in skin cancer appeared to track with a decrease in the steepness of the hierarchy (Driessens et al. 2012). Through the fate mapping/lineage-tracing experiments as well as with the use of animal models, it was additionally demonstrated that the stem cell frequency could be altered by genetic mutations in the stem cells or background (Vaillant et al. 2008; Curtis et al. 2010; Vermeulen et al. 2013) and that for some normal tissues and many tumors, the pool of stem cells could be replenished, if significantly depleted, via dedifferentiation of a previously non-self-renewing cell (Debeb et al. 2012; van Es et al. 2012;

Buczacki et al. 2013; Schwitalla et al. 2013). The latter challenged the idea that targeting cancer stem cells within bulk tumors would be curative since the remaining more differentiated cells could potentially replace the targeted pool and might be driven to do so by a shift in stem-differentiated cell equilibrium caused by therapy targeting one side of the equation. This demonstration of plasticity led to the concept that stem cells in fact represent a heterogeneous compartment into which cells readily transit and exit becoming temporarily primed for specific stem cell activity [reviewed in Blanpain and Simons (2013)]. It was clear that pressure on the tumor cells such as therapy could shift this equilibrium and that specific signaling pathways could be identified that mediated these transitions.

The most plastic of tumor cells were also presumed to transition between epithelial and mesenchymal states to escape from the primary soil into the circulation and beyond to reseed distant soil (Liu et al. 2014). It further became clear that the microenvironment, including a niche of cells that supported the stem cell state, contributed to maintaining this proposed transient stemness compartment [reviewed in Inman et al. (2015)]. As numerous normal cells were identified as niche conspirators, including macrophages and mesenchymal stem cells, distinct niches for active versus quiescent or dormant stem cells were proposed (Ehninger and Trumpp 2011), and subsequently, the possibility of end organ-specific niches, bone marrow versus lung versus brain, was added to the emerging complex picture.

Alongside the progress made through lineage-tracing experiments, progress in genetic analysis began to converge on the cancer stem cell field. Studies merging these fields led to a direct demonstration that the pressure of therapy to select surviving clones indeed did not in all cases select genetically hardy clones, but rather phenotypically hardy clones, supporting the cancer stem cell hypothesis (Kreso et al. 2013). It was further shown in this work transplanting 150 single cells from 10 colorectal cancer patients that there can be genetic variability within a clone derived from a single stem cell (Kreso et al. 2013). Kreso and Dick proposed a unified model drawing on the genetic and cancer stem cell data and hypothesized that the accumulation of cancer-promoting mutations in the most primitive normal stem cells at the top of the hierarchy led to the most undifferentiated and aggressive cancers, while mutations in more differentiated cells might confer self-renewal and therefore lead to less aggressive cancers (Kreso and Dick 2014). Consistent with this proposal, Tomasetti and Vogelstein report a strong correlation extending over five orders of magnitude between lifetime incidence of multiple cancers and the estimated number of normal stem cell divisions in the corresponding tissues over a lifetime. This suggests that random errors occurring during DNA replication in normal stem cells are a major contributing factor in cancer development (Tomasetti and Vogelstein 2015). Without question, the cancer stem cell model has matured making room for greater complexity.

2 Markers and Models

As above, the solid tumor cancer stem cell field was propelled forward by landmark papers in which tumorigenic breast and brain cancer cells were prospectively identified and distinguished from non-tumorigenic cells in the same cancer using membrane markers (Al-Hajj et al. 2003; Singh et al. 2004). The readout in these studies was tumor outgrowth in an orthotopic xenograft. This work led to a rapid increase in papers across many tumor types identifying marker sets that prospectively identified the tumorigenic population in human tumors and cell lines using outgrowth in a xenograft as the proof of stemness (Collins et al. 2005; Bao et al. 2006; Dalerba et al. 2007; Ginestier et al. 2007; Hermann et al. 2007; Li et al. 2007; O'Brien et al. 2007; Patrawala et al. 2007; Prince et al. 2007; Ricci-Vitiani et al. 2007; Eramoi et al. 2008; Curley et al. 2009; Li et al. 2009a; Piccirillo et al. 2009; Stewart et al. 2011; Wang et al. 2011; Chen et al. 2012; Charafe-Jauffret et al. 2013; Wu et al. 2013; Zhang et al. 2015) (Table 2). In sum, these studies demonstrated minority tumorigenic populations in multiple tumor types including breast, colon, pancreas, head and neck, sarcoma, lung, ovary, AML, and CML. These studies relied on immunocompromised mice to grow human tumors, and it was quickly recognized that mice with greater immune suppression yielded higher frequencies of tumorigenic cells in AML, ALL, melanoma, and lung cancer (Quintana et al. 2008; Taussig et al. 2008; Chiu et al. 2010; Ishizawa et al. 2010; Notta et al. 2011) raising the question of whether the apparent tumor hierarchy was an artifact of the assay or a clinical reality, although studies supporting the reality were also compelling(O'Brien et al. 2009; Ishizawa et al. 2010). It was further noted that not all murine growth factors cross-react with human receptors and that numerous tissue processing issues may impact the outgrowth in a transplantation assay (Bossen et al. 2006; Rongvaux et al. 2013). One approach to address the variability related to altered immunity was to examine tumors in syngeneic mice with intact immune systems. Consistent with the data from the human tumors, several tumor types examined in these studies supported the cancer stem cell model (Neering et al. 2007; Vaillant et al. 2008; Zhang et al. 2008; Read et al. 2009; Ward et al. 2009). These studies did not necessarily yield markers that are relevant in human cancers however, a difference may relate to the fact that many surface markers do not relate directly to stem cell function.

Following the identification of markers in various solid tumor types, there were numerous studies using these markers in vitro and in translational work to identify genetic signatures from these populations, to identify targets to eradicate them, and

Table 2 Markers reported to prospectively identify tumor initiation from human tumors

Prostate	CD44+		
Head and Neck	CD44+	SP	
Breast	CD44+ ESA+ CD24-	ALDH	GD2
Colon	CD44+ ESA+	CD133+	CD166
Pancreas	CD44+ ESA+ CD24+	CD133+ CXCR4+	
Glioma	CD133+*		
Lung	CD133+		
Ovary	CD133+	CA125	

[a]Controversial. Abbreviations: SP, side population; ALDH, aldehyde dehydrogenase activity; ESA, epithelial-specific antigen

Blue and *Green* colors denote their relevance across tumor types. *Bold* represent single markers

to demonstrate their relationship to prognosis. While these were supportive of the model in many cases, it was quickly demonstrated that the markers can depend on context [reviewed in Meacham and Morrison (2013)], that they are promiscuous, and that they are not necessarily related to function. In larger studies of patient samples, it was apparent that in some tumors, the tumorigenic potential may reside in varying minority populations, suggesting that functionally determining which cells were CSCs would need to be a component of individual patient sample analysis (Chiu et al. 2010; Eppert et al. 2011; Sarry et al. 2011). Certainly, it is clear stem cell markers identified and validated in one xenograft model cannot be assumed to identify CSCs in new systems or models where this has not been explicitly demonstrated. Further, it remains to be seen how widely results from cancer stem cell models will apply to the clinic, although various clinical studies have reported that the proportion of cells expressing CSC markers, such as ALDH1 or low proteasome activity, correlates with treatment outcome (Lagadec et al. 2014; Atkinson et al. 2013; Ginestier et al. 2007).

While marker studies furthered the field by identifying cells with tumorigenic potential under permissive circumstances, lineage-tracing studies including proliferation kinetics and clonal dynamics [reviewed in Blanpain and Simons (2013)] have allowed more direct examination of the clonal dynamics of the stem cells under more relevant contextual circumstances. Three techniques have been used to study proliferation kinetics in population-based assays. These are pulse-chase, continuous labeling, and label dilution experiments. These can be applied in vivo by targeting inducible reporter constructs with lineage-restricted promoters to a small number of cells and examining the distribution of labeled cells after elapsed time for the organ of interest to develop. Quantitative analysis is performed to assess the clonal dynamics based on the fixed tissue analysis. These approaches cannot definitively distinguish between population balance that is perfectly maintained through either asymmetric division of a single stem cell that results in a stem cell and a differentiated cell versus division of a stem cell into two stem cells. Importantly, although they have been used to demonstrate differences in multipotency among stem cells in their native context, further work to resolve the fate of individual cells is needed to determine whether lineage is specified early (bestowed on only a few cells early on) or instead involves a competition between equipotent precursors.

In the gut, lineage tracing identified two stem cell pools, one LGR5-expressing pool and a second BMI-1-expressing pool. It was further shown that on ablation of the LGR5 pool, the BMI-1 expressing stem cells can repopulate the crypt (Barker et al. 2007; Sangiorgi and Capecchi 2008; Barker et al. 2012). What is not clear, however, is whether these populations are mutually exclusive. Indeed recent studies have raised the possibility that this work may have targeted the same pool using different promoters (Itzkovitz et al. 2012; Munoz et al. 2012; Buczacki et al. 2013), and Blanpain et al. speculate that the stem cell pool may express all of the identified markers at different times specified by different contexts (Blanpain and Simons 2013). Quantitative studies using these models demonstrated that the number of label-retaining cells was maintained over time by increase in the size of remaining clones as the total number of surviving clones diminished and largely ruled out the likelihood that ingrained hierarchy accounts for self-renewal, demonstrating instead that neutral competition for limited access to the niche dominates this process (Lopez-Garcia et al. 2010; Snippert et al. 2010b). Similar to the findings in the gut, lineage tracing in the skin also revealed that clones are lost over time and that the constant label-retaining pool is accounted for at the population level by proliferation of the remaining pool (Clayton et al. 2007; Doupe et al. 2010). Quantitative studies here suggested that the tissue was maintained by a single progenitor population, which divided asymmetrically most of the time, but may also divide symmetrically or terminally differentiate to maintain balance. Studies of response after injury mentioned below in aggregate support the model in which the pool is maintained by progenitors and a slower cycling stem cell pool sit ready in response to injury (Ito et al. 2005; Levy et al. 2007; Jaks et al. 2008; Snippert et al. 2010a). The possibility that these progenitors revert into the slow-cycling stem cell pool as described in esophagus (Doupe et al. 2012) cannot easily be ascertained or ruled out. It was reported that location within the niche predetermines the likelihood of a given cell to remain uncommitted or to differentiate, but that committed cells can replenish the stem cell pool after depletion (Rompolas et al. 2013). Using genetic lineage-tracing strategies, similar dedifferentiation behavior as that described in the skin has been reported for the Delta-like 1-expressing cells in the mouse intestine where lineage tracing demonstrates these normally committed, differentiated cells can be recruited into the stem cell compartment if needed upon injury (van Es et al. 2012). Similarly committed Paneth cells can apparently repopulate the stem cell compartment when needed(Buczacki et al. 2013). This important role of position and context has also been demonstrated to regulate the proliferation or quiescence of cancer stem cells (Bissell and Inman 2008).

Fate mapping in tumors was similarly informative. Expression of a conditional reporter in a small population of benign papilloma cells confirmed a hierarchical organization, which became more shallow on progression to squamous cell carcinoma (Driessens et al. 2012). In intestinal adenomas, the previously identified stem cell marker Lgr5+ was tracked through the development of benign lesions using a multicolor lineage reporter. The marked normal stem cells gave rise to the adenomas, and these cells in the adenoma contributed extensively to the tumor growth. The preponderance of Lgr− progeny led to the speculation that the Lgr+ cells gave rise to largely non-proliferative Lgr− cells. Reflecting what is likely a clinical reality, similar studies of intestinal adenomas in different context yield a dissimilar story. Upon Wnt pathway activation, Vermeulen et al. found the Lgr− cells could contribute to the adenoma formation and Lgr− cells gave rise to Lgr+ cells (Vermeulen et al. 2013). It has not yet been established what fraction of adenomas have a hierarchical organization, and how it relates to progression to invasive cancer has not been studied. In glioma studies, the presumptive Nestin+ stem cell population was selectively depleted extending the animals' lives (Chen et al. 2012). Regrowth after therapy with temozolomide was attributed to the Nestin+ population correlating this population to cancer stem cell status although it was not conclusively demonstrated that Nestin− cells did not contribute (Chen et al. 2012).

3   Role of the Tumor Microenvironment

The stromal components and cell–cell interactions in a tumor play an important role in its growth and response to treatment. Stroma within a tumor includes the vasculature, various populations of cells derived from the bone marrow (BMDC) such as monocytes/macrophages and a variety of immune cell populations, cancer-associated fibroblasts, and non-cellular tissue components such as collagens, fibronectin, and laminin. Further, the poorly organized structure of the vasculature in most tumors (Vaupel et al. 1989) creates an environment in which there is substantial heterogeneity in the supply of nutrients such as oxygen or glucose and in the removal of catabolic products. This leads to regions of low oxygen tension (hypoxia), high levels of acidity due to lactic acid production, increased interstitial fluid pressure due to increased leakiness of the blood vessels, and poor removal of tissue fluid partly caused by lack of functional lymphatics. Specific microenvironmental factors, but also cell–cell interactions and genetically regulated cellular signals, are important determinants for stem cell maintenance and survival. As discussed above, different kinds of 'niches' have been described in which certain stromal cell populations may provide a supportive environment for CSCs and/or help to maintain the stem-like phenotype of tumor cells (Pajonk and Vlashi 2013). For example, in two mouse models of metastatic breast cancer, distinct endothelial sub-niches were shown to regulate disseminated tumor cell dormancy with vascular homeostasis maintaining quiescence but stimulation of vasculature causing outgrowth of the tumor cells (Bissell). It has also been reported that glioblastoma cells may sit in a perivascular niche involving endothelial cell contact (Heddleston et al. 2010) but it has also been reported that both glioblastoma and breast cancer CSCs may sit at a distance from functional vasculature and can be at low oxygen levels (i.e., in an hypoxic niche) (Heddleston et al. 2010; Liu et al. 2014; Peitzsch et al. 2014). Interestingly, hypoxia can suppress miRNA levels by repression of both the DICER and DROSHA enzymes, which are required for miRNA processing (van den Beucken et al. 2014). This leads to a significant decrease in overall levels of certain miRNA in hypoxic cells, which in turn can lead to the acquisition of stem and metastatic phenotypes. In a genetically engineered mouse model of soft tissue sarcoma, deletion of one allele of DICER can decrease miRNA expression and increase the rate of metastasis to the lung (Mito et al. 2013). In breast cancer, reduction in DICER results in a selective loss of the miR200 family of proteins, which stimulates an epithelial to mesenchymal transition (EMT) (van den Beucken et al. 2014). This transition has been associated with a CSC phenotype in breast cancer cells (Mani et al. 2008; Liu et al. 2014). Exposure to hypoxia has also been reported to result in changes in the methylation levels of certain genes, due to a requirement for oxygen by some of the enzymes that cause demethylation. This results in a more primitive phenotype similar to that of stem cells. Thus, exposure to hypoxia may cause various epigenetic changes that promote a stem cell phenotype.

4 Response to Therapy

There are many datasets which support a higher treatment resistance of CSC to both radiation and chemotherapeutic drugs compared to non-CSC (Krause et al. 2011; Alison et al. 2012; Sebens and Schafer 2012; Alisi et al. 2013; Holohan et al. 2013; Crowder et al. 2014; Rycaj and Tang 2014; Cui et al. 2015). The increased resistance to chemotherapy has been variably associated with the proliferative quiescence of CSCs and their resistance to DNA damage and reduced susceptibility to induction of apoptosis. A high expression of ABC transporters that can pump drugs out of cells has also been observed in CSCs. Early studies demonstrated an increase in the ex vivo fraction of CD133 positive cells, confirmed as CSC by transplantation assays, following in vivo irradiation of glioma xenografts. Interestingly, DNA damage checkpoints were preferentially activated in marker-positive versus marker-negative cells (Bao et al. 2006). Higher levels of antioxidant molecules have also been observed in CSCs suggesting increased ability to inactivate reactive oxygen species (ROS), a mediator of radiation damage in cells (Diehn et al. 2009). Compared to progenitor cells, breast CSCs have been shown in vitro to contain a lower level of ROS with higher expression of genes involved in ROS scavenging. Moreover, the initially higher post-irradiation clonogenic cell survival of breast CSC can be altered by pharmacological modulation of the ROS levels. Recent studies by Pajonk and colleagues have also reported that low proteasome activity is associated with a stem cell phenotype and that cells from tumors with low proteasome activity are more resistant to chemotherapy and radiation treatment (Lagadec et al. 2012, 2014; Vlashi and Pajonk 2015). However, a higher intrinsic resistance of CSC cannot be regarded as a general phenomenon, since heterogeneity seems to exist between individual tumors of the same histology (Zielske et al. 2011). Further, the early work of West et al. (West et al. 1993) reported a wide range of radiosensitivities for cells derived from different tumors of the cervix and head and neck that were capable of growing in in vitro clonogenic assays in agarose. This was a spheroid-like environment, although not the same as currently accepted stem cell assays.

A link between hypoxia and putative stem cells has also been shown by an increase in the fraction of CD133-positive cells in brain tumor cells exposed to hypoxia in vitro (Blazek et al. 2007; Platet et al. 2007) and the preferential expression of HIF2α- and HIF-regulated genes in glioma stem cells (Li et al. 2009b). This might be expected to affect their relative radiosensitivity, although it should be noted that the level of hypoxia in 'hypoxic' niches is not well defined and may represent a level of hypoxia more consistent with increased levels of HIF-1α and HIF-2α ($<\sim 10$–20 mm Hg) rather than the levels required for full hypoxia-induced radioresistance (<1–5 mm Hg) (Wilson and Hay 2011). Important in this context is that EMT (which as noted above can be induced by hypoxic exposure) has also been previously associated with increased radiation resistance (Theys et al. 2011; Bhat et al. 2013; Al-Assar et al. 2014; Zhang et al. 2014), as well as increased metastatic potential. The hypoxic niche has also been reported to protect colon cancer CSCs from chemotherapy (Mao et al. 2013). However, a recent study has reported that hypoxia does not affect the radiation survival of breast cancer stem cells cultured as mammospheres putatively because of their high levels of antioxidant molecules capable of scavenging reactive oxygen species (Lagadec et al. 2012). Thus, the potential role of hypoxia in modifying the treatment sensitivity of CSCs in vivo remains uncertain and may vary from tumor to tumor.

The number of CSCs in tumor is highly heterogeneous but will also play an important role in overall response to treatment. In animal models, it was demonstrated that the number of (putative) stem cells assessed by transplantation assays correlated with the single radiation dose required for tumor control (Hill and Milas 1989; Baumann et al. 2008). Similar results have been reported for experimental studies in animal models using fractionated radiation treatment (Yaromina et al. 2007) and the expression of the stem cell-related marker CD44 has been reported to correlate with local control in early laryngeal cancers treated with radiation (Baumann and Krause 2010). Two important considerations in the context of the analysis of the treatment sensitivity of CSC are the increasing evidence for the plasticity of the cancer stem cell phenotype and the method of assessment. The concept that early progenitor cells may regain stem cell properties induced by treatment would result in an effective increase in the number of CSCs in the tumor and hence the level of cell killing required to achieve tumor control (Pajonk and Vlashi 2013; Vlashi and Pajonk 2015). The results of Bao et al. (2006) mentioned above, in which radiation-treated gliomas demonstrated increased CSC content, may be explained by the concept that the radiation treatment induced progenitor cell populations in the tumor to reacquire stem cell properties, consistent with findings in normal tissues described above concerning rebalancing of stem and progenitor cell populations after traumatic injury. Assessing the sensitivity of CSCs in vivo using an experimental tumor response assay to determine treatment outcome rather than tumor control assay is also a concern. The essence of the CSC model is that it is the killing of these cells that is ultimately responsible for tumor control, whereas tumor response can reflect the sensitivity of both stem cells and progenitor cells (Baumann et al. 2008). This concern makes it particularly difficult to use experimental studies to assess the response of CSC to drug treatment in vivo, since such treatments are rarely capable of achieving tumor control on their own, and thus, they reflect the response of both stem and progenitor cells. Combination treatments with radiation can potentially address this concern, and such studies have indicated the failure of certain drugs to target stem cell populations (Baumann/Krause). A further complication is that these two considerations are independent of one another but may, of course, both occur during tumor treatments in vivo; thus in some cases, the interpretation of studies assessing the treatment sensitivity of CSC may be impacted by factors that do not directly relate to the sensitivity of the individual tumor cells. In vitro studies of the drug or radiation sensitivity of cells expressing putative stem cell markers can partially overcome this concern but the different environments found within tumors require that such observations are confirmed by in vivo studies.

5 Conclusion

Without question, the cancer stem cell model has been refined numerous times in the last decade and is far more complex than initially proposed. Heterogeneity within tumors and even in clonal populations within tumors, between tumors in the same patient, and between patients as well as across tumor types are the common themes that emerge across fields. The prognostic value of signatures from small populations of cells may imply that there are ways to clinically identify patients whose tumors are driven by a stem cell phenotype that may be amenable to directed therapy and get around the challenges of variation in prospective markers between patients as well as the limited feasibility in profiling each tumor for stemness markers in order to make treatment decisions. Nevertheless, real-time tumor profiling will likely be needed to select patients for therapy, and to date, there are still no trials selecting patients for treatment using such approaches and strategies to merge stem cell targeting with genetics-based targets are in their infancy. Certainly, advances in clinical imaging-based identification of stem cell-driven tumors would greatly enhance the translatability of these models as would liquid biopsy advances still very much unexplored in this area. Still, in spite of the work yet to do, the progress in the last decade has been rapid and continues on.

Acknowledgements Dr. Woodward is supported by the National Institutes of Health R01CA138239-01 and 1R01CA180061-01 and The State of Texas Grant for Rare and Aggressive Breast Cancer Research Program.

References

Al-Assar O, Demiciorglu F, Lunardi S, Gaspar-Carvalho MM, McKenna WG, Muschel RM, Brunner TB (2014) Contextual regulation of pancreatic cancer stem cell phenotype and radioresistance by pancreatic stellate cells. Radiother Oncol 111(2):243–251

Al-Hajj M, Wicha MS, Benito-Hernandez A, Morrison SJ, Clarke MF (2003) Prospective identification of tumorigenic breast cancer cells. Proc Natl Acad Sci U.S.A. 100(7):3983–3988

Alisi A, Cho WC, Locatelli F, Fruci D (2013) Multidrug resistance and cancer stem cells in neuroblastoma and hepatoblastoma. Int J Mol Sci 14(12):24706–24725

Alison MR, Lin WR, Lim SM, Nicholson LJ (2012) Cancer stem cells: in the line of fire. Cancer Treat Rev 38(6):589–598

Atkinson RL, Yang WT, Rosen DG, Landis MD, Wong H, Lewis MT, Creighton CJ, Sexton KR, Hilsenbeck SG, Sahin AA, Brewster AM, Woodward WA, Chang JC (2013) Cancer stem cell markers are enriched in normal tissue adjacent to triple negative breast cancer and inversely correlated with DNA repair deficiency. Breast Cancer Res 15(5):R77

Bao S, Wu Q, McLendon RE, Hao Y, Shi Q, Hjelmeland AB, Dewhirst MW, Bigner DD, Rich JN (2006) Glioma stem cells promote radioresistance by preferential activation of the DNA damage response. Nature 444(7120):756–760

Barker N, van Es JH, Kuipers J, Kujala P, van den Born M, Cozijnsen M, Haegebarth A, Korving J, Begthel H, Peters PJ, Clevers H (2007) Identification of stem cells in small intestine and colon by marker gene Lgr5. Nature 449(7165):1003–1007

Barker N, van Oudenaarden A, Clevers H (2012) Identifying the stem cell of the intestinal crypt: strategies and pitfalls. Cell Stem Cell 11(4):452–460

Bartholdy B, Christopeit M, Will B, Mo Y, Barreyro L, Yu Y, Bhagat TD, Okoye-Okafor UC, Todorova TI, Greally JM, Levine RL, Melnick A, Verma A, Steidl U (2014) HSC commitment-associated epigenetic signature is prognostic in acute myeloid leukemia. J Clin Invest 124(3):1158–1167

Baumann M, Krause M (2010) CD44: a cancer stem cell-related biomarker with predictive potential for radiotherapy. Clin Cancer Res 16(21):5091–5093

Baumann M, Krause M, Hill R (2008) Exploring the role of cancer stem cells in radioresistance. Nat Rev Cancer 8(7):545–554

Becker D, Sfakianakis I, Krupp M, Staib F, Gerhold-Ay A, Victor A, Binder H, Blettner M, Maass T, Thorgeirsson S, Galle PR, Teufel A (2012) Genetic signatures shared in embryonic liver development and liver cancer define prognostically relevant subgroups in HCC. Mol Cancer 11:55

Bhat KP, Balasubramaniyan V, Vaillant B, Ezhilarasan R, Hummelink K, Hollingsworth F, Wani K, Heathcock L, James JD, Goodman LD, Conroy S, Long L, Lelic N, Wang S, Gumin J, Raj D, Kodama Y, Raghunathan A, Olar A, Joshi K, Pelloski CE, Heimberger A, Kim SH, Cahill DP, Rao G, Den Dunnen WF, Boddeke HW, Phillips HS, Nakano I, Lang FF, Colman H, Sulman EP, Aldape K (2013) Mesenchymal differentiation mediated by NF-kappaB promotes radiation resistance in glioblastoma. Cancer Cell 24(3):331–346

Bissell MJ, Inman J (2008) Reprogramming stem cells is a microenvironmental task. Proc Natl Acad Sci U.S.A. 105(41):15637–15638

Blanpain C, Simons BD (2013) Unravelling stem cell dynamics by lineage tracing. Nat Rev Mol Cell Biol 14(8):489–502

Blazek ER, Foutch JL, Maki G (2007) Daoy medulloblastoma cells that express CD133 are radioresistant relative to CD133− cells, and the CD133+ sector is enlarged by hypoxia. Int J Radiat Oncol Biol Phys 67(1):1–5

Bossen C, Ingold K, Tardivel A, Bodmer JL, Gaide O, Hertig S, Ambrose C, Tschopp J, Schneider P (2006) Interactions of tumor necrosis factor (TNF) and TNF receptor family members in the mouse and human. J Biol Chem 281(20):13964–13971

Buczacki SJ, Zecchini HI, Nicholson AM, Russell R, Vermeulen L, Kemp R, Winton DJ (2013) Intestinal label-retaining cells are secretory precursors expressing Lgr5. Nature 495(7439):65–69

Charafe-Jauffret E, Ginestier C, Bertucci F, Cabaud O, Wicinski J, Finetti P, Josselin E, Adelaide J, Nguyen TT, Monville F, Jacquemier J, Thomassin-Piana J, Pinna G, Jalaguier A, Lambaudie E, Houvenaeghel G, Xerri L, Harel-Bellan A, Chaffanet M, Viens P, Birnbaum D (2013) ALDH1-positive cancer stem cells predict engraftment of primary breast tumors and are governed by a common stem cell program. Cancer Res 73(24):7290–7300

Chen J, Li Y, Yu TS, McKay RM, Burns DK, Kernie SG, Parada LF (2012) A restricted cell population propagates glioblastoma growth after chemotherapy. Nature 488(7412):522–526

Chen R, Nishimura MC, Bumbaca SM, Kharbanda S, Forrest WF, Kasman IM, Greve JM, Soriano RH, Gilmour LL, Rivers CS, Modrusan Z, Nacu S, Guerrero S, Edgar KA, Wallin JJ, Lamszus K, Westphal M, Heim S, James CD, VandenBerg SR, Costello JF, Moorefield S, Cowdrey CJ, Prados M, Phillips HS (2010) A hierarchy of self-renewing tumor-initiating cell types in glioblastoma. Cancer Cell 17(4):362–375

Chiu PP, Jiang H, Dick JE (2010) Leukemia-initiating cells in human T-lymphoblastic leukemia exhibit glucocorticoid resistance. Blood 116(24):5268–5279

Clarke MF, Dick JE, Dirks PB, Eaves CJ, Jamieson CH, Jones DL, Visvader J, Weissman IL, Wahl GM (2006) Cancer stem cells–perspectives on current status and future directions: AACR workshop on cancer stem cells. Cancer Res 66(19):9339–9344

Clayton E, Doupe DP, Klein AM, Winton DJ, Simons BD, Jones PH (2007) A single type of progenitor cell maintains normal epidermis. Nature 446(7132):185–189

Collins AT, Berry PA, Hyde C, Stower MJ, Maitland NJ (2005) Prospective identification of tumorigenic prostate cancer stem cells. Cancer Res 65(23):10946–10951

Crowder SW, Balikov DA, Hwang YS, Sung HJ (2014) Cancer stem cells under hypoxia as a chemoresistance factor in breast and brain. Curr Pathobiol Rep 2(1):33–40

Cui H, Zhang AJ, Chen M, Liu JJ (2015) ABC transporter inhibitors in reversing multidrug resistance to chemotherapy. Curr Drug Targets

Curley MD, Therrien VA, Cummings CL, Sergent PA, Koulouris CR, Friel AM, Roberts DJ, Seiden MV, Scadden DT, Rueda BR, Foster R (2009) CD133 expression defines a tumor initiating cell population in primary human ovarian cancer. Stem Cells 27(12):2875–2883

Curtis SJ, Sinkevicius KW, Li D, Lau AN, Roach RR, Zamponi R, Woolfenden AE, Kirsch DG, Wong KK, Kim CF (2010) Primary tumor genotype is an important determinant in identification of lung cancer propagating cells. Cell Stem Cell 7(1):127–133

Dalerba P, Dylla SJ, Park IK, Liu R, Wang X, Cho RW, Hoey T, Gurney A, Huang EH, Simeone DM, Shelton AA, Parmiani G, Castelli C, Clarke MF (2007) Phenotypic characterization of human colorectal cancer stem cells. Proc Natl Acad Sci U.S.A. 104 (24):10158–10163

Debeb BG, Lacerda L, Xu W, Larson R, Solley T, Atkinson R, Sulman EP, Ueno NT, Krishnamurthy S, Reuben JM, Buchholz TA, Woodward WA (2012) Histone deacetylase inhibitors stimulate dedifferentiation of human breast cancer cells through WNT/beta-catenin signaling. Stem Cells 30(11):2366–2377

Diehn M, Cho RW, Lobo NA, Kalisky T, Dorie MJ, Kulp AN, Qian D, Lam JS, Ailles LE, Wong M, Joshua B, Kaplan MJ, Wapnir I, Dirbas FM, Somlo G, Garberoglio C, Paz B, Shen J, Lau SK, Quake SR, Brown JM, Weissman IL, Clarke MF (2009) Association of reactive oxygen species levels and radioresistance in cancer stem cells. Nature 458(7239):780–783

Doupe DP, Alcolea MP, Roshan A, Zhang G, Klein AM, Simons BD, Jones PH (2012) A single progenitor population switches behavior to maintain and repair esophageal epithelium. Science 337(6098):1091–1093

Doupe DP, Klein AM, Simons BD, Jones PH (2010) The ordered architecture of murine ear epidermis is maintained by progenitor cells with random fate. Dev Cell 18(2):317–323

Driessens G, Beck B, Caauwe A, Simons BD, Blanpain C (2012) Defining the mode of tumour growth by clonal analysis. Nature 488(7412):527–530

Ehninger A, Trumpp A (2011) The bone marrow stem cell niche grows up: mesenchymal stem cells and macrophages move in. J Exp Med 208(3):421–428

Eppert K, Takenaka K, Lechman ER, Waldron L, Nilsson B, van Galen P, Metzeler KH, Poeppl A, Ling V, Beyene J, Canty AJ, Danska JS, Bohlander SK, Buske C, Minden MD, Golub TR, Jurisica I, Ebert BL, Dick JE (2011) Stem cell gene expression programs influence clinical outcome in human leukemia. Nat Med 17(9):1086–1093

Eramo A, Lotti F, Sette G, Pilozzi E, Biffoni M, Di Virgilio A, Conticello C, Ruco L, Peschle C, De Maria R (2008) Identification and expansion of the tumorigenic lung cancer stem cell population. Cell Death Differ 15(3):504–514

Feuring-Buske M, Gerhard B, Cashman J, Humphries RK, Eaves CJ, Hogge DE (2003) Improved engraftment of human acute myeloid leukemia progenitor cells in beta 2-microglobulin-deficient NOD/SCID mice and in NOD/SCID mice transgenic for human growth factors. Leukemia 17(4):760–763

Gentles AJ, Plevritis SK, Majeti R, Alizadeh AA (2010) Association of a leukemic stem cell gene expression signature with clinical outcomes in acute myeloid leukemia. JAMA 304(24):2706–2715

Ginestier C, Hur MH, Charafe-Jauffret E, Monville F, Dutcher J, Brown M, Jacquemier J, Viens P, Kleer CG, Liu S, Schott A, Hayes D, Birnbaum D, Wicha MS, Dontu G (2007) ALDH1 is a marker of normal and malignant human mammary stem cells and a predictor of poor clinical outcome. Cell Stem Cell 1(5):555–567

Glinsky GV, Berezovska O, Glinskii AB (2005) Microarray analysis identifies a death-from-cancer signature predicting therapy failure in patients with multiple types of cancer. J Clin Invest 115(6):1503–1521

Heddleston JM, Li Z, Lathia JD, Bao S, Hjelmeland AB, Rich JN (2010) Hypoxia inducible factors in cancer stem cells. Br J Cancer 102(5):789–795

Hermann PC, Huber SL, Herrler T, Aicher A, Ellwart JW, Guba M, Bruns CJ, Heeschen C (2007) Distinct populations of cancer stem cells determine tumor growth and metastatic activity in human pancreatic cancer. Cell Stem Cell 1(3):313–323

Hill RP, Milas L (1989) The proportion of stem cells in murine tumors. Int J Radiat Oncol Biol Phys 16(2):513–518

Holohan C, Van Schaeybroeck S, Longley DB, Johnston PG (2013) Cancer drug resistance: an evolving paradigm. Nat Rev Cancer 13(10):714–726

Inman JL, Robertson C, Mott JD, Bissell MJ (2015) Mammary gland development: cell fate specification, stem cells and the microenvironment. Development 142(6):1028–1042

Ishizawa K, Rasheed ZA, Karisch R, Wang Q, Kowalski J, Susky E, Pereira K, Karamboulas C, Moghal N, Rajeshkumar NV, Hidalgo M, Tsao M, Ailles L, Waddell TK, Maitra A, Neel BG, Matsui W (2010) Tumor-initiating cells are rare in many human tumors. Cell Stem Cell 7 (3):279–282

Ito M, Liu Y, Yang Z, Nguyen J, Liang F, Morris RJ, Cotsarelis G (2005) Stem cells in the hair follicle bulge contribute to wound repair but not to homeostasis of the epidermis. Nat Med 11 (12):1351–1354

Itzkovitz S, Lyubimova A, Blat IC, Maynard M, van Es J, Lees J, Jacks T, Clevers H, van Oudenaarden A (2012) Single-molecule transcript counting of stem-cell markers in the mouse intestine. Nat Cell Biol 14(1):106–114

Jaks V, Barker N, Kasper M, van Es JH, Snippert HJ, Clevers H, Toftgard R (2008) Lgr5 marks cycling, yet long-lived, hair follicle stem cells. Nat Genet 40(11):1291–1299

Krause M, Yaromina A, Eicheler W, Koch U, Baumann M (2011) Cancer stem cells: targets and potential biomarkers for radiotherapy. Clin Cancer Res 17(23):7224–7229

Kreso A, Dick JE (2014) Evolution of the cancer stem cell model. Cell Stem Cell 14(3):275–291

Kreso A, O'Brien CA, van Galen P, Gan OI, Notta F, Brown AM, Ng K, Ma J, Wienholds E, Dunant C, Pollett A, Gallinger S, McPherson J, Mullighan CG, Shibata D, Dick JE (2013) Variable clonal repopulation dynamics influence chemotherapy response in colorectal cancer. Science 339(6119):543–548

Lagadec C, Dekmezian C, Bauche L, Pajonk F (2012) Oxygen levels do not determine radiation survival of breast cancer stem cells. PLoS ONE 7(3):e34545

Lagadec C, Vlashi E, Bhuta S, Lai C, Mischel P, Werner M, Henke M, Pajonk F (2014) Tumor cells with low proteasome subunit expression predict overall survival in head and neck cancer patients. BMC Cancer 14:152. doi:10.1186/1471-2407-14-152

Levy V, Lindon C, Zheng Y, Harfe BD, Morgan BA (2007) Epidermal stem cells arise from the hair follicle after wounding. FASEB J 21(7):1358–1366

Li C, Heidt DG, Dalerba P, Burant CF, Zhang L, Adsay V, Wicha M, Clarke MF, Simeone DM (2007) Identification of pancreatic cancer stem cells. Cancer Res 67(3):1030–1037

Li C, Lee CJ, Simeone DM (2009a) Identification of human pancreatic cancer stem cells. Methods Mol Biol 568:161–173

Li Z, Bao S, Wu Q, Wang H, Eyler C, Sathornsumetee S, Shi Q, Cao Y, Lathia J, McLendon RE, Hjelmeland AB, Rich JN (2009b) Hypoxia-inducible factors regulate tumorigenic capacity of glioma stem cells. Cancer Cell 15(6):501–513

Liu J, Pascal LE, Isharwal S, Metzger D, Ramos Garcia R, Pilch J, Kasper S, Williams K, Basse PH, Nelson JB, Chambon P, Wang Z (2011) Regenerated luminal epithelial cells are derived from preexisting luminal epithelial cells in adult mouse prostate. Mol Endocrinol 25 (11):1849–1857

Liu JC, Voisin V, Bader GD, Deng T, Pusztai L, Symmans WF, Esteva FJ, Egan SE, Zacksenhaus E (2012) Seventeen-gene signature from enriched Her2/Neu mammary tumor-initiating cells predicts clinical outcome for human HER2+ :ERalpha- breast cancer. Proc Natl Acad Sci U.S.A. 109(15):5832–5837

Liu R, Wang X, Chen GY, Dalerba P, Gurney A, Hoey T, Sherlock G, Lewicki J, Shedden K, Clarke MF (2007) The prognostic role of a gene signature from tumorigenic breast-cancer cells. N Engl J Med 356(3):217–226

Liu S, Cong Y, Wang D, Sun Y, Deng L, Liu Y, Martin-Trevino R, Shang L, McDermott SP, Landis MD, Hong S, Adams A, D'Angelo R, Ginestier C, Charafe-Jauffret E, Clouthier SG, Birnbaum D, Wong ST, Zhan M, Chang JC, Wicha MS (2014) Breast cancer stem cells transition between epithelial and mesenchymal states reflective of their normal counterparts. Stem Cell Reports 2(1):78–91

Lopez-Garcia C, Klein AM, Simons BD, Winton DJ (2010) Intestinal stem cell replacement follows a pattern of neutral drift. Science 330(6005):822–825

Mani SA, Guo W, Liao MJ, Eaton EN, Ayyanan A, Zhou AY, Brooks M, Reinhard F, Zhang CC, Shipitsin M, Campbell LL, Polyak K, Brisken C, Yang J, Weinberg RA (2008) The epithelial-mesenchymal transition generates cells with properties of stem cells. Cell 133 (4):704–715

Mao Q, Zhang Y, Fu X, Xue J, Guo W, Meng M, Zhou Z, Mo X, Lu Y (2013) A tumor hypoxic niche protects human colon cancer stem cells from chemotherapy. J Cancer Res Clin Oncol 139(2):211–222

Meacham CE, Morrison SJ (2013) Tumour heterogeneity and cancer cell plasticity. Nature 501 (7467):328–337

Merlos-Suarez A, Barriga FM, Jung P, Iglesias M, Cespedes MV, Rossell D, Sevillano M, Hernando-Momblona X, da Silva-Diz V, Munoz P, Clevers H, Sancho E, Mangues R, Batlle E (2011) The intestinal stem cell signature identifies colorectal cancer stem cells and predicts disease relapse. Cell Stem Cell 8(5):511–524

Metzeler KH, Maharry K, Kohlschmidt J, Volinia S, Mrozek K, Becker H, Nicolet D, Whitman SP, Mendler JH, Schwind S, Eisfeld AK, Wu YZ, Powell BL, Carter TH, Wetzler M, Kolitz JE, Baer MR, Carroll AJ, Stone RM, Caligiuri MA, Marcucci G, Bloomfield CD (2013) A stem cell-like gene expression signature associates with inferior outcomes and a distinct microRNA expression profile in adults with primary cytogenetically normal acute myeloid leukemia. Leukemia 27(10):2023–2031

Mito JK, Min HD, Ma Y, Carter JE, Brigman BE, Dodd L, Dankort D, McMahon M, Kirsch DG (2013) Oncogene-dependent control of miRNA biogenesis and metastatic progression in a model of undifferentiated pleomorphic sarcoma. J Pathol 229(1):132–140

Munoz J, Stange DE, Schepers AG, van de Wetering M, Koo BK, Itzkovitz S, Volckmann R, Kung KS, Koster J, Radulescu S, Myant K, Versteeg R, Sansom OJ, van Es JH, Barker N, van Oudenaarden A, Mohammed S, Heck AJ, Clevers H (2012) The Lgr5 intestinal stem cell signature: robust expression of proposed quiescent '+4' cell markers. EMBO J 31(14):3079–3091

Neering SJ, Bushnell T, Sozer S, Ashton J, Rossi RM, Wang PY, Bell DR, Heinrich D, Bottaro A, Jordan CT (2007) Leukemia stem cells in a genetically defined murine model of blast-crisis CML. Blood 110(7):2578–2585

Notta F, Doulatov S, Dick JE (2010) Engraftment of human hematopoietic stem cells is more efficient in female NOD/SCID/IL-2Rgc-null recipients. Blood 115(18):3704–3707

Notta F, Mullighan CG, Wang JC, Poeppl A, Doulatov S, Phillips LA, Ma J, Minden MD, Downing JR, Dick JE (2011) Evolution of human BCR-ABL1 lymphoblastic leukaemia-initiating cells. Nature 469(7330):362–367

O'Brien CA, Kreso A, Dick JE (2009) Cancer stem cells in solid tumors: an overview. Semin Radiat Oncol 19(2):71–77

O'Brien CA, Pollett A, Gallinger S, Dick JE (2007) A human colon cancer cell capable of initiating tumour growth in immunodeficient mice. Nature 445(7123):106–110

Oakes SR, Gallego-Ortega D, Ormandy CJ (2014) The mammary cellular hierarchy and breast cancer. Cell Mol Life Sci 71(22):4301–4324

Pajonk F, Vlashi E (2013) Characterization of the stem cell niche and its importance in radiobiological response. Semin Radiat Oncol 23(4):237–241

Patrawala L, Calhoun-Davis T, Schneider-Broussard R, Tang DG (2007) Hierarchical organization of prostate cancer cells in xenograft tumors: the CD44+ alpha2beta1+ cell population is enriched in tumor-initiating cells. Cancer Res 67(14):6796–6805

Peitzsch C, Perrin R, Hill RP, Dubrovska A, Kurth I (2014) Hypoxia as a biomarker for radioresistant cancer stem cells. Int J Radiat Biol 90(8):636–652

Peng Z, Skoog L, Hellborg H, Jonstam G, Wingmo IL, Hjalm-Eriksson M, Harmenberg U, Cedermark GC, Andersson K, Ahrlund-Richter L, Pramana S, Pawitan Y, Nister M, Nilsson S, Li C (2014) An expression signature at diagnosis to estimate prostate cancer patients' overall survival. Prostate Cancer Prostatic Dis 17(1):81–90

Pfefferle AD, Spike BT, Wahl GM, Perou CM (2015) Luminal progenitor and fetal mammary stem cell expression features predict breast tumor response to neoadjuvant chemotherapy. Breast Cancer Res Treat 149(2):425–437

Phillips HS, Kharbanda S, Chen R, Forrest WF, Soriano RH, Wu TD, Misra A, Nigro JM, Colman H, Soroceanu L, Williams PM, Modrusan Z, Feuerstein BG, Aldape K (2006) Molecular subclasses of high-grade glioma predict prognosis, delineate a pattern of disease progression, and resemble stages in neurogenesis. Cancer Cell 9(3):157–173

Piccirillo SG, Combi R, Cajola L, Patrizi A, Redaelli S, Bentivegna A, Baronchelli S, Maira G, Pollo B, Mangiola A, DiMeco F, Dalpra L, Vescovi AL (2009) Distinct pools of cancer stem-like cells coexist within human glioblastomas and display different tumorigenicity and independent genomic evolution. Oncogene 28(15):1807–1811

Platet N, Liu SY, Atifi ME, Oliver L, Vallette FM, Berger F, Wion D (2007) Influence of oxygen tension on CD133 phenotype in human glioma cell cultures. Cancer Lett 258(2):286–290

Prince ME, Sivanandan R, Kaczorowski A, Wolf GT, Kaplan MJ, Dalerba P, Weissman IL, Clarke MF, Ailles LE (2007) Identification of a subpopulation of cells with cancer stem cell properties in head and neck squamous cell carcinoma. Proc Natl Acad Sci U.S.A. 104(3): 973–978

Quintana E, Shackleton M, Sabel MS, Fullen DR, Johnson TM, Morrison SJ (2008) Efficient tumour formation by single human melanoma cells. Nature 456(7222):593–598

Read TA, Fogarty MP, Markant SL, McLendon RE, Wei Z, Ellison DW, Febbo PG, Wechsler-Reya RJ (2009) Identification of CD15 as a marker for tumor-propagating cells in a mouse model of medulloblastoma. Cancer Cell 15(2):135–147

Rehe K, Wilson K, Bomken S, Williamson D, Irving J, den Boer ML, Stanulla M, Schrappe M, Hall AG, Heidenreich O, Vormoor J (2013) Acute B lymphoblastic leukaemia-propagating cells are present at high frequency in diverse lymphoblast populations. EMBO Mol Med 5 (1):38–51

Ricci-Vitiani L, Lombardi DG, Pilozzi E, Biffoni M, Todaro M, Peschle C, De Maria R (2007) Identification and expansion of human colon-cancer-initiating cells. Nature 445(7123): 111–115

Rios AC, Fu NY, Lindeman GJ, Visvader JE (2014) In situ identification of bipotent stem cells in the mammary gland. Nature 506(7488):322–327

Rompolas P, Mesa KR, Greco V (2013) Spatial organization within a niche as a determinant of stem-cell fate. Nature 502(7472):513–518

Rongvaux A, Takizawa H, Strowig T, Willinger T, Eynon EE, Flavell RA, Manz MG (2013) Human hemato-lymphoid system mice: current use and future potential for medicine. Annu Rev Immunol 31:635–674

Roy E, Neufeld Z, Livet J, Khosrotehrani K (2014) Concise review: understanding clonal dynamics in homeostasis and injury through multicolor lineage tracing. Stem Cells 32 (12):3046–3054

Rycaj K, Tang DG (2014) Cancer stem cells and radioresistance. Int J Radiat Biol 90(8):615–621

Sangiorgi E, Capecchi MR (2008) Bmi1 is expressed in vivo in intestinal stem cells. Nat Genet 40 (7):915–920

Sarry JE, Murphy K, Perry R, Sanchez PV, Secreto A, Keefer C, Swider CR, Strzelecki AC, Cavelier C, Recher C, Mansat-De Mas V, Delabesse E, Danet-Desnoyers G, Carroll M (2011) Human acute myelogenous leukemia stem cells are rare and heterogeneous when assayed in NOD/SCID/IL2Rgammac-deficient mice. J Clin Invest 121(1):384–395

Schepers AG, Snippert HJ, Stange DE, van den Born M, van Es JH, van de Wetering M, Clevers H (2012) Lineage tracing reveals Lgr5+ stem cell activity in mouse intestinal adenomas. Science 337(6095):730–735

Schwede M, Spentzos D, Bentink S, Hofmann O, Haibe-Kains B, Harrington D, Quackenbush J, Culhane AC (2013) Stem cell-like gene expression in ovarian cancer predicts type II subtype and prognosis. PLoS ONE 8(3):e57799

Schwitalla S, Fingerle AA, Cammareri P, Nebelsiek T, Goktuna SI, Ziegler PK, Canli O, Heijmans J, Huels DJ, Moreaux G, Rupec RA, Gerhard M, Schmid R, Barker N, Clevers H, Lang R, Neumann J, Kirchner T, Taketo MM, van den Brink GR, Sansom OJ, Arkan MC, Greten FR (2013) Intestinal tumorigenesis initiated by dedifferentiation and acquisition of stem-cell-like properties. Cell 152(1–2):25–38

Sebens S, Schafer H (2012) The tumor stroma as mediator of drug resistance–a potential target to improve cancer therapy? Curr Pharm Biotechnol 13(11):2259–2272

Shipitsin M, Campbell LL, Argani P, Weremowicz S, Bloushtain-Qimron N, Yao J, Nikolskaya T, Serebryiskaya T, Beroukhim R, Hu M, Halushka MK, Sukumar S, Parker LM, Anderson KS, Harris LN, Garber JE, Richardson AL, Schnitt SJ, Nikolsky Y, Gelman RS, Polyak K (2007) Molecular definition of breast tumor heterogeneity. Cancer Cell 11(3):259–273

Singh SK, Hawkins C, Clarke ID, Squire JA, Bayani J, Hide T, Henkelman RM, Cusimano MD, Dirks PB (2004) Identification of human brain tumour initiating cells. Nature 432(7015):396–401

Snippert HJ, Haegebarth A, Kasper M, Jaks V, van Es JH, Barker N, van de Wetering M, van den Born M, Begthel H, Vries RG, Stange DE, Toftgard R, Clevers H (2010a) Lgr6 marks stem cells in the hair follicle that generate all cell lineages of the skin. Science 327(5971):1385–1389

Snippert HJ, van der Flier LG, Sato T, van Es JH, van den Born M, Kroon-Veenboer C, Barker N, Klein AM, van Rheenen J, Simons BD, Clevers H (2010b) Intestinal crypt homeostasis results from neutral competition between symmetrically dividing Lgr5 stem cells. Cell 143(1):134–144

Stevenson M, Mostertz W, Acharya C, Kim W, Walters K, Barry W, Higgins K, Tuchman SA, Crawford J, Vlahovic G, Ready N, Onaitis M, Potti A (2009) Characterizing the clinical relevance of an embryonic stem cell phenotype in lung adenocarcinoma. Clin Cancer Res 15 (24):7553–7561

Stewart JM, Shaw PA, Gedye C, Bernardini MQ, Neel BG, Ailles LE (2011) Phenotypic heterogeneity and instability of human ovarian tumor-initiating cells. Proc Natl Acad Sci U.S. A. 108(16):6468–6473

Taussig DC, Miraki-Moud F, Anjos-Afonso F, Pearce DJ, Allen K, Ridler C, Lillington D, Oakervee H, Cavenagh J, Agrawal SG, Lister TA, Gribben JG, Bonnet D (2008) Anti-CD38 antibody-mediated clearance of human repopulating cells masks the heterogeneity of leukemia-initiating cells. Blood 112(3):568–575

Theys J, Jutten B, Habets R, Paesmans K, Groot AJ, Lambin P, Wouters BG, Lammering G, Vooijs M (2011) E-Cadherin loss associated with EMT promotes radioresistance in human tumor cells. Radiother Oncol 99(3):392–397

Tomasetti C, Vogelstein B (2015) Cancer etiology. Variation in cancer risk among tissues can be explained by the number of stem cell divisions. Science 347(6217):78–81

Vaillant F, Asselin-Labat ML, Shackleton M, Forrest NC, Lindeman GJ, Visvader JE (2008) The mammary progenitor marker CD61/beta3 integrin identifies cancer stem cells in mouse models of mammary tumorigenesis. Cancer Res 68(19):7711–7717

van Amerongen R (2014) Bipotent mammary stem cells: now in amazing 3D. Breast Cancer Res 16(6):480

van den Beucken T, Koch E, Chu K, Rupaimoole R, Prickaerts P, Adriaens M, Voncken JW, Harris AL, Buffa FM, Haider S, Starmans MH, Yao CQ, Ivan M, Ivan C, Pecot CV, Boutros PC, Sood AK, Koritzinsky M, Wouters BG (2014) Hypoxia promotes stem cell phenotypes and poor prognosis through epigenetic regulation of DICER. Nat Commun 5:5203

Van den Broeck A, Vankelecom H, Van Delm W, Gremeaux L, Wouters J, Allemeersch J, Govaere O, Roskams T, Topal B (2013) Human pancreatic cancer contains a side population expressing cancer stem cell-associated and prognostic genes. PLoS ONE 8(9):e73968 van Es JH, Sato T, van de Wetering M, Lyubimova A, Nee AN, Gregorieff A, Sasaki N, Zeinstra L, van den Born M, Korving J, Martens AC, Barker N, van Oudenaarden A, Clevers H (2012) Dll1+ secretory progenitor cells revert to stem cells upon crypt damage. Nat Cell Biol 14(10):1099–1104

Van Keymeulen A, Rocha AS, Ousset M, Beck B, Bouvencourt G, Rock J, Sharma N, Dekoninck S, Blanpain C (2011) Distinct stem cells contribute to mammary gland development and maintenance. Nature 479(7372):189–193

Vaupel P, Kallinowski F, Okunieff P (1989) Blood flow, oxygen and nutrient supply, and metabolic microenvironment of human tumors: a review. Cancer Res 49(23):6449–6465

Vermeulen L, Morrissey E, van der Heijden M, Nicholson AM, Sottoriva A, Buczacki S, Kemp R, Tavare S, Winton DJ (2013) Defining stem cell dynamics in models of intestinal tumor initiation. Science 342(6161):995–998

Vlashi E, Pajonk F (2015) Cancer stem cells, cancer cell plasticity and radiation therapy. Semin Cancer Biol 31:28–35

Wang J, Zhu HH, Chu M, Liu Y, Zhang C, Liu G, Yang X, Yang R, Gao WQ (2014) Symmetrical and asymmetrical division analysis provides evidence for a hierarchy of prostate epithelial cell lineages. Nat Commun 5:4758

Wang L, Park P, Zhang H, La Marca F, Lin CY (2011) Prospective identification of tumorigenic osteosarcoma cancer stem cells in OS99-1 cells based on high aldehyde dehydrogenase activity. Int J Cancer 128(2):294–303

Ward RJ, Lee L, Graham K, Satkunendran T, Yoshikawa K, Ling E, Harper L, Austin R, Nieuwenhuis E, Clarke ID, Hui CC, Dirks PB (2009) Multipotent CD15+ cancer stem cells in patched-1-deficient mouse medulloblastoma. Cancer Res 69(11):4682–4690

West CM, Davidson SE, Roberts SA, Hunter RD (1993) Intrinsic radiosensitivity and prediction of patient response to radiotherapy for carcinoma of the cervix. Br J Cancer 68(4):819–823

Wilson WR, Hay MP (2011) Targeting hypoxia in cancer therapy. Nat Rev Cancer 11(6):393–410

Wu CP, Zhou L, Xie M, Du HD, Tian J, Sun S, Li JY (2013) Identification of cancer stem-like side population cells in purified primary cultured human laryngeal squamous cell carcinoma epithelia. PLoS ONE 8(6):e65750

Yang XH, Li M, Wang B, Zhu W, Desgardin A, Onel K, de Jong J, Chen J, Chen L, Cunningham JM (2015) Systematic computation with functional gene-sets among leukemic and hematopoietic stem cells reveals a favorable prognostic signature for acute myeloid leukemia. BMC Bioinformatics 16(1):97

Yaromina A, Krause M, Thames H, Rosner A, Krause M, Hessel F, Grenman R, Zips D, Baumann M (2007) Pre-treatment number of clonogenic cells and their radiosensitivity are major determinants of local tumour control after fractionated irradiation. Radiother Oncol 83 (3):304–310

Yin ZQ, Liu JJ, Xu YC, Yu J, Ding GH, Yang F, Tang L, Liu BH, Ma Y, Xia YW, Lin XL, Wang HX (2014) A 41-gene signature derived from breast cancer stem cells as a predictor of survival. J Exp Clin Cancer Res 33:49

Zhang H, Yang Y, Wang Y, Gao X, Wang W, Liu H, He H, Liang Y, Pan K, Wu H, Shi J, Xue H, Liang L, Cai Z, Fan Y, Zhang Y (2015) Relationship of tumor marker CA125 and ovarian tumor stem cells: preliminary identification. J Ovarian Res 8(1):19

Zhang M, Behbod F, Atkinson RL, Landis MD, Kittrell F, Edwards D, Medina D, Tsimelzon A, Hilsenbeck S, Green JE, Michalowska AM, Rosen JM (2008) Identification of tumor-initiating cells in a p53-null mouse model of breast cancer. Cancer Res 68(12):4674–4682

Zhang P, Wei Y, Wang L, Debeb BG, Yuan Y, Zhang J, Yuan J, Wang M, Chen D, Sun Y, Woodward WA, Liu Y, Dean DC, Liang H, Hu Y, Ang KK, Hung MC, Chen J, Ma L (2014) ATM-mediated stabilization of ZEB1 promotes DNA damage response and radioresistance through CHK1. Nat Cell Biol 16(9):864–875

Zielske SP, Spalding AC, Wicha MS, Lawrence TS (2011) Ablation of breast cancer stem cells with radiation. Transl Oncol 4(4):227–233

Molecular Targeting of Growth Factor Receptor Signaling in Radiation Oncology

Shyhmin Huang, H. Peter Rodemann and Paul M. Harari

Abstract

Ionizing radiation has been shown to activate and interact with multiple growth factor receptor pathways that can influence tumor response to therapy. Among these receptor interactions, the epidermal growth factor receptor (EGFR) has been the most extensively studied with mature clinical applications during the last decade. The combination of radiation and EGFR-targeting agents using either monoclonal antibody (mAb) or small-molecule tyrosine kinase inhibitor (TKI) offers a promising approach to improve tumor control compared to radiation alone. Several underlying mechanisms have been identified that contribute to improved anti-tumor capacity after combined treatment. These include effects on cell cycle distribution, apoptosis, tumor cell repopulation, DNA damage/repair, and impact on tumor vasculature. However, as with virtually all cancer drugs, patients who initially respond to EGFR-targeted agents may eventually develop resistance and manifest cancer progression. Several

S. Huang · P.M. Harari (✉)
Department of Human Oncology, University of Wisconsin School
of Medicine and Public Health, 600 Highland Avenue K4/336 CSC,
Madison, WI 53792, USA
e-mail: harari@humonc.wisc.edu

S. Huang
Department of Human Oncology, University of Wisconsin Comprehensive Cancer Center,
WIMR 3136, 1111 Highland Ave Madison, Madison, WI 53705, USA
e-mail: huang@humonc.wisc.edu

H. Peter Rodemann
Division of Radiobiology and Molecular Environmental Research,
Department of Radiation Oncology, University of Tübingen, Röntgenweg,
72076 Tübingen, Germany
e-mail: hans-peter.rodemann@uni-tuebingen.de

© Springer-Verlag Berlin Heidelberg 2016
M. Baumann et al. (eds.), *Molecular Radio-Oncology*, Recent Results
in Cancer Research 198, DOI 10.1007/978-3-662-49651-0_3

potential mechanisms of resistance have been identified including mutations in EGFR and downstream signaling molecules, and activation of alternative member-bound tyrosine kinase receptors that bypass the inhibition of EGFR signaling. Several strategies to overcome the resistance are currently being explored in preclinical and clinical models, including agents that target the EGFR T790 M resistance mutation or target multiple EGFR family members, as well as agents that target other receptor tyrosine kinase and downstream signaling sites. In this chapter, we focus·primarily on the interaction of radiation with anti-EGFR therapies to summarize this promising approach and highlight newly developing opportunities.

Keywords
Radiation · Molecular targeting · Growth factor receptors

1 Interaction of Radiation and Growth Factor Receptors

Clinically relevant doses of ionizing radiation (2 Gy) are able to induce growth factor receptor signaling and ligand binding. Although precise mechanisms of radiation-induced receptor activation and stimulation of receptor-dependent downstream signaling are not fully understood, it is known that downstream pathways of stimulated receptors can mediate specific cellular radiation responses. For growth factor receptors such as the epidermal growth factor receptor (EGFR) family, preclinical data indicate a critical role of these receptors to influence intrinsic radiation sensitivity of tumor cells, as well as the DNA damage response (DDR) (Akimoto et al. 1999; Dent et al. 1999). In this chapter, specific aspects of the relevant EGFR-signaling events mediating these various radiation responses are discussed.

1.1 Epidermal Growth Factor Receptors

The EGFR/ErbB family of membrane-bound growth factor receptors is currently the most mature with regard to knowledge about radiation interaction and clinical trial development. This family consists of four distinct receptor isoforms, namely EGFR (ErbB1), ErbB2 (Neu, HER2), ErbB3 (HER3), and ErbB4 (Yarden and Pines 2012). These receptor molecules are transmembrane glycoproteins comprised of an extracellular ligand-binding domain and an intracellular tyrosine kinase domain (Fig. 1). Binding of the corresponding growth factors to the extracellular ligand-binding domain results in the dimerization of receptor monomers in the cell membrane. Upon dimerization, activation of the tyrosine kinase of the receptor occurs, which can stimulate various downstream signaling cascades, such as the

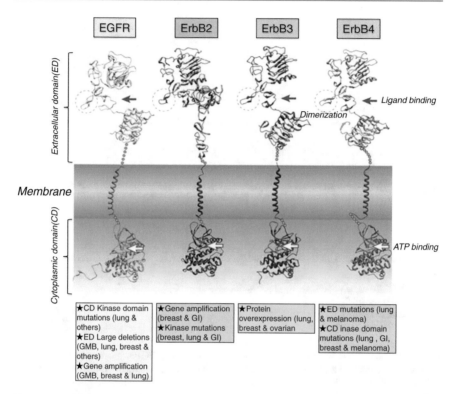

Fig. 1 EGFR/ErbB family members. The four EGFR/ErbB family members are represented by the crystal structures of their three major domains, the extracellular ligand-binding domain (ED), the transmembrane domain, and cytoplasmic kinase domain (CD). The ligand-binding clefts are marked by *black arrows* and the dimerization loops by *dashed circles*. ErbB2 harbors no ligand-binding cleft, but its dimerization loop is nevertheless extended. *White arrows* mark the ATP-binding clefts. The aberrations of EGFR family members in a variety of tumor types are shown in the *bottom*. Adapted with the permission from Yarden and Pines (2012)

Ras/Raf/MEK/ERK, PKC, STAT, and PI3 K/Akt pathways (Rodemann and Blaese 2007; Rodemann et al. 2007). It is well known that these cascades are involved in the regulation of various processes controlling stress sensitivity and survival, cell cycle progression and proliferation, differentiation and apoptosis, cell matrix interactions and cell motility, and transformation as well as oncogenesis and metastasis (Fig. 2).

Nearly 50 % of all human tumors present an overexpression of EGFR or a mutational activation of this receptor (Fig. 1). These receptor alterations play an important role in the treatment response of corresponding tumor cells. In many studies, it has been demonstrated that overexpression or mutational activation of EGFR is a major mechanism leading to resistance of tumor cells against both chemo- and radiotherapy, thereby contributing to poor prognosis (Ang et al. 2002; Krause et al. 2007; Das et al. 2007; Nakamura 2007; Gupta and Raina 2010). In

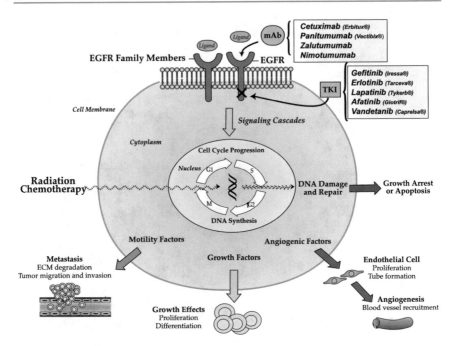

Fig. 2 Potential mechanisms of action for combined anti-EGFR therapy with radiation. Simplified schematic illustration of the EGFR pathway and potential downstream effects of EGFR-signaling inhibition combined with radiation [copied with the permission from Harari et al. (2007)]

addition, it has been well demonstrated that EGFR activity is inducible by ionizing radiation even in the absence of ligand binding (Dent et al. 2003; Yacoub et al. 2006). EGFR and several of the downstream signaling cascades are therefore the major components of a network of cellular radiation response pathways. Exposure of cells to ionizing radiation leads to an autophosphorylation and activation of the tyrosine kinase domain of EGFR, which subsequently stimulates downstream signaling cascades (Yacoub et al. 2001, 2006; Rodemann and Blaese 2007; Toulany et al. 2007; Toulany and Rodemann 2013). Both ligand and radiation-induced EGFR signaling are primarily involved in the control of DNA damage repair, cell proliferation, and survival as well as apoptosis as shown in Fig. 3. Mainly, the PI3 K-Akt and Ras-ERK pathways have been shown to be involved in resistance to chemo- and radiotherapy due to their regulatory role in stimulating cell survival by inhibiting apoptosis (PI3 K-AKT) and promoting cell proliferation (Ras-ERK) (Schmidt-Ullrich et al. 1997; Xing and Orsulic 2005; Kim et al. 2006; Tokunaga et al. 2006; Kriegs et al. 2010; Toulany et al. 2012).

DNA double-strand breaks (DSBs) are the most lethal of the various types of DNA damage (e.g., DNA single-strand breaks, base damages, and protein–DNA cross-links), induced by ionizing radiation (IR) as well as other cellular stressors, such as many chemotherapeutic agents or endogenously generated reactive oxygen

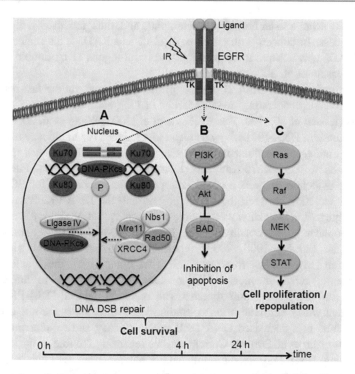

Fig. 3 Radiation induces EGFR activation and downstream signaling. A radioprotective role of EGFR is activated and separated into three phases as a function of time. **a** The early phase EGFR is translocated into the nucleus and activates repair signaling via binding with DNA-PK, Ku70, and Ku80 to control the rejoining of DNA double-strand breaks. **b** Activation of EGFR promotes PI3 K and Akt activation that results in the inhibition of radiation-induced apoptosis **c** EGFR activates the Ras/Raf/MEK/ERK and STAT pathways that promote cell survival. Copied with the permission from Lilleby et al. (2011)

species. Additionally, DNA DSBs are produced during S-phase when the DNA replication fork encounters, for example, DNA single-strand breaks. For accurate repair of DNA DSB, the damage must be sensed and recognized by specific proteins. Moreover, appropriate signaling to the cell cycle checkpoint control system enables recruitment of the DNA-repair machinery to sites of DSBs (Scott and Pandita 2006; Rodemann et al. 2007). Depending upon the cell cycle phase in which the DNA DSBs are initiated, the cell may select between two pathways of repair, namely non-homologous end joining (NHEJ) active predominantly not only in the G1-phase, but also in the S-phase and G2-phase and the homologous recombination (HR) active in late S-phase and G2-phase only. The key enzyme of the NHEJ mechanism is the catalytic subunit of the DNA-dependent protein kinase (DNA-PK), which for full activity forms a complex with Ku70/80 proteins that bind to the open 3'- and 5'-ends of the broken DNA double strand. Activated DNA-PK then recruits a variety of repair proteins, such as artemis, XRCC4, LIG4, and DNA-polymerase, to execute repair. In contrast, the HR repair pathway rejoins

DNA DSBs using a sister homolog as a template and, thus, facilitates a high-fidelity repair process. In concert with proteins BRCA2 and RAD54, the major player in HR is RAD51, which promotes repair of the homologous DNA double strand by HR (Shrivastav et al. 2008).

In mammalian cells, DNA DSBs are primarily repaired via the fast-responding NHEJ mechanism operating predominantly in G1-phase, for which DNA-PK is essential (Kasten et al. 1999; Kasten-Pisula et al. 2005; Wang et al. 2006). Even a small decrease in DNA-PK activity can lead to a reduced repair efficacy leading to a substantial increase in cellular radiation sensitivity. Normally, the vast majority of DNA-PK as well as Ku70/Ku80 are located within the nucleus. Interestingly, increasing evidence suggests a novel radioprotective mechanism for EGFR via a physical interaction between the EGFR protein and the DNA-PK. Based on con-focal imaging, Bandyopadhyay et al. note a colocalization of DNA-PK and EGFR in the cytoplasm (Bandyopadhyay et al. 1998). In several follow-up studies, Ditt-mann et al. (2005a, 2008, 2009) report that ionizing radiation triggers the translocation of EGFR from the cell membrane into the nucleus in a Src-kinase-dependent manner. In the nucleus, EGFR is able to interact with DNA-PK and this interaction correlates with radiation-induced DNA-PK activity. Pretreatment with cetuximab prior to irradiation downregulates the nuclear import of and results in a decreased DNA DSB repair efficacy and cellular radiosensiti-zation (Dittmann et al. 2005b). Current studies regarding the role of nuclear EGFR in mediating DNA DSB repair imply additional functions of nuclear EGFR in facilitating access of repair proteins to the sites of DNA DSB through opening and reorganizing heterochromatin structures (Dittmann et al. 2011).

Various molecular strategies to inhibit Akt (i.e., via siRNA and inhibitor approaches) provide strong evidence that Akt activity is necessary to stimulate efficient DNA DSB repair (Toulany et al. 2006, 2008, 2012; Toulany and Rode-mann 2010; Kang et al. 2012; Golding et al. 2009). Thus, EGFR-activated PI3 K-Akt signaling also plays a prominent role in the control and stimulation of radiation-induced DNA DSB repair. Although the detailed mechanism of how Akt is involved in the regulation of NHEJ-repair is still under investigation, recent reports demonstrate that Akt, especially the isoform Akt1, directly interacts with DNA-PK through its C-terminal domain by forming a functional complex after radiation exposure (Bozulic et al. 2008; Park et al. 2009; Toulany et al. 2012). As a consequence of this complex formation, Akt1 promotes DNA-PK accumulation at the DNA DSB site and stimulates DNA-PK kinase activity in a PI3 K-dependent manner (Toulany et al. 2012) (Fig. 4). Moreover, Akt1-dependent DNA-PK kinase activity results in DNA-PK autophosphorylation at S2056, which is essential for efficient repair (Chen et al. 2007) as well as the release of DNA-PK from the damage site (Toulany et al. 2012). Thus, Akt1 seems to be necessary for initiation, progression, and termination of the DNA-PK-dependent NHEJ-repair of DNA DSBs.

An alternative or concomitant pathway regulating DNA DSB repair via Akt is the upregulation of MRE11 expression after Akt activation through GSK3β/β-catenin/LEF-1 pathway (Bouchaert et al. 2012; Fraser et al. 2011).

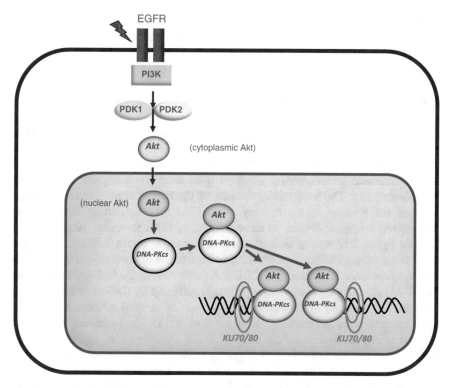

Fig. 4 PI3 K-dependent Akt regulation of DNA DSB. Akt activated via erbB-PI3 K signaling forms a complex with DNA-PKcs in the nucleus to stimulate initiation, progression, and termination of DNA DSB repair through the NHEJ mechanism

MRE11 is a central protein, which after radiation exposure of cells binds to the proteins RAD50 and NBS1 to form the MRN complex. This complex rapidly accumulates to damage site and appears to be the major sensor of DNA DSBs. At the DNA DSB site, MRN subsequently recruits, together with other proteins, the signaling protein ATM, which mediates cell cycle checkpoint control to allow DNA repair (Lavin 2007). Approximately, 85 % of DNA DSBs induced by ionizing radiation are repaired within the first 2–3 h post-irradiation via the so-called fast component of DNA DSB repair, which is independent of ATM function (Jeggo et al. 2011). The remaining 15 % of DNA DSBs mainly composed of complex lesions are repaired in an ATM-dependent manner via the so-called slow component (Goodarzi et al. 2010; Beucher et al. 2009). Inhibition of Akt leads to a downregulation of MRE11 protein; thus, Akt1 may function in the control of DNA repair additionally as a regulator of the slow components of DNA repair. This potential function would be complementary to the role of Akt in the DNA-PK-dependent fast repair process.

Thus, the importance of both EGFR signaling via signaling cascades and the nuclear translocation pathway of EGFR for the efficacy of DNA DSB repair through the DNA-PKcs-dependent NHEJ-repair mechanism underscores the efficacy of targeting the EGFR as well as the PI3 K-Akt pathway to improve outcome with radiation therapy.

1.2   Insulin Growth Factor Receptor 1

The insulin-like growth factor receptor 1 (IGF-1R) is another major growth factor receptor of relevance for mediating the radiation response of tumor cells (Larsson et al. 2005; Miller and Yee 2005; Riesterer et al. 2011). IGF-1R is a hetero-tetrameric protein with 2 identical α-subunits presenting the extracellular IGF-binding site. The intracellular domain of the two transmembrane β-subunits contains the tyrosine kinase activity responsible for transmitting the signal to intracellular cascades. Similar to the activation of ErbB receptors, binding of the specific ligand IGF results in conformational changes of the IGF-1R, autophosphorylation of specific tyrosine residues, and activation of downstream intracellular signaling cascades (Riesterer et al. 2011). As with EGFR, the Ras-Raf-MAPK and PI3 K-Akt cascades represent major pathways activated by IGF-1R resulting in the activation of a variety of cellular responses, such as survival, proliferation, differentiation, adhesion, and motility (Riesterer et al. 2011). The important function of IGF-1R as cell survival factor has been shown in a variety of cell types. Moreover, IGF-1R reduces the inducibility of apoptosis. Several lines of evidence suggest IGF-1R as a mediator of treatment resistance to cytotoxic agents and ionizing radiation (Macaulay et al. 2001; Peretz et al. 2001; Rochester et al. 2005). Downregulation of IGF-1R by antisense RNA impairs activation of the DNA damage sensor protein ATM kinase and can thus enhance cellular radiation sensitivity (Macaulay et al. 2001). In addition, several anti-IGF-1R antibodies including cixutumumab show to augment radiation response in a variety of preclinical models (Allen et al. 2007). Mechanistically, IGF-1R inhibition has been found to promote apoptosis and inhibit repair of radiation-induced DNA damage through interference with the expression of DSB repairing Ku-proteins and their binding to DNA (Cosaceanu et al. 2007).

2   EGFR-Targeting Agents

Despite gradual advancement in concurrent radiochemotherapy treatment regimens, the overall toxicity of treatment and relative lack of specificity for individual patients can limit the ultimate clinical effectiveness. These challenges have stimulated the development of molecular-targeted therapies that may provide more specific attack on tumor cells with less collateral impact on surrounding normal tissues. There are a rapidly expanding number of molecular-targeting agents against various growth factor receptors under development and in current clinical use. By targeting aberrant expression and/or mutations in growth factor receptor signaling pathways that are more prevalent in cancer cells, molecular-targeting agents offer the potential to improve therapeutic outcome. The EGFR-targeting agents have been a focus of research during the last two decades. Following the early work by Mendelsohn and colleagues (Mendelsohn 2003; Masui et al. 1984) who demonstrated the anti-tumor effect of a monoclonal antibody (mAb) to EGFR, two distinct classes of EGFR inhibitors, mAb and small-molecule tyrosine kinase inhibitor (TKI) against EGFR, have demonstrated preclinical and clinical promise and gained US Federal Drug Administration (FDA) approval in last 10 years (Table 1) (Harari and Huang 2004; Dassonville et al. 2007; Yarden and Pines 2012). Although both approaches can block EGFR activation, the mode of action and pharmacokinetic profile of mAbs and TKIs vary considerably (Table 2). Anti-EGFR mAbs block

Table 1 EGFR-targeting agents

Name	Manufacturer	Molecule	Specificity	Development status
Cetuximab *Erbitux®* *C225*	ImClone systems Inc. Bristol-Myers Squibb	Mouse-human Chimeric IgG1	EGFR	FDA approved for CRC patients with wt KRAS Approved for use in combination with radiotherapy in HNSCC patients
Panitumumab *Vectibix®* *ABX-EGF*	Amgen Abgenix	Human IgG2	EGFR	Approved for CRC patients with wt KRAS
Zalutumumab HuMax-EGFr	Genmab	Humab IgG1	EGFR	Approved for Fast Track by FDA in HNSCC patients who have failed standard therapies
Nimotuzumab *h-R3* *TheraCIM*	YM BioScience	Human IgG1	EGFR	Approved in Asia and Europe. In the USA, in late-stage development and testing for FDA review
Sym004	Symphogen A/S	A mixture of two chimeric IgG1 s	EGFR	Phases I and II in HNSCC and CRC
MEHD7945A	Genentech	Human bi-specific IgG1	EGFR HER3	Phases I and II in HNSCC and CRC
Gefitinib *Iressa®* *ZD1839*	AstraZeneca	Reversible TKI	EGFR	Approved for patients with advanced NSCLC
Erlotinib *Tarceva®* *OSI-774*	Genentech	Reversible TKI	EGFR	Approved for patients with advanced NSCLC patients Approved for use in combination with gemcitabine in patients with advanced pancreatic cancer
Vandetanib *Caprelsa®* ZD6474	AstraZeneca	Reversible TKI	EGFR VEGFR	Approved for patients with late-stage thyroid cancer

(continued)

Table 1 (continued)

Name	Manufacturer	Molecule	Specificity	Development status
Lapatinib *Tykerb®* GW572016	GlaxoSmithKline	Reversible TKI	EGFR HER2	Approved for use in combination with capecitabine in patients with breast cancer
Afatinib *Giotrif®* BIBW2992	Boehringer Ingelheim	Irreversible TKI	EGFR HER2	Phase III in breast and NSCLC Phase II in prostate and HNSCC
Neratinib HKI-272	Puma biotechnology	Irreversible TKI	EGFR HER2	Phases II and III in breast, brain and NSCLC patients
Dacomitinib PF-00299804	Pfizeer	Irreversible TKI	EGFR HER2 HER3 HER4	Phase II & III in HNSCC & NSCLC patients Phase II in patients with recurrent glioblastoma or advanced gastric cancer

Ab Antibody; *CRC* Colorectal cancer; *FDA* Food and drug administration; *HNSCC* Head and neck squamous cell carcinoma; *NSCLC* Non-small cell lung cancer; *TKI* Tyrosine kinase inhibitor

Table 2 mAb versus TKI

Parameter	mAb	TKI
Specificity	+++	+
Off-target activity	–	+
Size (kDa)	>150	<1
Administration	i.v (weekly)	Oral (daily)
Half-life	>4 days	<1 day
Receptor internalization	+	–
Block lateral receptor signaling	+	–
Immune response (ADCC, CDC)	+	–
Consistent pharmacokinetics	+	–
Nausea/Diarrhea	+	++
Acne-like rash	+++	++

ADCC Antibody-dependent cell-mediated cytotoxicity
CDC Complement-dependent cytotoxicity

ligand binding in the extracellular domain and TKIs directly inhibit the activation of cytosolic catalytic domain of the EGFR. Anti-EGFR mAbs are delivered intravenously since they are large molecules that are susceptible to degradation in GI tract and have a long half-life. There also exists the potential for stimulation of immunological responses with the use of mAbs. On the contrary, small-molecule TKIs are administrated orally due to their short half-life and effective absorption across the GI tract.

2.1   Anti-EGFR Antibody

A series of anti-EGFR mAbs have been used in the treatment of a variety of cancers as shown in Table 1. These antibodies have some potentially important differences in their structure and targeted EGFR epitope that may influence efficacy and toxicity. Among these, cetuximab (Erbitux®) and panitumumab (Vectibix®) are the most well-studied anti-EGFR mAbs with regard to mature clinical data. Cetuximab is a chimeric mAb with 65 % of human and 35 % of murine composition that received FDA approval in 2004 for the treatment of irinotecan-refractory colorectal cancer. Cetuximab is also the first EGFR-targeting agent approved to combine with radiotherapy in the treatment of HNSCC patients based on promising results from preclinical studies and phase III clinical trials (Nyati et al. 2006; Harari and Huang 2006; Bonner et al. 2006, 2010). The remaining portion of mouse immunoglobulin (IgG) in cetuximab might account for the low rate of infusional allergic reactions that have been described in the clinic with this drug. By contrast, panitumumab which is a fully human antibody may be less likely to elicit such host allergic responses. In addition, cetuximab may exhibit a potential therapeutic benefit to enhance antibody-dependent cellular cytotoxicity (ADCC) due to its IgG1 framework (Pahl et al. 2012; Kurai et al. 2007). Panitumumab, constructed on an IgG2 framework, does not possess this immune functionality. Ultimately, the comparative therapeutic efficacies of these two FDA-approved distinct anti-EGFR mAbs will be best evaluated in the context of controlled clinical trials.

2.2   EGFR Tyrosine Kinase Inhibitor

A second approach to disrupt EGFR function involves the use of synthetic quinazoline-derived TKIs that bind to the ATP-binding pocket of the EGFR tyrosine kinase domain and subsequently inhibit receptor activation. Gefitinib (Iressa®) and erlotinib (Tarceva®) are the first two EGFR-specific TKI to gain FDA approval for use in the treatment of chemotherapy-refractory NSCLC and advanced pancreatic cancer patients who have not received previous chemotherapy. Other FDA-approved drugs, such as vandetanib (Caprelsa®) and lapatinib (Tykerb®), inhibit multiple receptors in addition to EGFR, such as VEGFR and HER2. There are also several other promising multitargeted TKIs currently in the clinical trial seeking FDA approval such as afatinib, neratinib, and dacomitinib (Table 1).

To achieve a maximal therapeutic effect, the combination of an anti-EGFR mAb and a TKI has been explored as a potential cancer treatment strategy. Although these two classes of agents both target EGFR, they differ in their mode of action and carry distinct toxicity profiles as described above (Dassonville et al. 2007). By microarray analysis, Baselga and colleagues identified 45 genes that are differentially expressed after treatment with cetuximab versus gefitinib, including genes related to cellular proliferation and differentiation, DNA synthesis and repair, and angiogenesis and metastasis (Matar et al. 2004). Although the clinical significance of the differences in activity between anti-EGFR mAb and TKI is not yet clear, preclinical studies have demonstrated a synergistic effect in several xenograft model systems when cetuximab is administrated in combination with gefitinib or erlotinib compared with single agent treatment (Huang et al. 2004; Matar et al. 2004; Jimeno et al. 2005). These two agents given together are able to exert a superior induction in apoptosis and blockade of EGFR activation and downstream signaling. Interestingly, it is further shown that EGFR TKI can overcome acquired resistance to anti-EGFR mAb in cell culture and animal models (Huang et al. 2004; Regales et al. 2009; Brand et al. 2011). A phase I clinical trial confirms that treatments with cetuximab and gefitinib are feasible in patients with recurrent NSCLC and warrant further clinical investigation (Ramalingam et al. 2008).

3 Combination of EGFR-Targeting Agents with Radiation

3.1 Preclinical Studies—Biological Mechanisms of Action

A series of preclinical studies have provided proof-of-principle that blockade of EGFR can enhance radiation toxicity in a variety of tumor model systems (Krause et al. 2006; Baumann et al. 2007). Early studies identified the capacity of cetuximab to increase radiosensitivity in vitro and augment the effect of single dose and fractionated radiations in vivo (Huang et al. 1999; Milas et al. 2000). In addition, a more clinically relevant end point, improved local tumor control after single dose of irradiation in combination with cetuximab, was also reported in an animal model (Nasu et al. 2001). Thereafter, a series of anti-EGFR mAbs and TKIs were shown to augment radiation response in a variety of tumor models, including gefitinib, erlotinib, and panitumumab (Huang et al. 2002; Bianco et al. 2002; Chinnaiyan et al. 2005; Kruser et al. 2008). The potential underlying mechanisms for the radiosensitizing effect of EGFR inhibitors include radiation-induced repopulation, cell cycle arrest, senescence, apoptosis, DNA damage repair, and angiogenesis (Fig. 2).

3.1.1 Repopulation, Cell Cycle Progression, and Senescence
The negative impact of radiation-induced repopulation of cancer cells on the outcome of fractionated irradiation has been shown in preclinical and clinical studies, particularly for HNSCC. Preclinical data suggest that radiation-induced EGFR activation results in the accelerated repopulation of surviving clonogenic tumor cells and that EGFR inhibition counteracts this mechanism of radioresistance (Schmidt-Ullrich et al. 1997; Baumann et al. 2007). Simultaneous application of cetuximab during radiation with 30 fractions over 6 weeks in FaDu cancer cells improved local tumor control via the inhibition of tumor cell repopulation when compared to radiation alone (Krause et al. 2005). Further studies suggest that perturbations in cell cycle progression provide an underlying mechanism for the

anti-proliferation and radiosensitization effects of EGFR inhibitors (Ahsan et al. 2009).

Both anti-EGFR mAbs and TKIs have been shown to alter cell cycle distribution, with a 10–20 % shift from S-phase to G0/G1 arrest (Harari and Huang 2001; Huang et al. 2002; Chinnaiyan et al. 2005). Therefore, one hypothesis is that the radiosensitization effect of EGFR inhibitors may result from a decrease of the percentage of cells in S-phase, a relatively radioresistant phase, with concomitant increase in the more radiosensitive G1-phase of the cell cycle. Furthermore, the combined effects of G1 arrest induced by EGFR inhibitors, together with G2/M arrest induced by ionizing radiation, ultimately result in cell cycle checkpoint deregulation and subsequent apoptosis. In addition, EGFR inhibitors may trigger cellular senescence, an irreversible cell cycle arrest in response to double-strand break (DSB) produced by radiation. By screening 11 NSCLC cell lines in both in vitro and in vivo, a study showed that treatment with cetuximab or erlotinib led to pronounced cellular senescence but not apoptosis following radiation in 5 of 11 cell lines (Wang et al. 2011). Furthermore, EGFR inhibitor-induced senescence was associated with increased unrepaired DSB. These results recognize EGFR inhibitor-induced senescence as a meaningful contributor to the overall loss of tumor cell viability following radiation.

3.1.2 Apoptosis

EGFR inhibition may sensitize cells to apoptosis induced by radiation. In many preclinical studies, potentiation of apoptosis is shown to contribute to the radiosensitizing effect of EGFR inhibitors (Huang et al. 1999, 2002; Chinnaiyan et al. 2005; Kruser et al. 2008). The loss of EGFR alone is often insufficient to induce apoptosis completely. However, downregulation of EGFR-mediated survival signals has been shown to sensitize cells to apoptosis (Goel et al. 2007). EGFR inhibition downregulates Ras/Erk- or PI3 K/Akt-dependent survival pathways and is associated with a pro-apoptotic shift by inhibiting Bcl-2/Bcl-X_L and/or upregulating Bax/Bad (Gilmore et al. 2002; Sheng et al. 2007; Kruser et al. 2008). In addition, studies report that gefitinib can induce apoptosis through a p53-dependent signaling pathway, and p53 mutation in combination with p21 expression in colorectal cancer can serve as a predictor of resistance to gefitinib (Ogino et al. 2005; Rho et al. 2007; Chang et al. 2008). Recently, we found a loss of p53 in EGFR inhibitor-resistant cells that associate with a resistance phenotype to not only EGFR inhibitor, but also to radiation (Huang et al. 2011). Restoration of functional p53 in resistant cells can re-establish sensitivity to EGFR inhibitor and radiation via induction of cell cycle arrest, apoptosis, and DNA damage repair. Additional studies show that p53 is involved in the regulation of EGFR downstream PI3 K/AKT and ERK pathways (Singh et al. 2002; Bouali et al. 2009; Sauer et al. 2010; Zwang et al. 2011). All these results suggest that p53 may regulate sensitivity to EGFR inhibitors and radiation by modulating EGFR downstream signaling functionality and apoptosis induction.

3.1.3 DNA Damage Repair

Another mechanism of synergy between EGFR inhibition and radiation is through the inhibition of DNA DSB damage repair, mainly NHEJ (Szumiel 2006; Meyn et al. 2009; Lieber 2010). As described above, EGFR is shown to translocate into the nucleus after radiation to act either as a transcription factor or as a cofactor for the DNA-PK-Ku78/80 repair complex (Szumiel 2006; Chen and Nirodi 2007). When EGFR is blocked by cetuximab or gefitinib, a substantial amount of DNA-PK is retained in the cytosol due to a stalled nuclear import of the EGFR complex (Bandyopadhyay et al. 1998; Dittmann et al. 2005b; Friedmann et al. 2006). As a consequence, radiation-induced DNA-PK activation is abolished and leads to impaired repair as shown by increased numbers of γ-H2AX foci and significantly reduced clonogenic survival (Dittmann et al. 2005b). Additionally, a report indicates that gefitinib suppresses DNA-repair capacity via another DNA-repair protein NBS1, not DNA-PK (Tanaka et al. 2008) in NSCLC cells. In addition, erlotinib is shown to attenuate homologous recombinational repair of DSBs in breast cancer cells (Li et al. 2008b). The relationship between the EGFR signaling and the DNA-repair process has not been fully clarified, but these observations raise the possibility that impairment of DNA-repair processes, especially for DSB repair, may be involved in the modulation of radiosensitivity by EGFR inhibitors.

3.1.4 Angiogenesis

It is becoming clear that EGFR inhibitors can interfere with tumor–stromal interactions, such as angiogenesis, and this anti-angiogenic effect of EGFR inhibitors is considered as a potential underlying mechanism for EGFR inhibitor-mediated radiosensitization (Guillamo et al. 2009; Nijkamp et al. 2013). Although radiation oncologists have expressed caution about the induction of a radioresistant hypoxia environment from inhibition of angiogenesis, a body of preclinical and clinical data has emerged in support of combining angiogenesis inhibitors with radiation (O'Reilly 2006; Kleibeuker et al. 2012). An alternative hypothesis suggests that anti-angiogenic agents may serve to transiently "normalize" the abnormal structure and function of tumor vasculature to make it more efficient for oxygen and drug delivery (Jain 2005; Ma and Waxman 2008; Fukumura and Jain 2007). In addition, by determining the optimal scheduling and dose of anti-angiogenic agents, the combination of radiation with anti-angiogenic agents may improve therapeutic outcome via vessel normalization (Dings et al. 2007). Therefore, detailed investigation regarding the temporal changes of the tumor microenvironment appears important for our ultimate understanding of EGFR/radiation interactions.

Cetuximab or gefitinib have been extensively reported to suppress neovascularization in a variety of tumor xenografts (Huang and Harari 2000; Huang et al. 2001; She et al. 2003). The anti-angiogenic mechanism of EGFR inhibitors involves not only suppression of several angiogenic factors that are produced by tumor cells, but also direct inhibition of the proliferation and migration of endothelial cells, endothelial-associated pericytes, and perivascular cells (Al-Nedawi et al. 2009; Iivanainen et al. 2009). For example, simultaneous application of cetuximab during fractionated irradiation is found to improve reoxygenation of tumor xenografts that contributes to improved local control of FaDu tumors (Petersen et al. 2003; Krause et al. 2005). Further studies indicate that treatments with EGFR inhibitors result in a reduced expression of the hypoxia-related protein and hypoxia-inducible factor alpha (HIF-1 alpha) (Riesterer et al. 2009; Pore et al. 2006). Consistently, several studies confirm that EGFR inhibitors can modulate the microenvironment by vascular normalization to improve radiotherapy efficacy (Gan et al. 2009; Cerniglia et al. 2009; Qayum et al. 2009). Imaging studies further identify changes in vessel morphology in erlotinib-treated tumor xenografts accompanied by increased tumor blood flow, decreased vessel permeability, and reduced hypoxia that are typical characteristics of tumor vascular normalization. These changes correlate with improved drug delivery and increased response to radiation (Cerniglia et al. 2009). These findings suggest that improvement in blood flow leads to better drug delivery or increased tumor oxygenation and thereby offer a rationale for why EGFR inhibitors may enhance the radiation response of tumors.

3.2   Clinical Studies

3.2.1   Cetuximab + Radiotherapy

During the last 10 years, the combination of EGFR inhibitors with radiation has been actively tested in patients with a variety of tumors including HNSCC, NSCLC, colon, esophageal, breast, and brain (Al-Ejeh et al. 2013; Welsh et al. 2013). Results from phases I and II clinical trials indicate that combining EGFR inhibitors with radiotherapy or chemoradiotherapy is generally well tolerated with minimal overlapping toxicity (Table 3). In 2006, the first landmark multicenter phase III clinical trial was reported demonstrating that the administration of cetuximab to radiotherapy can provide a survival advantage for HNSCC patients. Bonner et al. compared the efficacy of radiotherapy alone to radiotherapy plus cetuximab in 424 patients with locoregionally advanced HNSCC. The benefit of the association of cetuximab with radiotherapy as compared to radiotherapy alone was demonstrated in terms of locoregional control (median duration: 24.4 vs. 14.9 months, $p = 0.005$), progression-free survival (3-year rate: 42 vs. 31 %, $p = 0.04$), and overall survival (median duration: 49 vs. 29.3 months, $p = 0.03$) (Bonner et al. 2006). Recently, the five-year follow-up report confirms stability of the advantage for the cetuximab arm with a 10 % improvement (45.6 vs. 36.4 %, $p = 0.018$) in overall survival compared to the radiation alone arm (Fig. 5) (Bonner et al. 2010). With the exception of the characteristic cutaneous toxicity of cetuximab (acneiform rash), the incidence of grade 3 toxicities was not significantly higher in the group treated with cetuximab. Moreover, the authors showed that for the patients treated with cetuximab, overall survival was significantly improved in those who experienced an acneiform rash of at least grade 2 severity compared with patients with no rash or grade. Importantly, this is the first trial showing that the outcomes of radiotherapy can be significantly improved by the addition of a

Table 3 Selected clinical trials combining EGFR inhibitors with radiation

Treatment	Phase	Cancer (N)	Response	Survival index	Reference
RT versus RT + cetuximab	III	H&N (424)	LRC: 14.9 versus 24.4 months OR: 64 versus 74 %	OS at 5 years: 29.3 versus 49 months	Bonner et al. (2006, 2010)
Platinum-based CRT versus platinum-based CRT + cetuximab	III (RTOG0522)	H&N (895)		OS at 2.5 years: 79.7 versus 82.6 months PFS: 64.3 versus 63.4 months	Ang et al. (2011)
Induction chemotherapy followed by CRT and cetuximab during sequential treatment	II	H&N (39)		OS at 3 years: 74 % PFS: 73 %	Argiris et al. (2010)
RT, cisplatin, 5-FU, and cetuximab (rapid alternating treatment)	II	H&N (45)	OR: 91 % CR: 71 %	OS at 3.5 years: 32.6 months PFS: 21 months	Merlano et al. (2011)
IMRT + cetuximab		NSCLC (49)	OR: 63 %	Median OS: 19.5 months Median PFS: 10.9 months	Jensen et al. (2011)
RT, carboplatin, pemetrexed versus RT, carboplatin, pemetrexed + cetuximab	II	NSCLC (101)		OS at 1.5 years: 58 versus 54 %	Govindan et al. (2011)
RT, CRT, and cetuximab	II	Esophagus (60)	CR:70 %		Safran et al. (2008)
RT, gemcitabine, oxiliplatin, and cetuximab	II	Pancreas (69)		Median OS: 19.2 months	Crane et al. (2011)
CRT, bevacizumab, erlotinib	II	H&N (48)	OR:77 %	OS at 3 years: 82 % PFS: 71 %	Hainsworth et al. (2011)
RT, cisplatin, erlotinib	I/II	H&N (31)	CR:74.2 %		Herchenhorn et al. (2010)
RT versus RT + erlotinib	II	NSCLC (23)	OR: 55.5 versus 83.3 %		Martinez et al. (2008)

(continued)

Table 3 (continued)

Treatment	Phase	Cancer (N)	Response	Survival index	Reference
RT, temozolomide, erlotinib	II	GBM (65)		Median OS: 19.3 months	Prados et al. (2009)
CRT, erlotinib	II	Esophagus (24)	CR:46 %		Li et al. (2010)
RT, 5-FU, hydroxyurea, gefitinib	II	H&N (69)	CR:90 %	OS at 4 years: 74 % PFS: 72 %	Cohen et al. (2010)
RT, gefitinib	II	H&N (23)		OS at 2 years: 72.1 % PFS: 63.6 %	Lewis et al. (2012)
RT + gefitinib	II (RTOG0211)	GBM (147)		Median OS:11.5 months DMC:32 versus 40 %	Chakravarti et al. (2013)
CRT versus CRT + gefitinib	II	Esophagus (80)		OS at 3 years: 28 versus 42 %	Rodriguez et al. (2010)

RT Radiotherapy; *CRT* Chemoradiation; *N* Number of patients; *LRC* Local regional control; *OR* Overall response; *CR* Complete response; *OS* Overall survival; *PFS* Progression-free survival; *IMRT* Intensity-modulated radiation therapy; *DMC* Distant metastatic control

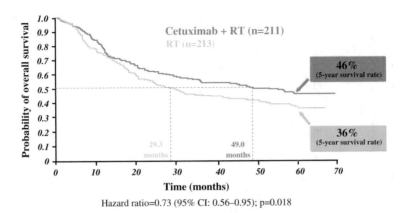

Fig. 5 Survival advantage of cetuximab in combination with radiotherapy from phase III clinical trial in HNSCC patients. Adapted with the permission from Bonner et al. (2010)

molecular-targeting agent without significantly increasing the radiation toxicity. Overall, results from this trial validate the preclinical models that predicted a significant improvement of tumor control based on the radiosensitizing and apoptosis-promoting effects of cetuximab (Huang et al. 1999).

Although the addition of cetuximab to radiotherapy improves locoregional control and survival in HNSCC, the addition of cetuximab to platinum-based chemoradiotherapy did not lead to an improved outcome based on the recent phase III trial, RTOG 0522 (Table 3) (Ang et al. 2011). This study evaluates the addition of cetuximab to a standard-of-care concurrent radiation/cisplatin regimen in 895 patients with stage III or IV nonmetastatic HNSCC. Following a median 2.4 years of follow-up, the initial results show that the addition of cetuximab to the radiation/cisplatin regimen did not improve progression-free (64.3 % without cetuximab and 63.4 % with cetuximab) or overall survival (79.7 vs. 82.6 %). The addition of cetuximab was associated with higher rates of mucositis and cetuximab-induced skin reactions. Further analysis is underway to determine whether tumor human papillomavirus status affects the relative efficacy of the chemoradiotherapy plus cetuximab regimen.

There are a number of clinical trials evaluating the safety and efficacy of cetuximab and other anti-EGFR agents in association with chemoradiotherapy, either as primary or as postoperative treatment in a spectrum of cancer patients (Table 3). For example, Argiris et al. conducted a trial of 39 patients with advanced HNSCC treated with induction docetaxel, cisplatin, and cetuximab followed by concurrent cisplatin and cetuximab with 70 Gy radiation. Preliminary reports from this study demonstrate that cetuximab-containing regimen results in excellent long-term survival and safety (Argiris et al. 2010). The progression-free survival and overall survival were 70 and 74 %, respectively. While most radiotherapy clinical trials were generally still using 2D techniques, one recent phase II study (NEAR trial) in NSCLC patients combined cetuximab with a 4D intensity-modulated radiation treatment (IMRT) that permits dose escalation while relatively sparing surrounding normal tissues (Jensen et al. 2011). The study showed encouraging preliminary results for safety, local regional control, and survival rate in patients treated with IMRT and cetuximab. Several other phase II studies also showed the efficacy and safety of the addition of cetuximab to chemoradiotherapy in other tumor sites such as esophageal and pancreatic cancer (Crane et al. 2011; Safran et al. 2008).

3.2.2   TKI + Radiotherapy

Beyond cetuximab, EGFR TKIs have also been evaluated in combination with radiotherapy in a number of cancer types (Table 3). Notable among these is a phase II study evaluating erlotinib plus temozolomide during and after radiation therapy in patients with glioblastoma multiforme or gliosarcoma (Prados et al. 2009). In addition to 75 mg/day of temozolomide, patients were given 100 mg/day of erlotinib and during radiation and were escalated after radiation therapy to 150 mg/day. The median survival was 5.2 months longer than that projected in comparison with historical controls patients without erlotinib. Interestingly, it was found that patients with methylguanine methyltransferase (MGMT) methylation had a better overall survival compared to patients without MGMT methylation (25.5 vs. 14.6 months). These findings provide information regarding patient selection for future clinical trials, though further studies are necessary to determine the importance of MGMT methylation in this patient cohort.

Several phase II trials have evaluated the combination of erlotinib and radiotherapy in the definitive treatment of HNSCC and NSCLC, although published data are limited (Mehta 2012). For example, a study evaluated the combination of erlotinib with a standard cisplatin-based chemoradiotherapy regimen in patients with stages III and IV HNSCC (Herchenhorn et al. 2010). At a median follow-up of 37 months, it was found that 3-year progression-free survival and overall survival rates were 61 and 72 %, respectively. Similar to cetuximab, further analysis revealed a trend toward superior overall survival in patients who developed acneiform rash compared with those who did not have rash. Because of the high complete response rate, the authors advocated further evaluation of this treatment regimen in phase III clinical trial. In addition, a prospective phase II study found that radiation and concurrent erlotinib used in the treatment of patients with NSCLC showed promising results without an increase in toxicity (Martinez et al. 2008). Patients with unresectable stage I to IIIA NSCLC received 3D thoracic radiotherapy with or without concomitant erlotinib. The addition of erlotinib did not appear to increase radiation-associated toxicities. Erlotinib-related adverse events included mild-to-moderate skin rash (61.5 %) and diarrhea (23 %). The response rate was 55.5 % in the radiotherapy arm compared with 83.3 % in the radiotherapy plus erlotinib arm. Thus, based on the evidence, further clinical investigation into the combination of radiotherapy with EGFR TKI appears warranted.

4   Resistance to EGFR-Targeted Therapy

Although the first generation of phase III clinical trials combining EGFR TKI with chemotherapy did not demonstrate a survival benefit (Giaccone et al. 2004; Herbst et al. 2004, 2005), the first major phase III trial combining cetuximab with radiation confirms a strong survival advantage for HNSCC patients. While this compelling clinical result provides powerful stimulus to better understand mechanisms underlying the favorable interaction between EGFR blockade and radiation, many patients who initially respond well to treatments still manifest tumor recurrence (Jackman et al. 2010; Sequist et al. 2011b). Moreover, the addition of EGFR inhibitors to chemoradiotherapy in several clinical trials, although feasible, does not lead to a clinical benefit. Both intrinsic and acquired resistance to EGFR inhibitors are now well-recognized occurrences in clinical trials and emerge as potential treatment barriers for the optimization of EGFR-targeted therapy (Jackman et al. 2010; Wheeler et al. 2010; Sequist et al. 2011b).

4.1   EGFR Mutations

Somatic mutations in the EGFR play a crucial role in regulating the efficacy of EGFR inhibitors. In 2004, a series of landmark studies identified several EGFR mutations in the tyrosine kinase domain that significantly correlate with clinical responsiveness to gefitinib or erlotinib in NSCLC cancer patients (Lynch et al. 2004; Paez et al. 2004; Pao et al. 2004; Pao and Miller 2005). These mutations included in-frame deletion of amino acids 746–750 in exon 19, and a point mutation in exon 21 (L858R) that are around the ATP-binding pocket of the tyrosine kinase domain. Similarly, a recent study in HNSCC identified a somatic mutation in the ligand-binding domain (P546S) that may contribute to increased sensitivity to cetuximab (Bahassi et al. 2013). Subsequently, it was found that patients with active EGFR mutation who initially responded to gefitinib or erlotinib developed acquired resistance after a median of 10–14 months on EGFR TKI treatment (Jackman et al. 2010; Zhou et al. 2011). It is now known that appropriately 50–60 % of patients with acquired resistance to gefitinib have a second-site mutation in T790 M (Pao et al. 2005). It can also be detected as a mechanism of primary resistance in patients with no prior exposure to EGFR TKI, and its presence has been significantly associated with poorer outcome on EGFR therapy (Rosell et al. 2011). Originally, it was first predicted that the T790 M mutation sterically hindered the binding of TKIs to the ATP pocket of EGFR due to the introduction of a bulky Met residue, thus resulting in drug resistance (Kobayashi et al. 2005). However, recent biochemical and structural studies reveal that TKI resistance associated with T790 M mutation is not attributable to steric blocking of TKI binding, as previously predicted, but rather to the increased affinity for ATP that dramatically decreases the potency of the drug at cellular concentration of ATP (Yun et al. 2008; Eck and Yun 2010; Yoshikawa et al. 2013). In addition to EGFR

T790 M mutation, several other mutations in EGFR kinase domain have also been associated with acquired resistance to EGFR TKI including the T854A in exon 21 (Bean et al. 2008), L747S (Costa et al. 2008), and D761Y (Balak et al. 2006) in exon 19. However, the frequency of these mutations appears to be much lower than T790 M mutation.

The discovery of these EGFR-activating mutations raises important questions about the response of mutant EGFR to ionizing radiation. In contrast to the radioresistance conferred by EGFR overexpression, several in vitro studies showed that the NSCLC cell lines bearing activating EGFR mutations were more sensitive to radiation, evidenced by poor clonogenic survival, incomplete DSB repair, and either induction of apoptosis or development of micronuclei in response to ionizing radiation (Das et al. 2006; Sato et al. 2012). Further mechanistic studies demonstrated that unlike wt EGFR, receptors with activating mutations were defective in radiation-induced translocation to the nucleus and failed to bind DNA-PK (Das et al. 2007). Interestingly, tumor cells with gefitinib-resistant T790 M mutant still exhibited enhanced sensitivity to radiation (Das et al. 2006). Thus, despite the differences in sensitivity to gefitinib, NSCLC cells with different kind of EGFR mutations show similar responses to radiation. Although the presence of EGFR mutations in NSCLC is associated with increased radiosensitivity in vitro, clinical studies regarding the radiosensitivity in NSCLC with mutant EGFR are currently under investigation. Early results are promising and show that patients with EGFR mutation have improved locoregional control and outcomes with radiotherapy (Lee et al. 2012; Mak et al. 2011).

Beyond the EGFR itself, mutations in several EGFR downstream signaling molecules could also influence the sensitivity to EGFR-targeting agents (Fig. 6). Among them, somatic KRAS mutations are found at high rates in leukemias, colon, pancreas, and lung cancers. KRAS mutation at codon 12 or 13 has been strongly correlated with resistance to cetuximab or panitumumab therapy in a number of large studies (Lievre et al. 2006; Massarelli et al. 2007; Jimeno et al. 2009; Ready et al. 2010). In the phase III CRYSTAL study for metastatic colorectal cancers, patients with the wt KRAS treated with cetuximab plus chemotherapy showed a response rate of up to 59 % compared to 43.2 % in those treated with chemotherapy alone (Van Cutsem et al. 2009). However, there is no clear benefit to cetuximab among patients with mutated KRAS tumors with a response rate of 36.2 % compared to the 40.2 % in chemotherapy alone arm. These results led to a recommendation by ASCO in 2009 that colon cancer patients with a KRAS mutation should not receive cetuximab or panitumumab therapy (Allegra et al. 2009).

Similarly, lung cancer patients who are positive for KRAS mutation have a low response rate to gefitinib or erlotinib estimated at 5 % or less (Suda et al. 2010). Among HNSCC patients, however, the frequency of KRAS mutation is very low (Sheikh Ali et al. 2008). There is no clinical recommendation for determining the KRAS mutation status in HNSCC before applying cetuximab or panitumumab. In a recent preclinical study in UT5R9 cells, acquired resistance to cetuximab is shown to associate with the overexpression of Ras family members and the loss of radiosensitivity (Saki et al. 2013). Moreover, radioresistant UT5R9 cells were not

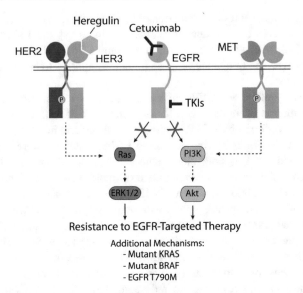

Fig. 6 Mechanisms of resistance to EGFR-targeted therapy. Acquired resistance to EGFR inhibitors may develop through MET amplification and activation of EGFR/HER family members that bypass EGFR inhibition. Additional mechanisms of resistance to EGFR-targeted therapies may exist due to the selected mutations of EGFR (T790 M) and downstream effectors, such as KRAS and BRAF. Adapted with the permission from Vlacich and Coffey (2011)

radiosensitized by cetuximab, but by manipulating KARS family members. Similarly, KRAS signaling through EGFR and HRAS was shown to promote radiation survival in pancreatic and colorectal carcinoma cells (Cengel et al. 2007). Based on these results, the inhibition of KRAS signaling is suggested to be an effective approach to overcome cetuximab- and radioresistance.

4.2   Other Potential Mechanisms

Acquired resistance to EGFR inhibitors may result from the activation of alternative membrane-bound receptor tyrosine kinases (RTK) that bypass EGFR pathway (Fig. 6) (Camp et al. 2005). Several RTKs, such as MET (hepatocyte growth factor receptor), platelet-derived growth factor (PDGF), vesicular growth factor receptor (VEGFR), and insulin-like growth factor receptor-1 (IGF-1R), can also activate the key downstream signals of EGFR including Erk and Akt pathways that may override the inhibitory effect of EGFR inhibitors. Among them, the amplification of MET was detected in 5–20 % of lung cancers that developed acquired resistance to EGFR inhibitors (Engelman and Settleman 2008). Although MET amplification can coexist with the EGFR T790 M mutation, approximately 60 % of MET amplification is independent of T790 M mutation (Bean et al. 2007). Mechanistic studies found that cells with EGFR TKI resistance relied on MET signaling to activate Akt through HER3-PI3 K signaling (Engelman et al. 2007; Engelman and Janne 2008). This activation of HER3-PI3 K-Akt signaling permits the cells to transmit the same downstream signaling in the presence of EGFR inhibitors. In addition, MET amplification was also found at a low frequency in patients with activating EGFR mutation prior to treatment and was associated with the subsequent development of acquired resistance to EGFR TKIs. It is very likely that EGFR inhibitor treatment may select for preexisting cells with MET amplification during the acquisition of resistance to EGFR inhibitors.

In general, EGFR T790 M and MET amplification account for ~60 % of acquired resistance to EGFR inhibitors. Other mechanisms of resistance that are operative in the remaining ~40 % of tumors are currently under active investigation. Among them, EGFR family members have been identified to play an important role in acquired resistance to EGFR inhibitors (Frolov et al. 2007; Baselga and Swain 2009; Wheeler et al. 2008) (Fig. 6). Following systematic screening of RTKs, a significant activation of HER3 was observed in cetuximab or erlotinib-resistant HNSCC and NSCLC cells in vitro (Wheeler et al. 2008). In the clinical scenario, HER3 overexpression, described in 30–80 % of primary or metastatic CRC, has also been associated with resistance to EGFR-targeting agents (Scartozzi et al. 2011). Further analysis indicates that acquired resistance to EGFR inhibitors might derive in part from activation of HER3 to effectively bypass the effect of EGFR inhibition (Jain et al. 2010). Depletion of HER3 by siRNA restores sensitivity to the EGFR inhibitors. Other than HER3, HER2 also appears to be involved in regulating acquired resistance to EGFR inhibitors (Baselga and Swain 2009; Vlacich and Coffey 2011). In HCC827 cells with acquired resistance to cetuximab, amplification of HER2 is identified as a mechanism of cetuximab resistance. Inhibition of HER2 activity or disruption of HER2/HER3 heterodimerization restores cetuximab sensitivity in both in vitro and in vivo models (Yonesaka et al. 2011). Other than these RTKs, IGF-1R and VEGFR have also been identified as crucial molecules to regulate acquired resistance to EGFR inhibitors (Viloria-Petit et al. 2001; Jones et al. 2004; Morgillo et al. 2007; Benavente et al. 2009). These findings suggest that combinations of molecular-targeted therapies blocking EGFR and other selected RTKs may offer a promising strategy to overcome acquired resistance and enhance the effectiveness of EGFR therapy.

5   Next-Generation EGFR-Targeting Approaches

Acquired resistance to the first generation of EGFR-targeting agents has prompted the design and development of new-generation EGFR inhibitors. Although the underlying mechanisms for acquired resistance to EGFR inhibitors are not fully understood, several strategies to overcome the resistance have been tested based on current findings on EGFR mutation and bypass mechanism. These include the next generation of EGFR-targeting agents that target the T790 M mutation or multiple

ErbB/HER family members (Yu and Riely 2013). Agents targeting other RTK or downstream signaling have also been extensively explored.

5.1 More Efficient EGFR-Targeting Agents

Next-generation EGFR-targeting agents include irreversible EGFR TKIs or pan-ErbB TKIs that simultaneously target multiple members of the EGFR family. The irreversible binding mechanism may increase TKI effectiveness by prolonging the inhibition of EGFR signaling and delaying the acquisition or growth of T790 M-mutant cells. Several irreversible pan-ErbB TKIs have been developed in recent years including neratinib (HKI-272), afatinib (BIBW2992), and dacomitinib (PF00299804) (see Table 1). These agents share a 4-anilinoquinazoline structure with the ability to form covalent bonds with Cys979 residue located directly at the ATP-binding cleft of EGFR protein and thus potentially preventing T790 M mutation-related resistance (Dienstmann et al. 2012; Giaccone and Wang 2011; Dziadziuszko and Jassem 2012; Ather et al. 2013). For instance, afatinib can inhibit NSCLC tumor cell growth with either wt or mutant forms of EGFR with a 100-fold greater activity than gefitinib against L858R/T790 M double mutants (Li et al. 2008a). Preclinical studies also show that afatinib synergizes with radiation to inhibit clonogenic survival and tumor xenograft growth of bladder tumor cells (Tsai et al. 2013). A recent phase III clinical trial (LUX-Lung 3) shows that afatinib improves progression-free survival compared with cisplatin and pemetrexed as first-line treatment for lung cancer patients with EGFR mutant (Sequist et al. 2013). However, the results of other trials (LUX-Lung 1, 4) demonstrate that single agent afatinib has minimal efficacy in patients previously treated with erlotinib or gefitinib (Miller et al. 2012; Katakami et al. 2013). This lack of efficacy may be due to the high potency of afatinib against EGFR with wt or activating mutation, leading to skin rash and gastrointestinal toxicity that limited administration of necessary doses for effective EGFR T790 M inhibition (Sequist et al. 2010). Ultimately, the development of T790 M-selective EGFR inhibitors appears to be a promising strategy to reduce on-target toxicity. Recent encouraging preclinical studies identify several potent inhibitors, such as WZ4002, Gö6976, and PKC412, that display improved selectivity against EGFR T790 M over wt EGFR (Zhou et al. 2009; Lee et al. 2013). The efficiency of these inhibitors in clinical practice is as yet undefined and will be better understood from the results of several ongoing phase II/III clinical trials. Nonetheless, afatinib was recently approved in July 2013 in the USA for the first-line treatment of patients with metastatic NSCLC who have tumors with activating EGFR mutations. Afatinib has also been approved in several countries in Asia and Europe.

Development of innovative mAbs with more efficient blocking ability to EGFR is another promising strategy to overcome resistance. When two mAbs against distinct epitopes of receptor are combined, a rapid and more efficient receptor internalization is observed and followed by EGFR degradation (Friedman et al. 2005). The antibody mixture is also more effective than single antibody in inhibiting signaling and tumor growth in tissue culture and animal models (Ben-Kasus et al. 2009; Spangler et al. 2010). Furthermore, antibody mixtures have been shown to activate complement-dependent cytotoxicity that contributes to a more effective anti-tumor capacity than single antibody (Dechant et al. 2008). Sym004 is a recently developed prototype following screening of >400 different anti-EGFR mAb combinations based on the highest anti-tumor capacity (Koefoed et al. 2011). Sym004 is a mixture of two anti-EGFR mAbs that targets non-overlapping epitopes (epitope 992 vs. 1024) in EGFR extracellular domain III. Preclinical studies demonstrate that Sym004 exhibits a superior anti-tumor capacity in comparison with cetuximab or panitumumab in both in vitro and in vivo models (Pedersen et al. 2010). Furthermore, Sym004 inhibits the growth of cancer cells with acquired resistance to cetuximab resulting from increased EGFR ligand production. Preclinical pharmacokinetic and safety studies in primates and humans indicate that Sym004 is well tolerated and does not induce unexpected toxicities (Skartved et al. 2011). A recent study shows that the powerful Sym004-induced EGFR downregulation can be translated into a profound augmentation of radiation response (Huang et al. 2013b). In HNSCC and NSCLC tumor xenografts, a superior anti-tumor capacity of Sym004 when combined with either single or fractionated radiation was observed. In addition, Sym004 demonstrated a stronger impact than cetuximab to inhibit DNA damage repair signaling and prompt the induction of apoptosis (Huang et al. 2013b). Several clinical trials are in progress to evaluate the clinical potential of Sym004 for patients with HNSCC and metastatic colorectal cancer with wt KRAS (Machiels et al. 2013; Dienstmann et al. 2013). With the known survival advantage for HNSCC patients treated with cetuximab with radiation in the phase III trial (Bonner et al. 2006), the more powerful impact of Sym004 compared to cetuximab provides a rationale to design clinical studies to test the impact of Sym004 with radiation for HNSCC patients in an effort to further improve overall outcome.

As described above, acquired resistance to EGFR inhibitors may derive in part from activation of HER2 or HER3 to effectively bypass the effect of EGFR inhibition. Dual-specific antibodies targeting both EGFR and HER3 or HER2 are currently under study. Among these, MEHD7945A is a recently developed dual-target antibody against EGFR and HER3 that shows a profound anti-tumor activity in vitro and in vivo across a variety of tumor cell types when compared to the respective monospecific antibodies (Schaefer et al. 2011). In addition, MEHD7945A is effective in facilitating antibody-dependent cell-mediated cytotoxicity, but appears to induce less skin toxicity in comparison with cetuximab in non-clinical studies (Kamath et al. 2012). Using established cetuximab- or erlotinib-resistant cells from NSCLC and HNSCC, it was found that MEHD7945A effectively regressed tumors that remain highly refractory to cetuximab or erlotinib (Huang et al. 2013a). In addition, MEHD7945A also overcomes cross-resistance to radiation in these EGFR inhibitor-resistant cells. A phase II, open-label, randomized study is currently ongoing to evaluate the efficacy and safety of MEHD7945A versus cetuximab in patients with recurrent/metastatic HNSCC who have progressed during or following platinum-based chemotherapy. (ClinicalTrials.gov Identifier NCT01577173).

5.2   Target Additional Pathways

Another area of intense clinical investigation resides in the combination of EGFR-targeting agents with agents targeting other pathways involved in regulating resistance to EGFR inhibitors, such as MET and VEGFR. There are a number of agents targeting MET in clinical trials that have come to fruition recently, such as rilotumumab, cabozantinib, tivantinib, crizotinib, MetMAb, and SU11274, (Peters and Adjei 2012; Sadiq and Salgia 2013; Scagliotti et al. 2013). Among these, tivantinib and MetMAb have shown positive signals in combination with erlotinib in phase II trials of lung cancer patients and are currently being tested in phase III trials (Sequist et al. 2011a; Spigel et al. 2011). In addition, preliminary results of a phase I/II trial in chemo-refractory colorectal cancer patients also demonstrate a 10 % improvement in overall response rate with the addition of rilotumumab to panitumumab (Eng et al. 2011). Given the encouraging findings from trials of several MET inhibitors to date, blocking both EGFR and MET in combination with radiotherapy is an attractive therapeutic strategy to overcome resistance to both EGFR inhibitors and radiation. Similar to EGFR, MET is also upregulated following radiation treatment (Bhardwaj et al. 2012; De Bacco et al. 2011). Preclinical studies show that inhibition of MET using small-molecule inhibitors or siRNA can radiosensitize cancer cells. The underlying mechanism of the radiosensitizing effect of MET inhibitor may include the inhibition of MET signaling, depolarization of the mitochondrial membrane potential, impairment of DNA damage repair, abrogation of cell cycle arrest, and enhancement of apoptotic cell death (Welsh et al. 2009; Yu et al. 2012; Bhardwaj et al. 2012; Sun et al. 2013).

Another promising approach to augment EGFR inhibitor impact is to combine with agents targeting VEGFR-regulated angiogenic pathway to potentiate anti-tumor effects of EGFR inhibitors as shown in a series of preclinical studies (Bozec et al. 2009a). Several studies have also established the resultant radiosensitizing effects by the dual inhibition of angiogenesis and EGFR pathways (Bozec et al. 2007, 2008, 2009b). For example, a synergistic effect is observed in an orthotopic H&N cancer model when combining cetuximab, radiation with anti-angiogenic agents, either bevacizumab or sunitinib (Bozec et al. 2008, 2009b). In addition, use of vandetanib, a dual-targeted agent targeting both EGFR and VEGFR, enhances the therapeutic efficiency of radiation in an orthotopic lung cancer model system (Shibuya et al. 2007; Wu et al. 2007).

Although various combinations of agents show activity in preclinical studies, the application of anti-angiogenic agents with EGFR and/or radiotherapy requires careful clinical evaluation since several trials with anti-angiogenic agents have proven disappointing due to toxicity (Spigel et al. 2010; Sliesoraitis and Tawfik 2011). The combination of VEGF and EGFR inhibitors was tested in NSCLC patients using concurrent bevacizumab, erlotinib, carboplatin, paxlitaxel, and RT51.

The addition of bevacizumab/erlotinib was determined not feasible due to pulmonary hemorrhage (Stinchcombe et al. 2011). However, a phase II trial in patients with HNSCC demonstrated that the combination of bevacizumab and cetuximab was active and the overall tolerance was acceptable despite some cases of bevacizumab-related toxicities (Argiris et al. 2011). In addition, bevacizumab or vandetanib was shown to be safely incorporated in conventional chemoradiotherapy and produced encouraging efficacy for patients with locally advanced HNSCC in two recent phase I studies (Harari et al. 2011; Papadimitrakopoulou et al. 2011). Similarly, the addition of bevacizumab and erlotinib to first-line chemoradiotherapy was also feasible and produced toxicity comparable to other effective combined modality regimens for HNSCC (Hainsworth et al. 2011). These inconsistent results suggest that the application of anti-angiogenic agents to EGFR and radiotherapy in the clinic will further the clinical evaluation in a systematic treatment schema in appropriate patient groups to identify potential clinical benefits (Citrin et al. 2006).

6   Conclusions

There are compelling reasons to explore the combination of radiation with agents that target growth factor receptors since radiation can activate receptor signaling. In particular, a beneficial impact of combining radiation with EGFR-targeting agents in cancer therapy has been established in recent years. This is particularly evident in HNSCC when there is phase III trial data showing a survival advantage when combining cetuximab with radiation. This clinical benefit validates preclinical data that projected a favorable interaction of anti-EGFR therapies with radiation. With over 50 % of cancer patients worldwide receiving radiation as an integral component of their treatment, this approach may provide significant stimulus to guide the combination of radiation not only with EGFR agents, but also with other molecular-targeting drugs for the improvement of cancer therapy. Many challenges remain since acquired resistance to EGFR inhibitors is emerging as a treatment barrier for optimizing EGFR-targeted therapy. With improved understanding of mechanisms of resistance, several next-generation EGFR-targeting agents have been developed and are currently being studied in preclinical and clinical models. Personalized cancer medicine based on molecular profiling of tumors is also a treatment strategy of the future. Improved selection of treatments for patients with activating or resistance mutations of EGFR or downstream effectors is central to improve the ultimate efficacy of EGFR-targeted therapies. The identification of reliable predictive markers for targeted therapies combined with radiation represents a worthy objective for the future.

Acknowledgements Supported in part by NIH/NCI Grant R01 CA 113448 to PMH

Disclosure PMH has held laboratory research agreements with industry sponsors developing EGFR and VEGFR inhibitors including Amgen, AstraZeneca, Genentech, ImClone, OSI, and Symphogen during the last 10 years.

References

Ahsan A, Hiniker SM, Davis MA, Lawrence TS, Nyati MK (2009) Role of cell cycle in epidermal growth factor receptor inhibitor-mediated radiosensitization. Cancer Res 69:5108–5114

Akimoto T, Hunter NR, Buchmiller L, Mason K, Ang KK, Milas L (1999) Inverse relationship between epidermal growth factor receptor expression and radiocurability of murine carcinomas. Clin Cancer Res 5:2884–2890

Al-Ejeh F, Shi W, Miranda M, Simpson PT, Vargas AC, Song S, Wiegmans AP, Swarbrick A, Welm AL, Brown MP, Chenevix-Trench G, Lakhani SR, Khanna KK (2013) Treatment of triple-negative breast cancer using anti-EGFR-directed radioimmunotherapy combined with radiosensitizing chemotherapy and PARP inhibitor. J Nucl Med 54:913–921

Allegra CJ, Jessup JM, Somerfield MR, Hamilton SR, Hammond EH, Hayes DF, McAllister PK, Morton RF, Schilsky RL (2009) American Society of clinical oncology provisional clinical opinion: testing for KRAS gene mutations in patients with metastatic colorectal carcinoma to predict response to anti-epidermal growth factor receptor monoclonal antibody therapy. J Clin Oncol 27:2091–2096

Allen GW, Saba C, Armstrong EA, Huang S-M, Benavente S, Ludwig DL, Hicklin DJ, Harari PM (2007) Insulin-like growth factor-i receptor signaling blockade combined with radiation. Cancer Res 67:1155–1162

Al-Nedawi K, Meehan B, Kerbel RS, Allison AC, Rak J (2009) Endothelial expression of autocrine VEGF upon the uptake of tumor-derived microvesicles containing oncogenic EGFR. Proc Natl Acad Sci USA 106:3794–3799

Ang KK, Berkey BA, Tu X, Zhang HZ, Katz R, Hammond EH, Fu KK, Milas L (2002) Impact of epidermal growth factor receptor expression on survival and pattern of relapse in patients with advanced head and neck carcinoma. Cancer Res 62:7350–7356

Ang KK, Zhang QE, Rosenthal DI, Nguyen-Tan P, Sherman EJ, Weber RS, Galvin JM, Schwartz DL, El-Naggar AK, Gillison ML, Jordan R, List MA, Konski AA, Thorstad WL, Trotti A, Beitler JJ, Garden AS, Spanos WJ, Yom SS, Axelrod RS (2011) A randomized phase III trial (RTOG 0522) of concurrent accelerated radiation plus cisplatin with or without cetuximab for stage III-IV head and neck squamous cell carcinomas (HNC). J Clin Oncol 29:5500

Argiris A, Heron DE, Smith RP, Kim S, Gibson MK, Lai SY, Branstetter BF, Posluszny DM, Wang L, Seethala RR, Dacic S, Gooding W, Grandis JR, Johnson JT, Ferris RL (2010) Induction docetaxel, cisplatin, and cetuximab followed by concurrent radiotherapy, cisplatin, and cetuximab and maintenance cetuximab in patients with locally advanced head and neck cancer. J Clin Oncol 28:5294–5300

Argiris A, kotsakis AP, Kim S, Worden FP, Savvides P, Gibson MK, Blumenschein GR, Chen HX, Grandis JR, Kies MS (2011) Phase II trial of cetuximab (C) and bevacizumab (B) in recurrent or metastatic squamous cell carcinoma of the head and neck (SCCHN): Final results. J Clin Oncol 29 Abstr 5564

Ather F, Hamidi H, Fejzo MS, Letrent S, Finn RS, Kabbinavar F, Head C, Wong SG (2013) Dacomitinib, an irreversible Pan-ErbB inhibitor significantly abrogates growth in head and neck cancer models that exhibit low response to cetuximab. PLoS ONE 8:e56112

Bahassi ELM, Li YQ, Wise-Draper TM, Deng L, Wang J, Darnell CN, Wilson KM, Wells SI, Stambrook PJ, Rixe O (2013) A patient-derived somatic mutation in the epidermal growth factor receptor ligand-binding domain confers increased sensitivity to cetuximab in head and neck cancer. Eur J Cancer 49:2345–2355

Balak MN, Gong Y, Riely GJ, Somwar R, Li AR, Zakowski MF, Chiang A, Yang G, Ouerfelli O, Kris MG, Ladanyi M, Miller VA, Pao W (2006) Novel D761Y and common secondary T790 M mutations in epidermal growth factor receptor-mutant lung adenocarcinomas with acquired resistance to kinase inhibitors. Clin Cancer Res 12:6494–6501

Bandyopadhyay D, Mandal M, Adam L, Mendelsohn J, Kumar R (1998) Physical interaction between epidermal growth factor receptor and DNA-dependent protein kinase in mammalian cells. J Biol Chem 273:1568–1573

Baselga J, Swain SM (2009) Novel anticancer targets: revisiting ERBB2 and discovering ERBB3. Nat Rev Cancer 9:463–475

Baumann M, Krause M, Dikomey E, Dittmann K, Dorr W, Kasten-Pisula U, Rodemann HP (2007) EGFR-targeted anti-cancer drugs in radiotherapy: preclinical evaluation of mechanisms. Radiother Oncol 83:238–248

Bean J, Brennan C, Shih JY, Riely G, Viale A, Wang L, Chitale D, Motoi N, Szoke J, Broderick S, Balak M, Chang WC, Yu CJ, Gazdar A, Pass H, Rusch V, Gerald W, Huang SF, Yang PC, Miller V, Ladanyi M, Yang CH, Pao W (2007) MET amplification occurs with or without T790 M mutations in EGFR mutant lung tumors with acquired resistance to gefitinib or erlotinib. Proc Natl Acad Sci USA 104:20932–20937

Bean J, Riely GJ, Balak M, Marks JL, Ladanyi M, Miller VA, Pao W (2008) Acquired resistance to epidermal growth factor receptor kinase inhibitors associated with a novel T854A mutation in a patient with EGFR-mutant lung adenocarcinoma. Clin Cancer Res 14:7519–7525

Benavente S, Huang S, Armstrong EA, Chi A, Hsu K-T, Wheeler DL, Harari PM (2009) Establishment and characterization of a model of acquired resistance to epidermal growth factor receptor targeting agents in human cancer cells. Clin Cancer Res 15:1585–1592

Ben-Kasus T, Schechter B, Lavi S, Yarden Y, Sela M (2009) Persistent elimination of ErbB-2/HER2-overexpressing tumors using combinations of monoclonal antibodies: relevance of receptor endocytosis. Proc Natl Acad Sci USA 106:3294–3299

Beucher A, Birraux J, Tchouandong L, Barton O, Shibata A, Conrad S, Goodarzi AA, Krempler A, Jeggo PA, Lobrich M (2009) ATM and Artemis promote homologous recombination of radiation-induced DNA double-strand breaks in G2. EMBO J 28:3413–3427

Bhardwaj V, Zhan Y, Cortez MA, Ang KK, Molkentine D, Munshi A, Raju U, Komaki R, Heymach JV, Welsh J (2012) C-Met inhibitor MK-8003 radiosensitizes c-Met-expressing non-small-cell lung cancer cells with radiation-induced c-Met-expression. J Thorac Oncol 7:1211–1217

Bianco C, Tortora G, Bianco R, Caputo R, Veneziani BM, Caputo R, Damiano V, Troiani T, Fontanini G, Raben D, Pepe S, Bianco AR, Ciardiello F (2002) Enhancement of antitumor activity of ionizing radiation by combined treatment with the selective epidermal growth factor receptor-tyrosine kinase inhibitor ZD1839 (Iressa). Clin Cancer Res 8:3250–3258

Bonner JA, Harari PM, Giralt J, Azarnia N, Shin DM, Cohen RB, Jones CU, Sur R, Raben D, Jassem J, Ove R, Kies MS, Baselga J, Youssoufian H, Amellal N, Rowinsky EK, Ang KK (2006) Radiotherapy plus cetuximab for squamous-cell carcinoma of the head and neck. N Engl J Med 354:567–578

Bonner JA, Harari PM, Giralt J, Cohen RB, Jones CU, Sur RK, Raben D, Baselga J, Spencer SA, Zhu J, Youssoufian H, Rowinsky EK, Ang KK (2010) Radiotherapy plus cetuximab for locoregionally advanced head and neck cancer: 5-year survival data from a phase 3 randomised trial, and relation between cetuximab-induced rash and survival. Lancet Oncol. 11:21–28

Bouali S, Chretien AS, Ramacci C, Rouyer M, Marchal S, Galenne T, Juin P, Becuwe P, Merlin JL (2009) P53 and PTEN expression contribute to the inhibition of EGFR downstream signaling pathway by cetuximab. Cancer Gene Ther 16:498–507

Bouchaert P, Guerif S, Debiais C, Irani J, Fromont G (2012) DNA-PKcs expression predicts response to radiotherapy in prostate cancer. Int J Radiat Oncol Biol Phys 84:1179–1185

Bozec A, Formento P, Lassalle S, Lippens C, Hofman P, Milano G (2007) Dual inhibition of EGFR and VEGFR pathways in combination with irradiation: antitumour supra-additive effects on human head and neck cancer xenografts. Br J Cancer 97:65–72

Bozec A, Sudaka A, Fischel JL, Brunstein MC, Etienne-Grimaldi MC, Milano G (2008) Combined effects of bevacizumab with erlotinib and irradiation: a preclinical study on a head and neck cancer orthotopic model. Br J Cancer 99:93–99

Bozec A, Peyrade F, Fischel JL, Milano G (2009a) Emerging molecular targeted therapies in the treatment of head and neck cancer. Expert Opin Emerg Drugs 14:299–310

Bozec A, Sudaka A, Toussan N, Fischel JL, Etienne-Grimaldi MC, Milano G (2009b) Combination of sunitinib, cetuximab and irradiation in an orthotopic head and neck cancer model. Ann Oncol 20:1703–1707

Bozulic L, Surucu B, Hynx D, Hemmings BA (2008) PKBalpha/Akt1 acts downstream of DNA-PK in the DNA double-strand break response and promotes survival. Mol Cell 30:203–213

Brand TM, Dunn EF, Iida M, Myers RA, Kostopoulos KT, Li C, Peet CR, Wheeler DL (2011) Erlotinib is a viable treatment for tumors with acquired resistance to cetuximab. Cancer Biol Ther 12:436–446

Camp ER, Summy J, Bauer TW, Liu W, Gallick GE, Ellis LM (2005) Molecular mechanisms of resistance to therapies targeting the epidermal growth factor receptor. Clin Cancer Res 11:397–405

Cengel KA, Voong KR, Chandrasekaran S, Maggiorella L, Brunner TB, Stanbridge E, Kao GD, McKenna WG, Bernhard EJ (2007) Oncogenic K-Ras signals through epidermal growth factor receptor and wild-type H-Ras to promote radiation survival in pancreatic and colorectal carcinoma cells. Neoplasia 9:341–348

Cerniglia GJ, Pore N, Tsai JH, Schultz S, Mick R, Choe R, Xing X, Durduran T, Yodh AG, Evans SM, Koch CJ, Hahn SM, Quon H, Sehgal CM, Lee WMF, Maity A (2009) Epidermal growth factor receptor inhibition modulates the microenvironment by vascular normalization to improve chemotherapy and radiotherapy efficacy. PLoS ONE 4:e6539

Chakravarti A, Wang M, Robins HI, Lautenschlaeger T, Curran WJ, Brachman DG, Schultz CJ, Choucair A, Dolled-Filhart M, Christiansen J, Gustavson M, Molinaro A, Mischel P, Dicker AP, Bredel M, Mehta M (2013) RTOG 0211: a phase 1/2 study of radiation therapy with concurrent gefitinib for newly diagnosed glioblastoma patients. Int J Radiat Oncol Biol Phys 85:1206–1211

Chang G-C, Yu C-TR, Tsai C-H, Tsai J-R, Chen J-C, Wu C-C, Wu W-J, Hsu S-L (2008) An epidermal growth factor inhibitor, Gefitinib, induces apoptosis through a p53-dependent upregulation of pro-apoptotic molecules and downregulation of anti-apoptotic molecules in human lung adenocarcinoma A549 cells. Eur J Pharmacol 600:37–44

Chen D, Nirodi C (2007) The epidermal growth factor receptor: a role in repair of radiation-induced DNA damage. Clin Cancer Res 13:6555–6560

Chen BP, Uematsu N, Kobayashi J, Lerenthal Y, Krempler A, Yajima H, Lobrich M, Shiloh Y, Chen DJ (2007) Ataxia telangiectasia mutated (ATM) is essential for DNA-PKcs phospho-rylations at the Thr-2609 cluster upon DNA double strand break. J Biol Chem 282:6582–6587

Chinnaiyan P, Huang S, Vallabhaneni G, Armstrong E, Varambally S, Tomlins SA, Chin-naiyan AM, Harari PM (2005) Mechanisms of enhanced radiation response following epidermal growth factor receptor signaling inhibition by erlotinib (Tarceva). Cancer Res 65:3328–3335

Citrin D, Menard C, Camphausen K (2006) Combining radiotherapy and angiogenesis inhibitors: clinical trial design. Int J Radiat Oncol Biol Phys 64:15–25

Cohen EE, Haraf DJ, Kunnavakkam R, Stenson KM, Blair EA, Brockstein B, Lester EP, Salama JK, Dekker A, Williams R, Witt ME, Grushko TA, Dignam JJ, Lingen MW,

Olopade OI, Vokes EE (2010) Epidermal growth factor receptor inhibitor gefitinib added to chemoradiotherapy in locally advanced head and neck cancer. J Clin Oncol 28:3336–3343

Cosaceanu D, Budiu RA, Carapancea M, Castro J, Lewensohn R, Dricu A (2007) Ionizing radiation activates IGF-1R triggering a cytoprotective signaling by interfering with Ku-DNA binding and by modulating Ku86 expression via a p38 kinase-dependent mechanism. Oncogene 26:2423–2434

Costa DB, Schumer ST, Tenen DG, Kobayashi S (2008) Differential responses to erlotinib in epidermal growth factor receptor (EGFR)-mutated lung cancers with acquired resistance to gefitinib carrying the L747S or T790 M secondary mutations. J Clin Oncol 26:1182–1184 (author reply 1184–1186)

Crane CH, Varadhachary GR, Yordy JS, Staerkel GA, Javle MM, Safran H, Haque W, Hobbs BD, Krishnan S, Fleming JB, Das P, Lee JE, Abbruzzese JL, Wolff RA (2011) Phase II trial of cetuximab, gemcitabine, and oxaliplatin followed by chemoradiation with cetuximab for locally advanced (T4) pancreatic adenocarcinoma: correlation of Smad4(Dpc4) immunostaining with pattern of disease progression. J Clin Oncol 29:3037–3043

Das AK, Sato M, Story MD, Peyton M, Graves R, Redpath S, Girard L, Gazdar AF, Shay JW, Minna JD, Nirodi CS (2006) Non-small cell lung cancers with kinase domain mutations in the epidermal growth factor receptor are sensitive to ionizing radiation. Cancer Res 66:9601–9608

Das AK, Chen BP, Story MD, Sato M, Minna JD, Chen DJ, Nirodi CS (2007) Somatic mutations in the tyrosine kinase domain of epidermal growth factor receptor (EGFR) abrogate EGFR-mediated radioprotection in non-small cell lung carcinoma. Cancer Res 67:5267–5274

Dassonville O, Bozec A, Fischel JL, Milano G (2007) EGFR targeting therapies: monoclonal antibodies versus tyrosine kinase inhibitors: similarities and differences. Crit Rev Oncol/Hemotol 62:53–61

de Bacco F, Luraghi P, Medico E, Reato G, Girolami F, Perera T, Gabriele P, Comoglio PM, Boccaccio C (2011) Induction of MET by ionizing radiation and its role in radioresistance and invasive growth of cancer. J Natl Cancer Inst 103:645–661

Dechant M, Weisner W, Berger S, Peipp M, Beyer T, Schneider-Merck T, van Bueren JJL, Bleeker WK, Parren PW, van de Winkel JG, Valerius T (2008) Complement-dependent tumor cell lysis triggered by combinations of epidermal growth factor receptor antibodies. Cancer Res 68:4998–5003

Dent P, Reardon DB, Park JS, Bowers G, Logsdon C, Valerie K, Schmidt-Ullrich R (1999) Radiation-induced release of transforming growth factor alpha activates the epidermal growth factor receptor and mitogen-activated protein kinase pathway in carcinoma cells, leading to increased proliferation and protection from radiation-induced cell death. Mol Biol Cell 10:2493–2506

Dent P, Yacoub A, Contessa J, Caron R, Amorino G, Valerie K, Hagan MP, Grant S, Schmidt-Ullrich R (2003) Stress and radiation-induced activation of multiple intracellular signaling pathways. Radiat Res 159:283–300

Dienstmann R, de Dosso S, Felip E, Tabernero J (2012) Drug development to overcome resistance to EGFR inhibitors in lung and colorectal cancer. Mol Oncol 6:15–26

Dienstmann R, Tabernero J, Cutsem EV, Cervantes-ruiperez A, Keranen SR, Viñuales MB, Kjær I, Pedersen MW, Skartved NJO, Flensburg MF, Horak ID, Garcia-carbonero R (2013) Proof-of-concept study of sym004, an anti-egfr monoclonal antibody (mab) mixture, in patients (pts) with anti-egfr mab-refractory kras wild-type (wt) metastatic colorectal cancer (mcrc). J Clin Oncol 31 (suppl; abstr 3551)

Dings RPM, Loren M, Heun H, McNiel E, Griffioen AW, Mayo KH, Griffin RJ (2007) Scheduling of radiation with angiogenesis inhibitors anginex and avastin improves therapeutic outcome via vessel normalization. Clin Cancer Res 13:3395–3402

Dittmann K, Mayer C, Fehrenbacher B, Schaller M, Raju U, Milas L, Chen DJ, Kehlbach R, Rodemann HP (2005a) Radiation-induced epidermal growth factor receptor nuclear import is linked to activation of DNA-dependent protein kinase. J Biol Chem 280:31182–31189

Dittmann K, Mayer C, Rodemann H (2005b) Inhibition of radiation-induced EGFR nuclear import by C225 (Cetuximab) suppresses DNA-PK activity. Radiother Oncol 76:157–161

Dittmann K, Mayer C, Kehlbach R, Rodemann HP (2008) Radiation-induced caveolin-1 associated EGFR internalization is linked with nuclear EGFR transport and activation of DNA-PK. Mol Cancer 7:69

Dittmann K, Mayer C, Kehlbach R, Rothmund M-C, Peter Rodemann H (2009) Radiation-induced lipid peroxidation activates src kinase and triggers nuclear EGFR transport. Radiother Oncol, in Press, corrected proof

Dittmann K, Mayer C, Fehrenbacher B, Schaller M, Kehlbach R, Rodemann HP (2011) Nuclear epidermal growth factor receptor modulates cellular radio-sensitivity by regulation of chromatin access. Radiother Oncol 99:317–322

Dziadziuszko R, Jassem J (2012) Epidermal growth factor receptor (EGFR) inhibitors and derived treatments. Ann Oncol 23(Suppl 10):x193–x196

Eck MJ, Yun CH (2010) Structural and mechanistic underpinnings of the differential drug sensitivity of EGFR mutations in non-small cell lung cancer. Biochim Biophys Acta 1804:559–566

Eng C, Van Cutsem E, Nowara E, Swieboda-Sadlej A, Tebbutt NC, Mitchell EP, Davidenko I, Oliner K, Chen L, Huang J, Mccaffery I, Loh E, Smethurst D, Tabernero J (2011) A randomized, phase Ib/II trial of rilotumumab (AMG 102; ril) or ganitumab (AMG 479; gan) with panitumumab (pmab) versus pmab alone in patients (pts) with wild-type (WT) KRAS metastatic colorectal cancer (mCRC): primary and biomarker analyses. J Clin Oncol 29 (suppl; abstr 3500)

Engelman JA, Janne PA (2008) Mechanisms of acquired resistance to epidermal growth factor receptor tyrosine kinase inhibitors in non-small cell lung cancer. Clin Cancer Res 14:2895–2899

Engelman JA, Settleman J (2008) Acquired resistance to tyrosine kinase inhibitors during cancer therapy. Curr Opin Genet Dev 18:73–79

Engelman JA, Zejnullahu K, Mitsudomi T, Song Y, Hyland C, Park JO, Lindeman N, Gale C-M, Zhao X, Christensen J, Kosaka T, Holmes AJ, Rogers AM, Cappuzzo F, Mok T, Lee C, Johnson BE, Cantley LC, Janne PA (2007) MET amplification leads to gefitinib resistance in lung cancer by activating ERBB3 signaling. Science 316:1039–1043

Fraser M, Harding SM, Zhao H, Coackley C, Durocher D, Bristow RG (2011) MRE11 promotes AKT phosphorylation in direct response to DNA double-strand breaks. Cell Cycle 10:2218–2232

Friedman LM, Rinon A, Schechter B, Lyass L, Lavi S, Bacus SS, Sela M, Yarden Y (2005) Synergistic down-regulation of receptor tyrosine kinases by combinations of mAbs: Implications for cancer immunotherapy. PNAS 102:1915–1920

Friedmann BJ, Caplin M, Savic B, Shah T, Lord CJ, Ashworth A, Hartley JA, Hochhauser D (2006) Interaction of the epidermal growth factor receptor and the DNA-dependent protein kinase pathway following gefitinib treatment. Mol Cancer Ther 5:209–218

Frolov A, Schuller K, Tzeng CW, Cannon EE, Ku BC, Howard JH, Vickers SM, Heslin MJ, Buchsbaum DJ, Arnoletti JP (2007) ErbB3 expression and dimerization with egfr influence pancreatic cancer cell sensitivity to Erlotinib. Cancer Biol Ther 6

Fukumura D, Jain RK (2007) Tumor microvasculature and microenvironment: targets for anti-angiogenesis and normalization. Microvasc Res 74:72–84

Gan HK, Lappas M, Cao DX, Cvrljevdic A, Scott AM, Johns TG (2009) Targeting a unique EGFR epitope with monoclonal antibody 806 activates NF-kappaB and initiates tumour vascular normalization. J Cell Mol Med 13:3993–4001

Giaccone G, Wang Y (2011) Strategies for overcoming resistance to EGFR family tyrosine kinase inhibitors. Cancer Treat Rev 37:456–464

Giaccone G, Herbst RS, Manegold C, Scagliotti G, Rosell R, Miller V, Natale RB, Schiller JH, von Pawel J, Pluzanska A, Gatzemeier U, Grous J, Ochs JS, Averbuch SD, Wolf MK, Rennie P, Fandi A, Johnson DH (2004) Gefitinib in combination with gemcitabine and cisplatin in advanced non-small-cell lung cancer: a phase III trial–INTACT 1. J Clin Oncol 22:777–784

Gilmore AP, Valentijn AJ, Wang P, Ranger AM, Bundred N, O'Hare MJ, Wakeling A, Korsmeyer SJ, Streuli CH (2002) Activation of BAD by therapeutic inhibition of epidermal growth factor receptor and transactivation by insulin-like growth factor receptor. J Biol Chem 277:27643–27650

Goel S, Hidalgo M, Perez-Soler R (2007) EGFR inhibitor-mediated apoptosis in solid tumors. J Exp Ther Oncol 6:305–320

Golding SE, Morgan RN, Adams BR, Hawkins AJ, Povirk LF, Valerie K (2009) Pro-survival AKT and ERK signaling from EGFR and mutant EGFRvIII enhances DNA double-strand break repair in human glioma cells. Cancer Biol Ther 8:730–738

Goodarzi AA, Jeggo P, Lobrich M (2010) The influence of heterochromatin on DNA double strand break repair: getting the strong, silent type to relax. DNA Repair (Amst) 9:1273–1282

Govindan R, Bogart J, Stinchcombe T, Wang X, Hodgson L, Kratzke R, Garst J, Brotherton T, Vokes EE (2011) Randomized phase II study of pemetrexed, carboplatin, and thoracic radiation with or without cetuximab in patients with locally advanced unresectable non-small-cell lung cancer: cancer and leukemia group B trial 30407. J Clin Oncol 29:3120–3125

Guillamo J-S, de Bouard S, Valable S, Marteau L, Leuraud P, Marie Y, Poupon M-F, Parienti J-J, Raymond E, Peschanski M (2009) Molecular mechanisms underlying effects of epidermal growth factor receptor inhibition on invasion, proliferation, and angiogenesis in experimental glioma. Clin Cancer Res 15:3697–3704

Gupta A, Raina V (2010) Geftinib. J Cancer Res Ther 6:249–254

Hainsworth JD, Spigel DR, Greco FA, Shipley DL, Peyton J, Rubin M, Stipanov M, Meluch A (2011) Combined modality treatment with chemotherapy, radiation therapy, bevacizumab, and erlotinib in patients with locally advanced squamous carcinoma of the head and neck: a phase II trial of the Sarah Cannon oncology research consortium. Cancer J 17:267–272

Harari PM, Huang S (2001) Radiation response modification following molecular inhibition of epidermal growth factor receptor signaling. Semin Radiat Oncol 11:281–289

Harari PM, Huang S-M (2004) Searching for reliable epidermal growth factor receptor response predictors: commentary re. Clin Cancer Res 10:428–432

Harari PM, Huang S (2006) Radiation combined With EGFR signal inhibitors: head and neck cancer focus. Semin Radiat Oncol 16:38–44

Harari PM, Allen GW, Bonner JA (2007) Biology of interactions: antiepidermal growth factor receptor agents. J Clin Oncol 25:4057–4065

Harari PM, Khuntia D, Traynor AM, Hoang T, Yang DT, Hartig GK, McCulloch TM, Jeraj R, Nyflot MJ, Wiederholt PA, Gentry LR (2011) Phase I trial of bevacizumab combined with concurrent chemoradiation for squamous cell carcinoma of the head and neck: preliminary outcome results. ASCO Meet Abstr 29:5518

Herbst RS, Giaccone G, Schiller JH, Natale RB, Miller V, Manegold C, Scagliotti G, Rosell R, Oliff I, Reeves JA, Wolf MK, Krebs AD, Averbuch SD, Ochs JS, Grous J, Fandi A, Johnson DH (2004) Gefitinib in combination with paclitaxel and carboplatin in advanced non-small-cell lung cancer: a phase III trial–INTACT 2. J Clin Oncol 22:785–794

Herbst RS, Prager D, Hermann R, Fehrenbacher L, Johnson BE, Sandler A, Kris MG, Tran HT, Klein P, Li X, Ramies D, Johnson DH, Miller VA (2005) TRIBUTE: a phase III trial of Erlotinib Hydrochloride (OSI-774) combined with carboplatin and paclitaxel chemotherapy in advanced non-small-cell lung cancer. J Clin Oncol 23:5892–5899

Herchenhorn D, Dias FL, Viegas CM, Federico MH, Araujo CM, Small I, Bezerra M, Fontao K, Knust RE, Ferreira CG, Martins RG (2010) Phase I/II study of erlotinib combined with cisplatin and radiotherapy in patients with locally advanced squamous cell carcinoma of the head and neck. Int J Radiat Oncol Biol Phys 78:696–702

Huang S-M, Harari PM (2000) Modulation of radiation response after epidermal growth factor receptor blockade in squamous cell carcinomas: inhibition of damage repair, cell cycle kinetics, and tumor angiogenesis. Clin Cancer Res 6:2166–2174

Huang S, Bock JM, Harari PM (1999) Epidermal growth factor receptor blockade with C225 modulates proliferation, apoptosis, and radiosensitivity in squamous cell carcinomas of the head and neck. Cancer Res 59:1935–1940

Huang S, Li J, Harari PM (2001) Modulation of radiation response and tumor-induced angiogenesis following EGFR inhibition by ZD1839 (Iressa) in human squamous cell carcinomas. Clin. Cancer Res 7:3705 s(A#259)

Huang S, Li J, Armstrong EA, Harari PM (2002) Modulation of radiation response and tumor-induced angiogenesis after epidermal growth factor receptor inhibition by ZD1839 (Iressa). Cancer Res 62:4300–4306

Huang S, Armstrong EA, Benavente S, Chinnaiyan P, Harari PM (2004) Dual-agent molecular targeting of the epidermal growth factor receptor (EGFR): combining anti-EGFR antibody with tyrosine kinase inhibitor. Cancer Res 64:5355–5362

Huang S, Benavente S, Armstrong EA, Li C, Wheeler DL, Harari PM (2011) p53 modulates acquired resistance to EGFR inhibitors and radiation. Cancer Res 71:7071–7079

Huang S, Li C, Armstrong EA, Peet CR, Saker J, Amler LC, Sliwkowski MX, Harari PM (2013a) Dual targeting of EGFR and HER3 with MEHD7945A overcomes acquired resistance to EGFR inhibitors and radiation. Cancer Res 73:824–833

Huang S, Peet CR, Saker J, Li C, Armstrong E, Kragh M, Pedersen MW, Harari PM (2013b) Sym004, a novel anti-EGFR antibody mixture augments radiation response in human lung and head and neck cancers. Mol Cancer Ther (in press)

Iivanainen E, Lauttia S, Zhang N, Tvorogov D, Kulmala J, Grenman R, Salven P, Elenius K (2009) The EGFR inhibitor gefitinib suppresses recruitment of pericytes and bone marrow-derived perivascular cells into tumor vessels. Microvasc Res, in press, corrected proof

Jackman D, Pao W, Riely GJ, Engelman JA, Kris MG, Janne PA, Lynch T, Johnson BE, Miller VA (2010) Clinical definition of acquired resistance to epidermal growth factor receptor tyrosine kinase inhibitors in non-small-cell lung cancer. J Clin Oncol 28:357–360

Jain RK (2005) Normalization of tumor vasculature: an emerging concept in antiangiogenic therapy. Science 307:58–62

Jain A, Penuel E, Mink S, Schmidt J, Hodge A, Favero K, Tindell C, Agus DB (2010) HER kinase axis receptor dimer partner switching occurs in response to EGFR tyrosine kinase inhibition despite failure to block cellular proliferation. Cancer Res 70:1989–1999

Jeggo PA, Geuting V, Lobrich M (2011) The role of homologous recombination in radiation-induced double-strand break repair. Radiother Oncol 101:7–12

Jensen AD, Munter MW, Bischoff HG, Haselmann R, Haberkorn U, Huber PE, Thomas M, Debus J, Herfarth KK (2011) Combined treatment of nonsmall cell lung cancer NSCLC stage III with intensity-modulated RT radiotherapy and cetuximab: the NEAR trial. Cancer 117:2986–2994

Jimeno A, Rubio-Viqueira B, Amador ML, Oppenheimer D, Bouraoud N, Kulesza P, Sebastiani V, Maitra A, Hidalgo M (2005) Epidermal growth factor receptor dynamics influences response to epidermal growth factor receptor targeted agents. Cancer Res 65:3003–3010

Jimeno A, Messersmith WA, Hirsch FR, Franklin WA, Eckhardt SG (2009) KRAS mutations and sensitivity to epidermal growth factor receptor inhibitors in colorectal cancer: practical application of patient selection. J Clin Oncol 27:1130–1136

Jones HE, Goddard L, Gee JMW, Hiscox S, Rubini M, Barrow D, Knowlden JM, Williams S, Wakeling AE, Nicholson RI (2004) Insulin-like growth factor-I receptor signalling and acquired resistance to gefitinib (ZD1839; Iressa) in human breast and prostate cancer cells. Endocr Relat Cancer 11:793–814

Kamath AV, Lu D, Gupta P, Jin D, Xiang H, Wong A, Leddy C, Crocker L, Schaefer G, Sliwkowski MX, Damico-Beyer LA (2012) Preclinical pharmacokinetics of MEHD7945A, a novel EGFR/HER3 dual-action antibody, and prediction of its human pharmacokinetics and efficacious clinical dose. Cancer Chemother Pharmacol 69:1063–1069

Kang KB, Zhu C, Wong YL, Gao Q, Ty A, Wong MC (2012) Gefitinib radiosensitizes stem-like glioma cells: inhibition of epidermal growth factor receptor-Akt-DNA-PK signaling, accompanied by inhibition of DNA double-strand break repair. Int J Radiat Oncol Biol Phys 83:e43–e52

Kasten U, Plottner N, Johansen J, Overgaard J, Dikomey E (1999) Ku70/80 gene expression and DNA-dependent protein kinase (DNA-PK) activity do not correlate with double-strand break (dsb) repair capacity and cellular radiosensitivity in normal human fibroblasts. Br J Cancer 79:1037–1041

Kasten-Pisula U, Tastan H, Dikomey E (2005) Huge differences in cellular radiosensitivity due to only very small variations in double-strand break repair capacity. Int J Radiat Biol 81:409–419

Katakami N, Atagi S, Goto K, Hida T, Horai T, Inoue A, Ichinose Y, Koboyashi K, Takeda K, Kiura K, Nishio K, Seki Y, Ebisawa R, Shahidi M, Yamamoto N (2013) LUX-lung 4: a phase II trial of afatinib in patients with advanced non-small-cell lung cancer who progressed during prior treatment with Erlotinib, Gefitinib, or both. J Clin Oncol

Kim TJ, Lee JW, Song SY, Choi JJ, Choi CH, Kim BG, Lee JH, Bae DS (2006) Increased expression of pAKT is associated with radiation resistance in cervical cancer. Br J Cancer 94:1678–1682

Kleibeuker EA, Griffioen AW, Verheul HM, Slotman BJ, Thijssen VL (2012) Combining angiogenesis inhibition and radiotherapy: a double-edged sword. Drug Resist Updat 15:173–182

Kobayashi S, Boggon TJ, Dayaram T, Janne PA, Kocher O, Meyerson M, Johnson BE, Eck MJ, Tenen DG, Halmos B (2005) EGFR mutation and resistance of non-small-cell lung cancer to gefitinib. N Engl J Med 352:786–792

Koefoed K, Steinaa L, Soderberg JN, Kjaer I, Jacobsen HJ, Meijer PJ, Haurum JS, Jensen A, Kragh M, Andersen PS, Pedersen MW (2011) Rational identification of an optimal antibody mixture for targeting the epidermal growth factor receptor. MAbs 3:584–595

Krause M, Ostermann G, Petersen C, Yaromina A, Hessel F, Harstrick A, van der Kogel AJ, Thames HD, Baumann M (2005) Decreased repopulation as well as increased reoxygenation contribute to the improvement in local control after targeting of the EGFR by C225 during fractionated irradiation. Radiother Oncol 76:162–167

Krause M, Zips D, Thames HD, Kummermehr J, Baumann M (2006) Preclinical evaluation of molecular-targeted anticancer agents for radiotherapy. Radiother Oncol 80:112–122

Krause M, Prager J, Zhou X, Yaromina A, Dorfler A, Eicheler W, Baumann M (2007) EGFR-TK inhibition before radiotherapy reduces tumour volume but does not improve local control: differential response of cancer stem cells and nontumourigenic cells? Radiother Oncol 83:316–325

Kriegs M, Kasten-Pisula U, Rieckmann T, Holst K, Saker J, Dahm-Daphi J, Dikomey E (2010) The epidermal growth factor receptor modulates DNA double-strand break repair by regulating non-homologous end-joining. DNA Repair 9:889–897

Kruser TJ, Armstrong EA, Ghia AJ, Huang S, Wheeler DL, Radinsky R, Freeman DJ, Harari PM (2008) Augmentation of radiation response by panitumumab in models of upper aerodigestive tract cancer. Int J Radiat Oncol Biol Phys 72:534–542

Kurai J, Chikumi H, Hashimoto K, Yamaguchi K, Yamasaki A, Sako T, Touge H, Makino H, Takata M, Miyata M, Nakamoto M, Burioka N, Shimizu E (2007) Antibody-dependent cellular cytotoxicity mediated by cetuximab against lung cancer cell lines. Clin Cancer Res 13:1552–1561

Larsson O, Girnita A, Girnita L (2005) Role of insulin-like growth factor 1 receptor signalling in cancer. Br J Cancer 92:2097–2101

Lavin MF (2007) ATM and the Mre11 complex combine to recognize and signal DNA double-strand breaks. Oncogene 26:7749–7758

Lee H-L, Chung T-S, Ting L-L, Tsai J-T, Chen S-W, Chiou J-F, Leung H, Liu H (2012) EGFR mutations are associated with favorable intracranial response and progression-free survival following brain irradiation in non-small cell lung cancer patients with brain metastases. Radiat Oncol 7:181

Lee HJ, Schaefer G, Heffron TP, Shao L, Ye X, Sideris S, Malek S, Chan E, Merchant M, La H, Ubhayakar S, Yauch RL, Pirazzoli V, Politi K, Settleman J (2013) Noncovalent wild-type-sparing inhibitors of EGFR T790 M. Cancer Discov 3:168–181

Lewis CM, Glisson BS, Feng L, Wan F, Tang X, Wistuba II, El-Naggar AK, Rosenthal DI, Chambers MS, Lustig RA, Weber RS (2012) A phase II study of gefitinib for aggressive cutaneous squamous cell carcinoma of the head and neck. Clin Cancer Res 18:1435–1446

Li D, Ambrogio L, Shimamura T, Kubo S, Takahashi M, Chirieac LR, Padera RF, Shapiro GI, Baum A, Himmelsbach F, Rettig WJ, Meyerson M, Solca F, Greulich H, Wong KK (2008a) BIBW2992, an irreversible EGFR/HER2 inhibitor highly effective in preclinical lung cancer models. Oncogene 27:4702–4711

Li L, Wang H, Yang ES, Arteaga CL, Xia F (2008b) Erlotinib attenuates homologous recombinational repair of chromosomal breaks in human breast cancer cells. Cancer Res 68:9141–9146

Li G, Hu W, Wang J, Deng X, Zhang P, Zhang X, Xie C, Wu S (2010) Phase II study of concurrent chemoradiation in combination with erlotinib for locally advanced esophageal carcinoma. Int J Radiat Oncol Biol Phys 78:1407–1412

Lieber MR (2010) The mechanism of double-strand DNA break repair by the nonhomologous DNA end-joining pathway. Annu Rev Biochem 79:181–211

Lievre A, Bachet J-B, le Corre D, Boige V, Landi B, Emile J-F, Cote J-F, Tomasic G, Penna C, Ducreux M, Rougier P, Penault-Llorca F, Laurent-Puig P (2006) KRAS mutation status is predictive of response to cetuximab therapy in colorectal cancer. Cancer Res 66:3992–3995

Lilleby W, Solca F, Røe K (2011) Radiotherapy and inhibition of the EGF family as treatment strategies for prostate cancer: combining theragnostics with theragates. Oncol Rev 5:119–128

Lynch TJ, Bell DW, Sordella R, Gurubhagavatula S, Okimoto RA, Brannigan BW, Harris PL, Haserlat SM, Supko JG, Haluska FG, Louis DN, Christiani DC, Settleman J, Haber DA (2004) Activating mutations in the epidermal growth factor receptor underlying responsiveness of non-small-cell lung cancer to gefitinib. N Engl J Med 350:2129–2139

Ma J, Waxman DJ (2008) Combination of antiangiogenesis with chemotherapy for more effective cancer treatment. Mol Cancer Ther 7:3670–3684

Macaulay VM, Salisbury AJ, Bohula EA, Playford MP, Smorodinsky NI, Shiloh Y (2001) Downregulation of the type 1 insulin-like growth factor receptor in mouse melanoma cells is associated with enhanced radiosensitivity and impaired activation of Atm kinase. Oncogene 20:4029–4040

Machiels J-PH, Specenier PM, Krauss J, Dietz A, Kaminsky M-C, Lalami Y, Henke M, Keilholz U, Knecht R, Skartved NJO, Horak ID, Flensburg MF, Gauler TC (2013) Sym004, a novel strategy to target EGFR with an antibody mixture, in patients with advanced SCCHN progressing after anti-EGFR monoclonal antibody: a proof of concept study. J Clin Oncol 31 (suppl; abstr 6002)

Mak RH, Doran E, Muzikansky A, Kang J, Neal JW, Baldini EH, Choi NC, Willers H, Jackman DM, Sequist LV (2011) Outcomes after combined modality therapy for EGFR-mutant and wild-type locally advanced NSCLC. Oncologist 16:886–895

Martinez E, Martinez M, Viñolas N, Casas F, De la Torre A, Valcarcel F, Minguez J, Paredes A, Perez Casas A, Dómine M (2008) Feasibility and tolerability of the addition of erlotinib to 3D thoracic radiotherapy (RT) in patients (p) with unresectable NSCLC: a prospective randomized phase II study. J Clin Oncol 26 abstr#7563

Massarelli E, Varella-Garcia M, Tang X, Xavier AC, Ozburn NC, Liu DD, Bekele BN, Herbst RS, Wistuba II (2007) KRAS mutation is an important predictor of resistance to therapy with epidermal growth factor receptor tyrosine kinase inhibitors in non-small-cell lung cancer. Clin Cancer Res 13:2890–2896

Masui H, Kawamoto T, Sato JD, Wolf B, Sato G, Mendelsohn J (1984) Growth inhibition of human tumor cells in athymic mice by anti-epidermal growth factor receptor monoclonal antibodies. Cancer Res 44:1002–1007

Matar P, Rojo F, Cassia R, Moreno-Bueno G, di Cosimo S, Tabernero J, Guzman M, Rodriguez S, Arribas J, Palacios J, Baselga J (2004) Combined epidermal growth factor receptor targeting with the tyrosine kinase inhibitor Gefitinib (ZD1839) and the monoclonal antibody Cetuximab (IMC-C225): superiority over single-agent receptor targeting. Clin Cancer Res 10:6487–6501

Mehta VK (2012) Radiotherapy and erlotinib combined: review of the preclinical and clinical evidence. Front Oncol 2

Mendelsohn J (2003) Antibody-mediated EGF receptor blockade as an anticancer therapy: from the laboratory to the clinic. Cancer Immunol Immunother 52:342–346

Merlano M, Russi E, Benasso M, Corvo R, Colantonio I, Vigna-Taglianti R, Vigo V, Bacigalupo A, Numico G, Crosetto N, Gasco M, Lo Nigro C, Vitiello R, Violante S, Garrone O (2011) Cisplatin-based chemoradiation plus cetuximab in locally advanced head and neck cancer: a phase II clinical study. Ann Oncol 22: 712–717

Meyn RE, Munshi A, Haymach JV, Milas L, Ang KK (2009) Receptor signaling as a regulatory mechanism of DNA repair. Radiotherapy and Oncology, in press, corrected proof

Milas L, Mason K, Hunter N, Petersen S, Yamakawa M, Ang K, Mendelsohn J, Fan Z (2000) In vivo enhancement of tumor radioresponse by C225 antiepidermal growth factor receptor antibody. Clin Cancer Res 6:701–708

Miller BS, Yee D (2005) Type I Insulin-like growth factor receptor as a therapeutic target in cancer. Cancer Res 65:10123–10127

Miller VA, Hirsh V, Cadranel J, Chen YM, Park K, Kim SW, Zhou C, Su WC, Wang M, Sun Y, Heo DS, Crino L, Tan EH, Chao TY, Shahidi M, Cong XJ, Lorence RM, Yang JC (2012) Afatinib versus placebo for patients with advanced, metastatic non-small-cell lung cancer after failure of erlotinib, gefitinib, or both, and one or two lines of chemotherapy (LUX-Lung 1): a phase 2b/3 randomised trial. Lancet Oncol 13:528–538

Morgillo F, Kim W-Y, Kim ES, Ciardiello F, Hong WK, Lee H-Y (2007) Implication of the insulin-like growth factor-ir pathway in the resistance of non-small cell lung cancer cells to treatment with Gefitinib. Clin Cancer Res 13:2795–2803

Nakamura JL (2007) The epidermal growth factor receptor in malignant gliomas: pathogenesis and therapeutic implications. Expert Opin Ther Targets 11:463–472

Nasu S, Ang KK, Fan Z, Milas L (2001) C225 antiepidermal growth factor receptor antibody enhances tumor radiocurability. Int J Radiat Oncol Biol Phys 51:474–477

Nijkamp MM, Span PN, Bussink J, Kaanders JH (2013) Interaction of EGFR with the tumour microenvironment: Implications for radiation treatment. Radiother Oncol

Nyati MK et al (2004) Radiosensitization by Pan-ErbB inhibitor CI-1033 in vitro and in vivo. Clin Cancer Res 10:691–700

Nyati MK, Morgan MA, Feng FY, Lawrence TS (2006) Integration of EGFR inhibitors with radiochemotherapy. Nat Rev Cancer 6:876–885

Ogino S, Meyerhardt JA, Cantor M, Brahmandam M, Clark JW, Namgyal C, Kawasaki T, Kinsella K, Michelini AL, Enzinger PC, Kulke MH, Ryan DP, Loda M, Fuchs CS (2005) Molecular alterations in tumors and response to combination chemotherapy with gefitinib for advanced colorectal cancer. Clin Cancer Res 11:6650–6656

O'Reilly MS (2006) Radiation combined with antiangiogenic and antivascular agents. Semin Radiat Oncol 16:45–50

Paez JG, Janne PA, Lee JC, Tracy S, Greulich H, Gabriel S, Herman P, Kaye FJ, Lindeman N, Boggon TJ, Naoki K, Sasaki H, Fujii Y, Eck MJ, Sellers WR, Johnson BE, Meyerson M (2004) EGFR mutations in lung cancer: correlation with clinical response to gefitinib therapy. Science 304:1497–1500

Pahl JHW, Ruslan SEN, Buddingh EP, Santos SJ, Szuhai K, Serra M, Gelderblom H, Hogendoorn PCW, Egeler RM, Schilham MW, Lankester AC (2012) Anti-EGFR antibody cetuximab enhances the cytolytic activity of natural killer cells toward osteosarcoma. Clin Cancer Res 18:432–441

Pao W, Miller VA (2005) Epidermal growth factor receptor mutations, small-molecule kinase inhibitors, and non-small-cell lung cancer: current knowledge and future directions. J Clin Oncol 23:2556–2568

Pao W, Miller V, Zakowski M, Doherty J, Politi K, Sarkaria I, Singh B, Heelan R, Rusch V, Fulton L, Mardis E, Kupfer D, Wilson R, Kris M, Varmus H (2004) EGF receptor gene mutations are common in lung cancers from "never smokers" and are associated with sensitivity of tumors to gefitinib and erlotinib. Proc Natl Acad Sci USA 101:13306–13311

Pao W, Miller VA, Politi KA, Riely GJ, Somwar R, Zakowski MF, Kris MG, Varmus H (2005) Acquired resistance of lung adenocarcinomas to gefitinib or erlotinib is associated with a second mutation in the EGFR kinase domain. PLoS Med 2:1–11

Papadimitrakopoulou V, Heymach J, Frank SJ, Myers J, Lin H, Tran HT, Chen C, Hirsch FR, Langmuir PB, Vasselli JR, Lippman SM, Raben D (2011) Updated clinical and biomarker results from a phase I study of vandetanib with radiation therapy (RT) with or without cisplatin in locally advanced head and neck squamous cell carcinoma (HNSCC). ASCO Meet Abstr 29:5510

Park J, Feng J, Li Y, Hammarsten O, Brazil DP, Hemmings BA (2009) DNA-dependent protein kinase-mediated phosphorylation of protein kinase B requires a specific recognition sequence in the C-terminal hydrophobic motif. J Biol Chem 284:6169–6174

Pedersen MW, Jacobsen HJ, Koefoed K, Hey A, Pyke C, Haurum JS, Kragh M (2010) Sym004: a novel synergistic anti-epidermal growth factor receptor antibody mixture with superior anticancer efficacy. Cancer Res 70:588–597

Peretz S, Jensen R, Baserga R, Glazer PM (2001) ATM-dependent expression of the insulin-like growth factor-I receptor in a pathway regulating radiation response. Proc Natl Acad Sci USA 98:1676–1681

Peters S, Adjei AA (2012) MET: a promising anticancer therapeutic target. Nat Rev Clin Oncol 9:314–326

Petersen C, Eicheler W, Frommel A, Krause M, Balschukat S, Zips D, Baumann M (2003) Proliferation and micromilieu during fractionated irradiation of human FaDu squamous cell carcinoma in nude mice. Int J Radiat Biol 79:469–477

Pore N, Jiang Z, Gupta A, Cerniglia G, Kao GD, Maity A (2006) EGFR tyrosine kinase inhibitors decrease VEGF expression by both hypoxia-inducible factor (HIF)-1-independent and HIF-1-dependent mechanisms. Cancer Res 66:3197–3204

Prados MD, Chang SM, Butowski N, Deboer R, Parvataneni R, Carliner H, Kabuubi P, Ayers-Ringler J, Rabbitt J, Page M, Fedoroff A, Sneed PK, Berger MS, McDermott MW, Parsa AT, Vandenberg S, James CD, Lamborn KR, Stokoe D, Haas-Kogan DA (2009) Phase II study of erlotinib plus temozolomide during and after radiation therapy in patients with newly diagnosed glioblastoma multiforme or gliosarcoma. J Clin Oncol 27:579–584

Qayum N, Muschel RJ, Im JH, Balathasan L, Koch CJ, Patel S, Mckenna WG, Bernhard EJ (2009) Tumor vascular changes mediated by inhibition of oncogenic signaling. Cancer Res 0008-5472.CAN-09-0657

Ramalingam SMD, Forster JRNBSN, Naret CBA, Evans TMD, Sulecki MMD, Lu HP, Teegarden PMS, Weber MRMD, Belani CPMD (2008). Dual inhibition of the epidermal growth factor receptor with cetuximab, an IgG1 monoclonal antibody, and gefitinib, a tyrosine kinase inhibitor, in patients with refractory non-small cell lung cancer (NSCLC): A phase i study. J Thorac Oncol 3:258–264

Ready N, Janne PA, Bogart J, Dipetrillo T, Garst J, Graziano S, Gu L, Wang X, Green MR, Vokes EE (2010) Chemoradiotherapy and gefitinib in stage III non-small cell lung cancer with epidermal growth factor receptor and KRAS mutation analysis: cancer and leukemia group B (CALEB) 30106, a CALGB-stratified phase II trial. J Thorac Oncol 5:1382–1390

Regales L, Gong Y, Shen R, De Stanchina E, Vivanco I, Goel A, Koutcher JA, Spassova M, Ouerfelli O, Mellinghoff IK, Zakowski MF, Politi KA, Pao W (2009) Dual targeting of EGFR can overcome a major drug resistance mutation in mouse models of EGFR mutant lung cancer. J Clin Invest 119:3000–3010

Rho JK, Choi YJ, Ryoo B-Y, Na III, Yang SH, Kim CH, Lee JC (2007) p53 enhances gefitinib-induced growth inhibition and apoptosis by regulation of fas in non-small cell lung cancer. Cancer Res 67:1163–1169

Riesterer O, Mason KA, Raju U, Yang Q, Wang L, Hittelman WN, Ang KK, Milas L (2009) Enhanced response to C225 of A431 tumor xenografts growing in irradiated tumor bed. Radiother Oncol, in press, corrected proof

Riesterer O, Yang Q, Raju U, Torres M, Molkentine D, Patel N, Valdecanas D, Milas L, Ang KK (2011) Combination of anti-IGF-1R antibody A12 and ionizing radiation in upper respiratory tract cancers. Int J Radiat Oncol Biol Phys 79:1179–1187

Rochester MA, Riedemann J, Hellawell GO, Brewster SF, Macaulay VM (2005) Silencing of the IGF1R gene enhances sensitivity to DNA-damaging agents in both PTEN wild-type and mutant human prostate cancer. Cancer Gene Ther 12:90–100

Rodemann HP, Blaese MA (2007) Responses of normal cells to ionizing radiation. Semin Radiat Oncol 17:81–88

Rodemann H, Dittmann K, Toulany M (2007) Radiation-induced EGFR-signaling and control of DNA-damage repair. Int J Radiat Biol 83:781–791

Rodriguez CP, Adelstein DJ, Rice TW, Rybicki LA, Videtic GM, Saxton JP, Murthy SC, Mason DP, Ives DI (2010) A phase II study of perioperative concurrent chemotherapy, gefitinib, and hyperfractionated radiation followed by maintenance gefitinib in locoregionally advanced esophagus and gastroesophageal junction cancer. J Thorac Oncol 5:229–235

Rosell R, Molina MA, Costa C, Simonetti S, Gimenez-Capitan A, Bertran-Alamillo J, Mayo C, Moran T, Mendez P, Cardenal F, Isla D, Provencio M, Cobo M, Insa A, Garcia-Campelo R, Reguart N, Majem M, Viteri S, Carcereny E, Porta R, Massuti B, Queralt C, de Aguirre I, Sanchez JM, Sanchez-Ronco M, Mate JL, Ariza A, Benlloch S, Sanchez JJ, Bivona TG, Sawyers CL, Taron M (2011) Pretreatment EGFR T790M mutation and BRCA1 mRNA expression in erlotinib-treated advanced non-small-cell lung cancer patients with EGFR mutations. Clin Cancer Res 17:1160–1168

Sadiq AA, Salgia R (2013) MET as a possible target for non-small-cell lung cancer. J Clin Oncol 31:1089–1096

Safran H, Suntharalingam M, Dipetrillo T, Ng T, Doyle LA, Krasna M, Plette A, Evans D, Wanebo H, Akerman P, Spector J, Kennedy N, Kennedy T (2008) Cetuximab with concurrent chemoradiation for esophagogastric cancer: assessment of toxicity. Int J Radiat Oncol Biol Phys 70:391–395

Saki M, Toulany M, Rodemann HP (2013) Acquired resistance to cetuximab is associated with the overexpression of Ras family members and the loss of radiosensitization in head and neck cancer cells. Radiother Oncol

Sato Y, Ebara T, Sunaga N, Takahashi T, Nakano T (2012) Interaction of radiation and gefitinib on a human lung cancer cell line with mutant EGFR gene in vitro. Anticancer Res 32:4877–4881

Sauer L, Gitenay D, Vo C, Baron VT (2010) Mutant p53 initiates a feedback loop that involves Egr-1/EGF receptor/ERK in prostate cancer cells. Oncogene 29:2628–2637

Scagliotti GV, Novello S, von Pawel J (2013) The emerging role of MET/HGF inhibitors in oncology. Cancer Treat Rev 39:793–801

Scartozzi M, Mandolesi A, Giampieri R, Bittoni A, Pierantoni C, Zaniboni A, Galizia E, Giustini L, Silva RR, Bisonni R, Berardi R, Biscotti T, Biagetti S, Bearzi I, Cascinu S (2011) The role of HER-3 expression in the prediction of clinical outcome for advanced colorectal cancer patients receiving irinotecan and cetuximab. Oncologist 16:53–60

Schaefer G, Haber L, Crocker LM, Shia S, Shao L, Dowbenko D, Totpal K, Wong A, Lee CV, Stawicki S, Clark R, Fields C, Lewis Phillips GD, Prell RA, Danilenko DM, Franke Y, Stephan J-P, Hwang J, Wu Y, Bostrom J, Sliwkowski MX, Fuh G, Eigenbrot C (2011) A two-in-one antibody against HER3 and EGFR has superior inhibitory activity compared with monospecific antibodies. Cancer Cell 20: 472–486

Schmidt-Ullrich RK, Mikkelsen RB, Dent P, Todd DG, Valerie K, Kavanagh BD, Contessa JN, Rorrer WK, Chen PB (1997) Radiation-induced proliferation of the human A431 squamous carcinoma cells is dependent on EGFR tyrosine phosphorylation. Oncogene 15:1191–1197

Scott SP, Pandita TK (2006) The cellular control of DNA double-strand breaks. J Cell Biochem 99:1463–1475

Sequist LV, Besse B, Lynch TJ, Miller VA, Wong KK, Gitlitz B, Eaton K, Zacharchuk C, Freyman A, Powell C, Ananthakrishnan R, Quinn S, Soria JC (2010) Neratinib, an irreversible pan-ErbB receptor tyrosine kinase inhibitor: results of a phase II trial in patients with advanced non-small-cell lung cancer. J Clin Oncol 28:3076–3083

Sequist LV, von Pawel J, Garmey EG, Akerley WL, Brugger W, Ferrari D, Chen Y, Costa DB, Gerber DE, Orlov S, Ramlau R, Arthur S, Gorbachevsky I, Schwartz B, Schiller JH (2011a) Randomized phase II study of erlotinib plus tivantinib versus erlotinib plus placebo in previously treated non-small-cell lung cancer. J Clin Oncol 29:3307–3315

Sequist LV, Waltman BA, Dias-Santagata D, Digumarthy S, Turke AB, Fidias P, Bergethon K, Shaw AT, Gettinger S, Cosper AK, Akhavanfard S, Heist RS, Temel J, Christensen JG, Wain JC, Lynch TJ, Vernovsky K, Mark EJ, Lanuti M, Iafrate AJ, Mino-Kenudson M, Engelman JA (2011b) Genotypic and histological evolution of lung cancers acquiring resistance to EGFR inhibitors. Sci Transl Med 3:75ra26

Sequist LV, Yang JC, Yamamoto N, O'byrne K, Hirsh V, Mok T, Geater SL, Orlov S, Tsai CM, Boyer M, Su WC, Bennouna J, Kato T, Gorbunova V, Lee KH, Shah R, Massey D, Zazulina V, Shahidi M, Schuler M (2013) Phase III study of afatinib or cisplatin plus pemetrexed in patients with metastatic lung adenocarcinoma with EGFR mutations. J Clin Oncol

She YH, Lee F, Chen J, Haimovitz-Friedman A, Miller VA, Rusch VR, Kris MG, Sirotnak FM (2003) The epidermal growth factor receptor tyrosine kinase inhibitor ZD1839 selectively potentiates, radiation response of human tumors in nude mice, with a marked improvement in therapeutic index. Clin Cancer Res 9:3773–3778

Sheikh Ali MA, Gunduz M, Nagatsuka H, Gunduz E, Cengiz B, Fukushima K, Beder LB, Demircan K, Fujii M, Yamanaka N, Shimizu K, Grenman R, Nagai N (2008) Expression and mutation analysis of epidermal growth factor receptor in head and neck squamous cell carcinoma. Cancer Sci 99:1589–1594

Sheng G, Guo J, Warner BW (2007) Epidermal growth factor receptor signaling modulates apoptosis via p38Œ ± MAPK-dependent activation of Bax in intestinal epithelial cells. Am J Physiol—Gastrointest Liver Physiol 293:G599–G606

Shibuya K, Komaki R, Shintani T, Itasaka S, Ryan A, Jurgensmeier JM, Milas L, Ang K, Herbst RS, O'Reilly MS (2007) Targeted therapy against VEGFR and EGFR with ZD6474 enhances the therapeutic efficacy of irradiation in an orthotopic model of human non-small-cell lung cancer. Int J Radiat Oncol Biol Phys 69:1534–1543

Shrivastav M, de Haro LP, Nickoloff JA (2008) Regulation of DNA double-strand break repair pathway choice. Cell Res 18:134–147

Singh B, Reddy PG, Goberdhan A, Walsh C, Dao S, Ngai I, Chou TC, Pornchai OC, Levine AJ, Rao PH, Stoffel A (2002) p53 regulates cell survival by inhibiting PIK3CA in squamous cell carcinomas. Genes Dev 16: 984–993

Skartved NJØ, Jacobsen HJ, Pedersen MW, Jensen PF, Sen JW, Jørgensen TK, Hey A, Kragh M (2011) Preclinical pharmacokinetics and safety of Sym004: a synergistic antibody mixture directed against epidermal growth factor receptor. Clin Cancer Res 17:5962–5972

Sliesoraitis S, Tawfik B (2011) Bevacizumab-induced bowel perforation. J Am Osteopath Assoc 111:437–441

Spangler JB, Neil JR, Abramovitch S, Yarden Y, White FM, Lauffenburger DA, Wittrup KD (2010) Combination antibody treatment down-regulates epidermal growth factor receptor by inhibiting endosomal recycling. Proc Natl Acad Sci USA 107:13252–13257

Spigel DR, Hainsworth JD, Yardley DA, Raefsky E, Patton J, Peacock N, Farley C, Burris HA, 3rd, Greco FA (2010) Tracheoesophageal fistula formation in patients with lung cancer treated with chemoradiation and bevacizumab. J Clin Oncol 28: 43–48

Spigel DR, Ervin TJ, Ramlau R, Daniel DB, Goldschmidt JH, Blumenschein GR, Krzakowski MJ, Robinet G, Clement-Duchene C, Barlesi F, Govindan R, Patel T, Orlov SV, Wertheim MS, Zha J, Pandita A, Yu W, Yauch RL, Patel PH, Peterson AC (2011) Final efficacy results from OAM4558 g, a randomized phase II study evaluating MetMAb or placebo in combination with erlotinib in advanced NSCLC. J Clin Oncol 29, (suppl; abstr 7505)

Stinchcombe T, Socinski MA, Moore DT, Gettinger SN, Decker RH, Petty WJ, Blackstock AW, Schwartz GK, Lankford S, Morris DE (2011) Phase I/II trial of bevacizumab (B) and erlotinib (E) with induction (IND) and concurrent (CON) carboplatin (Cb)/paclitaxel (P) and 74 Gy of thoracic conformal radiotherapy (TCRT) in stage III non-small cell lung cancer (NSCLC). J Clin Oncol 29, abstr 7016

Suda K, Tomizawa K, Mitsudomi T (2010) Biological and clinical significance of KRAS mutations in lung cancer: an oncogenic driver that contrasts with EGFR mutation. Cancer Metastasis Rev 29:49–60

Sun Y, Nowak KA, Zaorsky NG, Winchester CL, Dalal K, Giacalone NJ, Liu N, Werner-Wasik M, Wasik MA, Dicker AP, Lu B (2013) ALK inhibitor PF02341066 (crizotinib) increases sensitivity to radiation in non-small cell lung cancer expressing EML4-ALK. Mol Cancer Ther 12:696–704

Szumiel I (2006) Epidermal growth factor receptor and DNA double strand break repair: the cell's self-defence. Cell Signal 18:1537–1548

Tanaka T, Munshi A, Brooks C, Liu J, Hobbs ML, Meyn RE (2008) Gefitinib radiosensitizes non-small cell lung cancer cells by suppressing cellular DNA repair capacity. Clin Cancer Res 14:1266–1273

Tokunaga E, Kataoka A, Kimura Y, Oki E, Mashino K, Nishida K, Koga T, Morita M, Kakeji Y, Baba H, Ohno S, Maehara Y (2006) The association between Akt activation and resistance to hormone therapy in metastatic breast cancer. Eur J Cancer 42:629–635

Toulany M, Rodemann HP (2010) Membrane receptor signaling and control of DNA repair after exposure to ionizing radiation. Nuklearmedizin 49(Suppl 1):S26–S30

Toulany M, Rodemann HP (2013) Potential of Akt mediated DNA repair in radioresistance of solid tumors overexpressing erbB-PI3 K-Akt pathway. 2013, 2

Toulany M, Kasten-Pisula U, Brammer I, Wang S, Chen J, Dittmann K, Baumann M, Dikomey E, Rodemann H (2006) Blockage of epidermal growth factor receptor-phosphatidylinositol 3-kinase-AKT signaling increases radiosensitivity of K-RAS mutated human tumor cells in vitro by affecting DNA repair. Clin Cancer Res 12:4119–4126

Toulany M, Baumann M, Rodemann H (2007) Stimulated PI3 K-AKT signaling mediated through ligand or radiation-induced EGFR depends indirectly, but not directly, on constitutive K-Ras activity. Mol Cancer Res 5:863–872

Toulany M, Kehlbach R, Florczak U, Sak A, Wang S, Chen J, Lobrich M, Rodemann HP (2008) Targeting of AKT1 enhances radiation toxicity of human tumor cells by inhibiting DNA-PKcs-dependent DNA double-strand break repair. Mol Cancer Ther 7:1772–1781

Toulany M, Lee KJ, Fattah KR, Lin YF, Fehrenbacher B, Schaller M, Chen BP, Chen DJ, Rodemann HP (2012) Akt promotes post-irradiation survival of human tumor cells through initiation, progression, and termination of DNA-PKcs-dependent DNA double-strand break repair. Mol Cancer Res 10:945–957

Tsai Y-C, Yeh C-H, Tzen K-Y, Ho P-Y, Tuan T-F, Pu Y-S, Cheng A-L, Cheng JC-H (2013) Targeting epidermal growth factor receptor/human epidermal growth factor receptor 2 signalling pathway by a dual receptor tyrosine kinase inhibitor afatinib for radiosensitisation in murine bladder carcinoma. Eur J Cancer 49:1458–1466

Van Cutsem E, Köhne C-H, Hitre E, Zaluski J, Chang Chien C-R, Makhson A, D'haens G, Pintér TS, Lim R, Bodoky GR, Roh JK, Folprecht G, Ruff P, Stroh C, Tejpar S, Schlichting M,

Nippgen J, Rougier P (2009) Cetuximab and chemotherapy as initial treatment for metastatic colorectal cancer. N Eng J Med 360: 1408–1417

Viloria-Petit A, Crombet T, Jothy S, Hicklin D, Bohlen P, Schlaeppi JM, Rak J, Kerbel RS (2001) Acquired resistance to the antitumor effect of epidermal growth factor receptor-blocking antibodies in vivo: a role for altered tumor angiogenesis. Cancer Res 61:5090–5101

Vlacich G, Coffey RJ (2011) Resistance to EGFR-targeted therapy: A family affair. Cancer Cell 20:423–425

Wang M, Wu W, Rosidi B, Zhang L, Wang H, Iliakis G (2006) PARP-1 and Ku compete for repair of DNA double strand breaks by distinct NHEJ pathways. Nucleic Acids Res 34:6170–6182

Wang M, Morsbach F, Sander D, Gheorghiu L, Nanda A, Benes C, Kriegs M, Krause M, Dikomey E, Baumann M, Dahm-Daphi J, Settleman J, Willers H (2011) EGF receptor inhibition radiosensitizes NSCLC cells by inducing senescence in cells sustaining DNA double-strand breaks. Cancer Res 71:6261–6269

Welsh JW, Mahadevan D, Ellsworth R, Cooke L, Bearss D, Stea B (2009) The c-Met receptor tyrosine kinase inhibitor MP470 radiosensitizes glioblastoma cells. Radiat Oncol 4:69

Welsh JW, Komaki R, Amini A, Munsell MF, Unger W, Allen PK, Chang JY, Wefel JS, McGovern SL, Garland LL, Chen SS, Holt J, Liao Z, Brown P, Sulman E, Heymach JV, Kim ES, Stea B (2013) Phase II trial of erlotinib plus concurrent whole-brain radiation therapy for patients with brain metastases from non-small-cell lung cancer. J Clin Oncol 31:895–902

Wheeler DL, Huang S, Kruser TJ, Nechrebecki MM, Armstrong EA, Benavente S, Gondi V, Hsu KT, Harari PM (2008) Mechanisms of acquired resistance to cetuximab: role of HER (ErbB) family members. Oncogene 27:3944–3956

Wheeler DL, Dunn EF, Harari PM (2010) Understanding resistance to EGFR inhibitors[mdash] impact on future treatment strategies. Nat Rev Clin Oncol 7:493–507

Wu W, Onn A, Isobe T, Itasaka S, Langley RR, Shitani T, Shibuya K, Komaki R, Ryan AJ, Fidler IJ, Herbst RS, O'Reilly MS (2007) Targeted therapy of orthotopic human lung cancer by combined vascular endothelial growth factor and epidermal growth factor receptor signaling blockade. Mol Cancer Ther 6:471–483

Xing D, Orsulic S (2005) A genetically defined mouse ovarian carcinoma model for the molecular characterization of pathway-targeted therapy and tumor resistance. Proc Natl Acad Sci USA 102:6936–6941

Yacoub A, Park JS, Qiao L, Dent P, Hagan MP (2001) MAPK dependence of DNA damage repair: ionizing radiation and the induction of expression of the DNA repair genes XRCC1 and ERCC1 in DU145 human prostate carcinoma cells in a MEK1/2 dependent fashion. Int J Radiat Biol 77:1067–1078

Yacoub A, Miller A, Caron RW, Qiao L, Curiel DA, Fisher PB, Hagan MP, Grant S, Dent P (2006) Radiotherapy-induced signal transduction. Endocr Relat Cancer 13(Suppl 1):S99–S114

Yarden Y, Pines G (2012) The ERBB network: at last, cancer therapy meets systems biology. Nat Rev Cancer, advance online publication

Yonesaka K, Zejnullahu K, Okamoto I, Satoh T, Cappuzzo F, Souglakos J, Ercan D, Rogers A, Roncalli M, Takeda M, Fujisaka Y, Philips J, Shimizu T, Maenishi O, Cho Y, Sun J, Destro A, Taira K, Takeda K, Okabe T, Swanson J, Itoh H, Takada M, Lifshits E, Okuno K, Engelman JA, Shivdasani RA, Nishio K, Fukuoka M, Varella-Garcia M, Nakagawa K, Jänne PA (2011) Activation of ERBB2 signaling causes resistance to the EGFR-directed therapeutic antibody cetuximab. Sci Transl Med 3: 99ra86

Yoshikawa S, Kukimoto-Niino M, Parker L, Handa N, Terada T, Fujimoto T, Terazawa Y, Wakiyama M, Sato M, Sano S, Kobayashi T, Tanaka T, Chen L, Liu ZJ, Wang BC, Shirouzu M, Kawa S, Semba K, Yamamoto T, Yokoyama S (2013) Structural basis for the altered drug sensitivities of non-small cell lung cancer-associated mutants of human epidermal growth factor receptor. Oncogene 32:27–38

Yu HA, Riely GJ (2013) Second-generation epidermal growth factor receptor tyrosine kinase inhibitors in lung cancers. J Natl Compr Canc Netw 11:161–169

Yu H, Li X, Sun S, Gao X, Zhou D (2012) c-Met inhibitor SU11274 enhances the response of the prostate cancer cell line DU145 to ionizing radiation. Biochem Biophys Res Commun 427:659–665

Yun CH, Mengwasser KE, Toms AV, Woo MS, Greulich H, Wong KK, Meyerson M, Eck MJ (2008) The T790 M mutation in EGFR kinase causes drug resistance by increasing the affinity for ATP. Proc Natl Acad Sci USA 105:2070–2075

Zhou W, Ercan D, Chen L, Yun CH, Li D, Capelletti M, Cortot AB, Chirieac L, Iacob RE, Padera R, Engen JR, Wong KK, Eck MJ, Gray NS, Janne PA (2009) Novel mutant-selective EGFR kinase inhibitors against EGFR T790M. Nature 462:1070–1074

Zhou C, Wu YL, Chen G, Feng J, Liu XQ, Wang C, Zhang S, Wang J, Zhou S, Ren S, Lu S, Zhang L, Hu C, Luo Y, Chen L, Ye M, Huang J, Zhi X, Zhang Y, Xiu Q, Ma J, You C (2011) Erlotinib versus chemotherapy as first-line treatment for patients with advanced EGFR mutation-positive non-small-cell lung cancer (OPTIMAL, CTONG-0802): a multicentre, open-label, randomised, phase 3 study. Lancet Oncol 12:735–742

Zwang Y, Sas-Chen A, Drier Y, Shay T, Avraham R, Lauriola M, Shema E, Lidor-Nili E, Jacob-Hirsch J, Amariglio N, Lu Y, Mills GB, Rechavi G, Oren M, Domany E, Yarden Y (2011) Two phases of mitogenic signaling unveil roles for p53 and EGR1 in elimination of inconsistent growth signals. Mol Cell 42:524–535

Molecular Targeting of Integrins and Integrin-Associated Signaling Networks in Radiation Oncology

Anne Vehlow, Katja Storch, Daniela Matzke and Nils Cordes

Abstract

Radiation and chemotherapy are the main pillars of the current multimodal treatment concept for cancer patients. However, tumor recurrences and resistances still hamper treatment success regardless of advances in radiation beam application, particle radiotherapy, and optimized chemotherapeutics. To specifically intervene at key recurrence- and resistance-promoting molecular processes, the development of potent and specific molecular-targeted agents is demanded for an efficient, safe, and simultaneous integration into current standard of care regimens. Potential targets for such an approach are integrins conferring structural and biochemical communication between cells and their microenvironment. Integrin binding to extracellular matrix activates intracellular signaling for regulating essential cellular functions such as survival, proliferation, differentiation, adhesion, and cell motility. Tumor-associated characteristics such as invasion, metastasis, and radiochemoresistance also highly depend on integrin function. Owing to their dual functionality and their overexpression in the majority of human malignancies, integrins present ideal and accessible targets for cancer therapy. In the following chapter, the current knowledge on aspects of the tumor microenvironment, the molecular regulation of integrin-dependent radiochemoresistance and current approaches to integrin targeting are summarized.

A. Vehlow · K. Storch · D. Matzke · N. Cordes (✉)
OncoRay—National Center for Radiation Research in Oncology,
Faculty of Medicine, University Hospital Carl Gustav Carus,
Technische Universität Dresden, Dresden, Germany
e-mail: nils.cordes@oncoray.de

N. Cordes
Institute of Radiooncology, Helmholtz-Zentrum
Dresden-Rossendorf, Dresden, Germany

© Springer-Verlag Berlin Heidelberg 2016
M. Baumann et al. (eds.), *Molecular Radio-Oncology*, Recent Results
in Cancer Research 198, DOI 10.1007/978-3-662-49651-0_4

Keywords
Integrins · Focal adhesion signaling · Radiochemosensitization · Molecular
targeting

1   Introduction

Radiotherapy, chemotherapy, surgery, and molecular therapeutics are essential
components of current interdisciplinary treatment concepts, which are individually
adapted to clinical tumor characteristics such as tumor entity, tumor volume, and
metastases (Niyazi et al. 2011; Higgins et al. 2015; Searle et al. 2014; Arias 2011). In
the past decades, great efforts have been made to optimize and design new irradiation
techniques, which have been translated to or are on the way to clinical application (Shi
et al. 2014; Allison et al. 2014). However, the success of radiation oncology will also
depend on the discovery of novel molecular therapeutics that are given to patients in
combination with standard radiochemotherapy. Key to a successful development of
such new therapies is a deep understanding of the genetic, epigenetic, proteomic, and
metabolomic tumor traits including the tumor microenvironment.

   Similar to normal cells within the organism, tumor cells are constantly commu-
nicating with specialized cell types and the extracellular matrix (ECM) in their
vicinity (Fig. 1). Hence, it is not surprising that the tumor microenvironment elicits
tumor progression, metastatic spread, and therapy resistance (Clark and Vignjevic

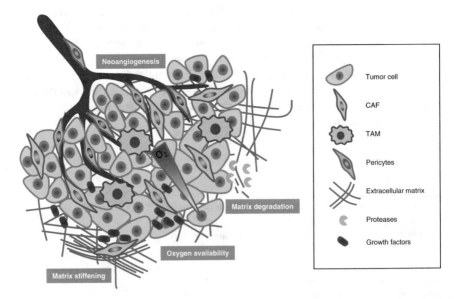

Fig. 1 Cellular and noncellular factors of the tumor microenvironment impact on therapy
resistance. *CAF*, cancer-associated fibroblasts; *TAM*, tumor-associated macrophages; O_2, oxygen

2015; Wei and Yang 2015; Barker et al. 2015; Klemm and Joyce 2014; Eke and Cordes 2015; Hanahan and Weinberg 2011). In fact, it is well known that cell adhesion to the ECM confers cell adhesion-mediated radioresistance (CAM-RR) (Cordes and Meineke 2003; Sandfort et al. 2007), and cell adhesion-mediated drug resistance (CAM-DR) (Damiano et al. 1999; Hazlehurst et al. 2000, 2006; Eke and Cordes 2011; Shishido et al. 2014; Damiano et al. 2001) for hematopoietic and solid tumors. This paradigm has recently been expanded to the whole cellular environment entitled environment-mediated drug resistance (EM-DR) (Meads et al. 2009).

Interactions of cells with ECM molecules are mainly mediated via the integrin family of heterodimeric transmembrane receptors (Hynes 2002) and regulate cell survival, cell proliferation, and cell motility (Legate et al. 2009; Harburger and Calderwood 2009). Integrins are composed of one of the 18 different α and 8 different β chains that are non-covalently associated (Hynes 2002), and their ECM specificity is dictated by the 24 possible α/β pairings (Humphries et al. 2006). Together with growth factor receptors, such as the epidermal growth factor receptor (EGFR), integrins translate extracellular cues to intracellular signals in specialized cell membrane areas, so-called focal adhesions (FA) (Geiger and Yamada 2011; Storch and Cordes 2012; Geiger et al. 2009). By this mechanism, integrins not only function to provide mechanical anchorage and chemical signals to cells (outside-in activation), but also to respond to intracellular stimuli by changing their conformation and ECM ligand affinity (inside-out activation) (Calderwood 2004). These two functionalities are mediated by a multiplicity of intracellular adaptor and signaling proteins that are collectively termed the "adhesome" (Zaidel-Bar et al. 2007; Geiger and Zaidel-Bar 2012). Importantly, adaptor proteins such as talin and kindlin directly bind to the cytoplasmic tails of integrins and recruit further signaling mediators to the FA (Morse et al. 2014). Among these, the focal adhesion kinase (FAK) and the IPP complex consisting integrin-linked kinase (ILK), particularly

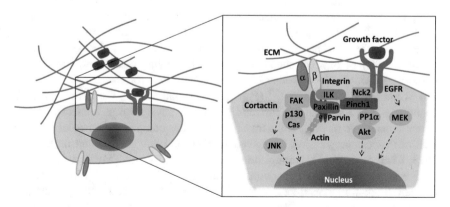

Fig. 2 Molecular insight in integrin and epidermal growth factor receptor (EGFR) signaling pathways involved in radiochemoresistance. *FAK*, focal adhesion kinase; *PINCH1*, particularly interesting new cysteine-histidine-rich protein 1; *ILK*, integrin-linked kinase; *AKT*, alpha serine/threonine-protein kinase; *p130Cas*, p130 Crk-associated substrate; *MEK*, mitogen-activated protein kinase kinase; *JNK*, c-Jun N-terminal kinase; *PP1α*, protein phosphatase 1α; *Nck2*, non-catalytic region of tyrosine kinase 2

interesting new cysteine-histidine-rich protein 1 (PINCH1) and α-parvin, bridge the gap to intracellular signaling cascades and recruit and modulate actin filaments trough Rho GTPases (Legate et al. 2006; Iwamoto and Calderwood 2015) (Fig. 2).

The significance of the ECM-integrin connection as determinant of tumor cell radio- and chemosensitivity and the potential of integrins as biomarkers and prognostic factors have made them potential cancer targets (Cordes and Park 2007; Hehlgans et al. 2007; Goodman and Picard 2012; Vehlow and Cordes 2013). Understanding the molecular mechanisms underlying FA hub signaling with regard to therapy sensitivity will foster the development of feasible multimodal treatment strategies. In the following chapters, current knowledge of the tumor microenvironment and the impact of integrin signaling on treatment resistance are reviewed.

2 The Microenvironment and the Modulation of Radiochemoresistance

During the past decade, a multitude of big-scale high-throughput screens has been performed to identify new drugs for combination with conventional radiochemotherapy to cure cancer patients (Collins and Workman 2006). However, potent anticancer drugs frequently fail in clinical trails because these preclinical screens are mainly performed without consideration of the tumor microenvironment (TME) (Jain 2013). Recent evidence suggests that the TME determines the success of radiochemotherapy by promoting therapy resistances (Barker et al. 2015; Barcellos-Hoff and Cordes 2009; Tavora et al. 2014; Nakasone et al. 2012). The underlying molecular mechanisms remain unclear.

Certainly, a tumor is more than an accumulation of malignant cells, it resembles a complex tissue consisting of different cell types such as stromal (e.g., cancer-associated fibroblasts (CAF) and pericytes), endothelial, and immune cells (e.g., tumor-associated macrophages and lymphocytes) (Hanahan and Weinberg 2011; Gandellini et al. 2015; Egeblad et al. 2010). In addition to these cellular components, the TME is furthermore defined by several noncellular factors such as the availability of oxygen, chemokines, growth factors, metabolites, and the surrounding ECM, which altogether create a unique niche for cancer cells (Hanahan and Weinberg 2011; Jain 2013) (Fig. 1). In normal tissues, the stroma provides connective and structural support and maintains physiological homeostasis in a tumor suppressive manner. Once transformation has commenced, stromal cells can facilitate cancer progression (Rønnov-Jessen et al. 1996; Junttila and de Sauvage 2013; Chen et al. 2015). During the neoplastic process, the TME is infiltrated by CAF and myofibroblasts (Gandellini et al. 2015; Chen et al. 2015; Micke and Ostman 2005; Kalluri and Zeisberg 2006; Sanchez-Lopez et al. 2015) leading to ECM stiffening and remodeling by the secretion of ECM proteins such as collagens and matrix metalloproteinase (MMP) enzymes (Egeblad et al. 2010; Kessenbrock et al. 2010; Levental et al. 2009). Thereby, the biochemical ECM properties are dramatically altered resulting in a biophysical, stiffness-related plasticity fundamentally different from the corresponding normal tissue (Levental et al. 2009;

Frantz et al. 2010; Butcher et al. 2009). These perturbations are known to facilitate tumorigenesis and metastasis by altering the mechanotransductive equilibrium between cells and their surrounding matrix (Plodinec et al. 2012; Kumar and Weaver 2009). Therefore, novel targeting strategies should not only reflect the complexity of different cell types within the TME but also their interaction with TME components to gain profound clinical benefits (Paulsson and Micke 2014). Further efforts are necessary to identify new potential targets that help to normalize the TME and simultaneously sensitize tumor cells.

3 The Modulation of Radiochemoresistance by Integrins and Focal Adhesion Signaling Networks

In contrast to normal tissues, the expression of many integrins is altered in tumor cells of different entities as well as tumor-associated endothelial cells or CAFs, leading to changes in cellular behavior and an aggressive tumor phenotype (Barker et al. 2015; Danen 2005; Guo and Giancotti 2004; Desgrosellier and Cheresh 2010). Facilitating tumor cell adhesion and invasion as obligate part of most of the integrin heterodimers, altered $\beta 1$ integrin expression is detected in breast carcinoma (Zutter et al. 1993), colon carcinoma (Koretz et al. 1991; Stallmach et al. 1992; Fujita et al. 1995), pancreatic carcinoma (Shimoyama et al. 1995; Hall et al. 1991), head and neck squamous cell carcinoma (HNSCC) (Jones et al. 1993; Eriksen et al. 2004), and glioblastoma mulitforme (GBM) (Paulus et al. 1993). Interestingly, integrin receptors containing the $\beta 4$, $\beta 5$, $\beta 6$, and $\beta 8$ subunits are often associated with a metastatic potential (Stallmach et al. 1992; Hall et al. 1991; Eriksen et al. 2004; Koukoulis et al. 1991; Vogetseder et al. 2013; Gui et al. 1996; Previtali et al. 1996), while overexpressed $av\beta 3$ and $\alpha v\beta 5$ critically function in angiogenesis and metastasis to distant organs (Koukoulis et al. 1991; Vogetseder et al. 2013; Gui et al. 1996; Weis and Cheresh 2011; Gingras et al. 1995).

Apart from tumor-associated integrin alterations, irradiation has been shown to increase integrin expression levels in a dose-dependent manner in several cancer entities such as GBM (Cordes and Meineke 2003; Wild-bode et al. 2001; Wick et al. 2002; Rieken et al. 2011; Eke et al. 2012a; Cordes et al. 2003), breast cancer (Park et al. 2003, 2006), NSCLC (Cordes et al. 2002), colon carcinoma (Meineke et al. 2002) and pancreatic carcinoma (Cordes and Meineke 2003). This phenomenon facilitates tumor cell survival and anti-invasion after X-ray exposure and corresponds to increased radiochemoresistance, pinpointing a critical function of integrins in the tumor cell response to irradiation (Damiano et al. 1999; Hazlehurst et al. 2000; Shishido et al. 2014; Damiano et al. 2001; Hazlehurst et al. 2006; Cordes and Meineke 2003). How exactly integrin expression is regulated upon irradiation is not well understood. Different independent studies suggest a positive feedback mechanism between nuclear factor kappa-light-chain-enhancer of activated B-cells (NF-κB) and integrin expression that can be targeted to enhance the tumor cell therapy response (Ritchie et al. 2000; Bradbury et al. 2001; Ahmed et al. 2013). Taken together, current data support the concept of therapeutic integrin targeting as

tumor-associated and radiation-dependent changes in integrin expression are critically linked to different stages of tumor progression, radiochemoresistances, and the
clinical outcome (Cordes and Park 2007; Goodman and Picard 2012; Eke and
Cordes 2015; Hehlgans et al. 2007).

3.1 Integrin-Dependent Radiochemoresistance

Among the 24 possible integrin heterodimers, especially those receptors containing
the β1 subunit and associated signaling hubs are the key components regulating
resistance to therapy (Eke and Cordes 2015; Cordes and Park 2007; Janes and Watt
2006). In HNSCC, several recent studies demonstrate that β1 integrin targeting with
inhibitory antibodies or siRNA results in radiosensitization of tumor cells in vitro and
in vivo (Eke and Cordes 2015; Dickreuter et al. 2015; Eke et al. 2012b, c). Especially
in three-dimensionally (3D) grown tumor HNSCC cells, β1 integrin targeting reduces
proliferation and the repair of radiogenic DNA double-strand breaks (Dickreuter et al.
2015; Eke et al. 2012c) by deactivation of FAK signaling as early key mechanistic
event (Dickreuter et al. 2015). Also cells from GBM respond to an inhibition of β1
integrin with reduced clonogenic survival upon irradiation (Eke et al. 2012a; Cordes
and Meineke 2003) by a hampered DNA double-strand break repair (Eke et al. 2012a).
Other preclinical studies show that β1 integrin is one of the mediators of glioblastoma
cell invasion (Vehlow and Cordes 2013; Cordes and Meineke 2003; Carbonell et al.
2013) and exerts its function via the regulation of different pro-invasive signaling
modules such as MMP-2 activity and FAK (Cordes and Meineke 2003; Carbonell
et al. 2013). Similar results are shown for breast carcinoma cells. Here, β1 integrin
inhibition decreases 3D tumor cell proliferation and induces apoptosis by downreg-
ulating the Akt signaling pathway without affecting nonmalignant cells (Park et al.
2006, 2008). In addition, β1 integrin inhibition allows a reduction of the irradiation
dose to achieve comparable tumor growth inhibition and apoptosis in breast carcinoma xenografts (Park et al. 2008), suggesting a possible therapeutic benefit.

Apart from β1 integrin, much attention has been focussed on αvβ3 and αvβ5
integrin heterodimers due to their prominent role in angiogenesis and neovascularization of tumors (Brooks et al. 1994; Eliceiri and Cheresh 2000). In GBM, these
integrins are linked to tumor progression correlating with the histological tumor
grade (Gingras et al. 1995; Gladson and Cheresh 1991; Bello et al. 2001; Schnell
et al. 2008) and a poor overall survival (Ducassou et al. 2013). Importantly, it has
been shown that the inhibition of both heterodimers induces radiosensitization of
glioblastoma cells in vitro by the induction of mitotic catastrophy (Monferran et al.
2008). This radiosensitizing effect further involves ILK signaling leading to the
activation of the small GTPase RhoB (Monferran et al. 2008). Also additional
preclinical studies suggest a positive effect of αvβ3 and αvβ5 therapeutic antagonists. Application of the αvβ3 peptide antagonist S247 enhances anti-angiogenic
and anti-tumor effects in combination with fractionated radiotherapy (Abdollahi
et al. 2005). Cilengitide, an αvβ3 and αvβ5 integrin antagonizing arginine–glycine–
aspartic acid (RGD) peptide, modulates adhesion and viability of glioblastoma cells

in vitro and increases animal survival in a schedule-dependent manner in combination with irradiation (Maurer et al. 2009; Mikkelsen et al. 2009). The data suggest that this effect of cilengitide is partially determined by an induction of apoptosis of endothelial and glioblastoma cells and can be further enhanced when combined with temozolomide (TMZ) therapy (Oliveira-Ferrer et al. 2008).

In addition to a plethora of studies investigating β integrins as potential anti-cancer targets, only little attention has been focused on the α integrin subunits (Kurokawa et al. 2008; Nam et al. 2010; Nagata et al. 2013; Shirakihara et al. 2013; Zhou et al. 2014; Steglich et al. 2015). Similar to β subunits, α subunits are also highly upregulated in HNSCC, GBM, and other entities (Vehlow and Cordes 2013; Estilo et al. 2009; Peng et al. 2011). Intruigingly, from the four α integrin subunits (α2, α3, α5, and α6) coprecipitated with inhibited β1 integrin, only targeting of α3 integrin resulted in enhanced radiosensitivity of HNSCC cell lines (Steglich et al. 2015). A partial independence of α3 integrin from β1 integrin signaling was obvious by radiosensitization when β1 and α3 integrins were co-targeted (Steglich et al. 2015). In the future, more research is warranted to clarify how therapy resistance mechanisms are induced by different α and β integrins and whether these can be circumvented by therapeutic interventions.

3.2 Adhesome Components and Radiochemoresistance

As integrin receptors are devoid of own enzymatic activity, the association with adaptor proteins in FA is critical to translate information from the extracellular microenvironment into intracellular signaling cues (Legate et al. 2009) (Fig. 2). By activating specific pro-survival signaling mechanisms, integrins essentially contribute to the evasion of apoptotic cell death and the acquisition of resistance to radiation and chemotherapy.

As main mediator of integrin signaling, several studies have implicated FAK as the most prominent regulator of tumor progression and radioresistance (Eke et al. 2012b; Tilghman and Parsons 2008). In fact, overexpression of FAK has been linked to poor prognosis in several tumor entities (Miyazaki et al. 2003; Fujii et al. 2004; Lark et al. 2005). FAK is recruited to FA upon binding of integrins to the ECM, and its kinase activity is activated by autophosphorylation on tyrosine 397 (Schaller 1992, Parsons 2003). Interaction with various signaling proteins such as p130 Crk-associated substrate (p130Cas) facilitates further intracellular signal transduction events (Polte and Hanks 1995). Targeting of FAK for cancer therapy is a promising approach as siRNA or small molecule inhibitors induce apoptosis and tumor growth delay of HNSCC (Eke and Cordes 2011; Hehlgans et al. 2009), GBM (Golubovskaya et al. 2013; Roberts et al. 2008), NSCLC (Roberts et al. 2008), and pancreatic carcinoma (Hochwald et al. 2009). Moreover, FAK inhibition elicits radiosensitization (Eke and Cordes 2011; Eke et al. 2012b; Hehlgans et al. 2009; Hehlgans et al. 2012). Effector molecules of FAK that regulate its radiosensitizing potential include the Akt/mitogen-activated protein kinase kinase 1/2 (MEK1/2) (Hehlgans et al. 2012), Cortactin/c-Jun N-terminal kinase (JNK) (Eke et al. 2012b), and PINCH1/protein phosphatase 1α (PP1α) signaling axes (Eke et al. 2010). Also the inactivation of FAK in endothelial cells seems a promising approach as this strategy increased chemosensitivity by suppressing NF-κB-dependent cytokine secretion (Tavora et al. 2014).

In addition to FAK, integrins link to a ternary protein complex consisting of ILK, PINCH1, and α-parvin (Legate et al. 2006), which transmits integrin outside-in signals (Legate et al. 2006). Recent studies suggest that ILK mainly serves as adaptor protein as evidence for enzymatic function is lacking in vivo (Wickström et al. 2010; Qin and Wu 2012). Regarding cellular radiosensitivity, ILK clearly plays a pro-survival role in tumor cells and is dispensable for radiation survival of fibroblasts (Hehlgans et al. 2008). In addition, overexpression of wildtype ILK or ILK mutants results in radioresistance of leukemia and NSCLC.

In contrast to ILK, knockdown of PINCH1 using siRNA technology generally radiosensitizes tumor cells from several cancer entities including colorectal, lung, pancreatic, and cervix cancer (Eke et al. 2010; Sandfort et al. 2010). Great part of the underlying mechanism has been identified indicating direct PINCH1 interactions with PP1α as key determinant of Akt pro-survival signaling. Thus, PINCH1 is considered a promising cancer target (Eke et al. 2010).

Another function of the IPP complex is the functional linkage of integrin-associated signaling pathways to receptor tyrosine kinases, such as the EGFR (Legate et al. 2006). Both signaling hubs cooperatively regulate survival, proliferation, adhesion, and migration of cells (Yamada and Even-Ram 2002) and significantly contribute to HNSCC radiochemotherapy resistance (Eke and Cordes 2015; Eke et al. 2013, 2015; Rossow et al. 2015). The exact interaction of both classes of cell surface receptors is still unclear, but evidence suggest that certain adaptor proteins, such as non-catalytic region of tyrosine kinase 2 (Nck2) connect integrins and EGFR via the IPP complex on the molecular level (Legate et al. 2006) and stimulate the repair of therapy-induced DNA double-strand breaks (Rossow et al. 2015). In addition, recent data from 3D lrECM grown HNSCC cells show that integrin signaling attenuates the effects of an EGFR targeted therapy with Cetuximab through bypassing JNK interacting protein 4 (JIP4) and JNK2 signaling (Eke et al. 2013). These data clearly indicate crosstalk of both receptor classes. Furthermore, preclinical research apparently demonstrates that co-targeting of β1 integrin and EGFR in combination with radiotherapy is a potent strategy to overcome resistance in HNSCC by modulating a protein complex consisting of FAK and extracellular signal-regulated kinase (Erk) and associated signaling hubs (Eke and Cordes 2015).

4   Clinical Trials Involving Molecular-Targeted Drugs for Integrins and Adhesome Components

Owing to their increased expression on tumor cells and fundamental functions in tumor-associated normal cells, integrins are considered encouraging cancer targets. Another tremendous advantage of integrins is their cell surface localization, making them accessible targets for function-blocking monoclonal antibodies and antagonistic peptides for abolishing pro-survival signaling mechanisms upon binding to the integrin extracellular domain. Whereas integrin targeting is already successfully implemented in the therapy of some human diseases such as multiple sclerosis (natalizumab, α4 integrin) and ischemia (abciximab, β3 integrin) (Salzler et al. 2015; Gensicke et al. 2012; Horsley et al. 2015; Coles 2015), potential anti-integrin components are still tested in clinical trials to clarify the overall effectiveness as anti-cancer therapeutics. In total, 65 inhibitory anti-integrin compounds have been generated for therapy of human diseases; however, only five entered late phase clinical trials on cancer (Table 1). Noteworthy, all of these inhibitors target RGD-binding integrins either by blocking specific integrin receptors or integrin heterodimers containing the αv subunit (Goodman and Picard 2012).

Etaracizumab (MEDI-522) is one of the first humanized αvβ3 antagonists, and its precursor vitaxin has been tested in phase I and phase II clinical trials (Gutheil 2000; Delbaldo et al. 2008; Hersey et al. 2010; McNeel 2005). Besides anti-angiogenic properties and low toxicity (Gutheil 2000), some patients with advanced solid tumors, i.e., renal cell carcinoma (RCC) and melanoma, benefited from a disease stabilization after vitaxin treatment (Delbaldo et al. 2008; Hersey et al. 2010; McNeel 2005). However, inhibition of αv-containing integrins with the monoclonal antibody intetumumab did not improve progression-free survival of stage IV melanoma patients alone or in combination with the standard treatment using dacarbazine (O'Day et al. 2011). Nevertheless, a slight but not significant enhancement of overall survival of stage IV melanoma patients was apparent after intetumumab administration requesting for further clarification in larger cohorts (O'Day et al. 2011). Cilengitide is the first integrin antagonist tested in a phase III clinical trial. After early disappointing results in pancreatic cancer, melanoma, and HNSCC, a promising antitumor activity in newly diagnosed and recurrent GBM patients was shown in phase I and phase II clinical studies applying cilengitide (Reardon et al. 2008). Finally, the subsequent phase III CENTRIC study shows no improvement of patient survival by cilengitide on top of standard radiochemotherapy (Stupp et al. 2014) questioning the general clinical impact of αv integrin antagonists.

Table 1 Integrin inhibitors in phase II and phase III clinical trials for cancer therapy

Clinical phase	Target	Drug	Tumor entity	References
Phase II	α5β1	ATN-161	HNSCC, GBM	Barkan and Chambers (2011)
		Volociximab	Melanoma, RCC, ovarian cancer, peritoneal neoplasms	Goodman and Picard (2012; Bell-McGuinn et al. (2011)
	αvβx	Intetumumab	Melanoma	O'Day et al. (2011)
	αvβ3	Etaracizumab	Melanoma, RCC, other solid tumors	Hersey et al. (2010), McNeel (2005)
Phase III	αvβ3, αvβ5	Cilengitide	GBM	(Reardon et al. (2008), Stupp et al. (2014)

Volociximab, a function-blocking antibody and inhibitor of the α5β1 fibronectin receptor, had no toxicity in a clinical phase I study involving patients with melanoma and renal cell carcinomas (Ricart et al. 2008; Heng et al. 2010). Volociximab failed in combination with chemotherapy in a later phase II trial on ovarian and primary peritoneal cancer patients, and the study was terminated due to a lack of efficacy (Goodman and Picard 2012; Bell-McGuinn et al. 2011). Another inhibitor of α5β1 integrin is the non-RGD-based peptide ATN-161, which showed no risks in phase I clinical trials (Cianfrocca et al. 2006). To clarify whether ATN-161 has any effects in combination with radio- and chemotherapy, further phase II trials in HNSCC and GBM patients are planned (Thundimadathil 2012; Barkan and Chambers 2011).

Despite our knowledge of integrin function in tumor development, progression, resistance, and metastasis, targeting integrins was not a clear success story until now. One might ask why and take into consideration a number of causes. For example, integrins might be influenced by other transmembrane receptors, integrin expression might be more cytoplasmic than membranous, receptor tyrosine kinase and cytoplasmic protein kinase bypass signaling might be fostered by the inhibition of specific integrins, ineffective inhibitor binding to integrins, and so on. An alternative to block integrins is the deactivation of integrin-associated signaling mediators using small molecules. As the key molecule transducing integrin signals, FAK can be targeted by either inhibiting its activity, its autophosphorylation, or scaffold function. Whereas a couple of preclinical trials with inhibitors for FAK enzymatic activity showed a decreased tumor cell growth in pancreatic (Liu et al. 2008) and head and neck cancers (Hehlgans et al. 2009), first FAK inhibitors are currently tested in phase I clinical trials.[1] Clinical application of the FAK inhibitor PF-562,271, for example, resulted in stable disease in patients with pancreatic cancer supporting the notion of FAK as auspicious therapeutic target (Infante et al. 2012). Many more FAK kinase inhibitors are currently in clinical trials for which results are long awaited.

Taken together, despite intensive development during the last decades, there is currently no therapeutic available that effectively targets integrins or adhesome components with profound clinical benefit. It seems clear that integrin inhibitors will not be curative by themselves provoking them as adjuvants to conventional cancer regimens.

5   Future Perspectives

With the increasing desire for individualized therapy regimens, the need for the identification of new biomarkers becomes apparent. In this regard, integrins and adhesome components have been demonstrated to substantially contribute to tumor development, progression, and resistance as well as correlated to reduced therapy sensitivity of certain tumor cell subpopulations and clinical outcome. Therefore,

---

[1]ClinicalTrials.gov. https://clinicaltrials.gov/.

novel targeting strategies may take into consideration and reflect the high complexity of cellular and noncellular components faced in a solid cancer. Currently, coherent data on integrins and adhesome expression, functionality and involvement in progression of different tumor entities are lacking and need to be determined using a combination of high sophisticated approaches such as phosphoproteomics and proteomics, metabolomics, epigenetics, and system biology. For the development of novel integrin-based therapeutic strategies, clinicopathological and treatment data require our attention to obtain a comprehensive understanding of integrin and adhesome regulation during tumor progression and therapy.

References

Abdollahi A, Griggs DW, Zieher H et al (2005) Inhibition of alpha(v)beta3 integrin survival signaling enhances antiangiogenic and antitumor effects of radiotherapy. Clin Cancer Res 11:6270–6279. doi:10.1158/1078-0432.CCR-04-1223

Ahmed KM, Zhang H, Park CC (2013) NF-B regulates radioresistance mediated by 1-integrin in three-dimensional culture of breast cancer cells. Cancer Res 73:3737–3748. doi:10.1158/0008-5472.CAN-12-3537

Allison RR, Patel RM, McLawhorn RA (2014) Radiation oncology: physics advances that minimize morbidity. Future Oncol 10:2329–2344. doi:10.2217/fon.14.176

Arias JL (2011) Drug targeting strategies in cancer treatment: an overview. Mini-Rev Med Chem 11:1–17. doi:10.2174/138955711793564024

Barcellos-Hoff MH, Cordes N (2009) Resistance to radio- and chemotherapy and the tumour microenvironment. Int J Radiat Biol 85:920–922. doi:10.3109/09553000903274043

Barkan D, Chambers AF (2011) β1-integrin: a potential therapeutic target in the battle against cancer recurrence. Clin Cancer Res 17:7219–7223. doi:10.1158/1078-0432.CCR-11-0642

Barker HE, Paget JTE, Khan AA, Harrington KJ (2015) The tumour microenvironment after radiotherapy: mechanisms of resistance and recurrence. Nat Rev Cancer 15:409–425. doi:10.1038/nrc3958

Bell-McGuinn KM, Matthews CM, Ho SN et al (2011) A phase II, single-arm study of the anti-α5β1 integrin antibody volociximab as monotherapy in patients with platinum-resistant advanced epithelial ovarian or primary peritoneal cancer. Gynecol Oncol 121:273–279. doi:10.1016/j.ygyno.2010.12.362

Bello L, Francolini M, Marthyn P, et al. (2001) Alpha(v)beta3 and alpha(v)beta5 integrin expression in glioma periphery. Neurosurgery 49:380–839; discussion 390

Bradbury CM, Markovina S, Wei SJ et al (2001) Indomethacin-induced radiosensitization and inhibition of ionizing radiation-induced NF-κB activation in HeLa cells occur via a mechanism involving p38 MAP kinase. Indomethacin-induced Radiosensitization and Inhibition of Ionizing via a Mechanism Involvi, pp 7689–7696

Brooks PC, Clark RA, Cheresh DA (1994) Requirement of vascular integrin alpha v beta 3 for angiogenesis. Science 264:569–571

Butcher DT, Alliston T, Weaver VM (2009) A tense situation: forcing tumour progression. Nat Rev Cancer 9:108–122. doi:10.1038/nrc2544

Calderwood DA (2004) Integrin activation. J Cell Sci 117:657–666. doi:10.1242/jcs.01014

Carbonell WS, DeLay M, Jahangiri A et al (2013) β1 integrin targeting potentiates antiangiogenic therapy and inhibits the growth of bevacizumab-resistant glioblastoma. Cancer Res 73:3145–3154. doi:10.1158/0008-5472.CAN-13-0011

Chen F, Zhuang X, Lin L et al (2015) New horizons in tumor microenvironment biology: challenges and opportunities. BMC Med 13:45. doi:10.1186/s12916-015-0278-7

Cianfrocca ME, Kimmel KA, Gallo J et al (2006) Phase 1 trial of the antiangiogenic peptide ATN-161 (Ac-PHSCN-NH(2)), a beta integrin antagonist, in patients with solid tumours. Br J Cancer 94:1621–1626. doi:10.1038/sj.bjc.6603171

Clark AG, Vignjevic DM (2015) Modes of cancer cell invasion and the role of the microenvironment. Curr Opin Cell Biol 36:13–22. doi:10.1016/j.ceb.2015.06.004

Coles A (2015) Newer therapies for multiple sclerosis. Ann Indian Acad Neurol 18:S30–S34. doi:10.4103/0972-2327.164824

Collins I, Workman P (2006) New approaches to molecular cancer therapeutics. Nat Chem Biol 2:689–700. doi:10.1038/nchembio840

Cordes N, Meineke V (2003) Cell adhesion-mediated radioresistance (CAM-RR). Extracellular matrix-dependent improvement of cell survival in human tumor and normal cells in vitro. Strahlenther Onkol 179:337–344. doi:10.1007/s00066-003-1074-4

Cordes N, Park CC (2007) B 1 Integrin as a molecular therapeutic target. Int J Radiat Biol 83:753–760. doi:10.1080/09553000701639694

Cordes N, Blaese MA, Meineke V, Van Beuningen D (2002) Ionizing radiation induces up-regulation of functional b1-integrin in human lung tumour cell lines in vitro. Int J Radiat Biol 78:347–357. doi:10.1080/0955300011011734

Cordes N, Hansmeier B, Beinke C et al (2003) Irradiation differentially affects substratum-dependent survival, adhesion, and invasion of glioblastoma cell lines. Br J Cancer 89:2122–2132. doi:10.1038/sj.bjc.6601429

Damiano JS, Cress AE, Hazlehurst LA et al (1999) Cell adhesion mediated drug resistance (CAM-DR): role of integrins and resistance to apoptosis in human myeloma cell lines. Blood 93:1658–1667

Damiano JS, Hazlehurst LA, Dalton WS (2001) Cell adhesion-mediated drug resistance (CAM-DR) protects the K562 chronic myelogenous leukemia cell line from apoptosis induced by BCR/ABL inhibition, cytotoxic drugs, and gamma-irradiation. Leukemia 15:1232–1239

Danen EHJ (2005) Integrins: regulators of tissue function and cancer progression. Curr Pharm Des 11:881–891

Delbaldo C, Raymond E, Vera K et al (2008) Phase I and pharmacokinetic study of etaracizumab (Abegrin), a humanized monoclonal antibody against alphavbeta3 integrin receptor, in patients with advanced solid tumors. Invest New Drugs 26:35–43. doi:10.1007/s10637-007-9077-0

Desgrosellier JS, Cheresh DA (2010) Integrins in cancer: biological implications and therapeutic opportunities. Nat Rev Cancer 10:9–22. doi:10.1038/nrc2748

Dickreuter E, Eke I, Krause M et al (2015) Targeting of β1 integrins impairs DNA repair for radiosensitization of head and neck cancer cells. Oncogene. doi:10.1038/onc.2015.212

Ducassou A, Uro-Coste E, Verrelle P et al (2013) αvβ3 Integrin and Fibroblast growth factor receptor 1 (FGFR1): Prognostic factors in a phase I-II clinical trial associating continuous administration of Tipifarnib with radiotherapy for patients with newly diagnosed glioblastoma. Eur J Cancer 49:2161–2169. doi:10.1016/j.ejca.2013.02.033

Egeblad M, Nakasone ES, Werb Z (2010) Tumors as organs: complex tissues that interface with the entire organism. Dev Cell 18:884–901. doi:10.1016/j.devcel.2010.05.012

Eke I, Cordes N (2011) Dual targeting of EGFR and focal adhesion kinase in 3D grown HNSCC cell cultures. Radiother Oncol 99:279–286. doi:10.1016/j.radonc.2011.06.006

Eke I, Cordes N (2015) Focal adhesion signaling and therapy resistance in cancer. Semin Cancer Biol 31C:65–75. doi:10.1016/j.semcancer.2014.07.009

Eke I, Koch U, Hehlgans S et al (2010) PINCH1 regulates Akt1 activation and enhances radioresistance by inhibiting PP1alpha. J Clin Invest 120:2516–2527. doi:10.1172/JCI41078

Eke I, Storch K, Kästner I et al (2012a) Three-dimensional invasion of human glioblastoma cells remains unchanged by X-ray and carbon ion irradiation in vitro. Int J Radiat Oncol Biol Phys 84:e515–e523. doi:10.1016/j.ijrobp.2012.06.012

Eke I, Deuse Y, Hehlgans S et al (2012b) beta(1)Integrin/FAK/cortactin signaling is essential for human head and neck cancer resistance to radiotherapy. J Clin Invest 122:1529–1540. doi:10.1172/jci61350

Eke I, Dickreuter E, Cordes N (2012c) Enhanced radiosensitivity of head and neck squamous cell carcinoma cells by beta1 integrin inhibition. Radiother Oncol 104:235–242. doi:10.1016/j. radonc.2012.05.009

Eke I, Schneider L, Förster C et al (2013) EGFR/JIP-4/JNK2 signaling attenuates cetuximab-mediated radiosensitization of squamous cell carcinoma cells. Cancer Res 73:297–306. doi:10.1158/0008-5472.CAN-12-2021

Eke I, Zscheppang K, Dickreuter E et al (2015) Simultaneous β1 integrin-EGFR targeting and radiosensitization of human head and neck cancer. J Natl Cancer Inst. doi:10.1093/jnci/dju419

Eliceiri BP, Cheresh DA (2000) Role of alpha v integrins during angiogenesis. Cancer J 6(Suppl 3):S245–S249

Eriksen JG, Steiniche T, Søgaard H, Overgaard J (2004) Expression of integrins and E-cadherin in squamous cell carcinomas of the head and neck. Apmis 112:560–568. doi:10.1111/j.1600-0463.2004.apm1120902.x

Estilo CL, O-charoenrat P, Talbot S et al (2009) Oral tongue cancer gene expression profiling: Identification of novel potential prognosticators by oligonucleotide microarray analysis. BMC Cancer 9:11. doi:10.1186/1471-2407-9-11

Frantz C, Stewart KM, Weaver VM (2010) The extracellular matrix at a glance. J Cell Sci 123:4195–4200. doi:10.1242/jcs.023820

Fujii T, Koshikawa K, Nomoto S et al (2004) Focal adhesion kinase is overexpressed in hepatocellular carcinoma and can be served as an independent prognostic factor. J Hepatol 41:104–111. doi:10.1016/j.jhep.2004.03.029

Fujita S, Watanabe M, Kubota T, et al. (1995) Alteration of expression in integrin beta 1-subunit correlates with invasion and metastasis in colorectal cancer. Cancer Lett 91:145–149. doi:030438359503735F [pii]

Gandellini P, Andriani F, Merlino G et al (2015) Complexity in the tumour microenvironment: cancer associated fibroblast gene expression patterns identify both common and unique features of tumour-stroma crosstalk across cancer types. Semin Cancer Biol 35:96–106. doi:10. 1016/j.semcancer.2015.08.008

Geiger B, Yamada KM (2011) Molecular architecture and function of matrix adhesions. Cold Spring Harb Perspect Biol 3:1–21. doi:10.1101/cshperspect.a005033

Geiger T, Zaidel-Bar R (2012) Opening the floodgates: proteomics and the integrin adhesome. Curr Opin Cell Biol 24:562–568. doi:10.1016/j.ceb.2012.05.004

Geiger B, Spatz JP, Bershadsky AD (2009) Environmental sensing through focal adhesions. Nat Rev Mol Cell Biol 10:21–33. doi:10.1038/nrm2593

Gensicke H, Leppert D, Yaldizli Ö et al (2012) Monoclonal antibodies and recombinant immunoglobulins for the treatment of multiple sclerosis. CNS Drugs 26:11–37. doi:10.2165/ 11596920-000000000-00000

Gingras MC, Roussel E, Bruner JM et al (1995) Comparison of cell adhesion molecule expression between glioblastoma multiforme and autologous normal brain tissue. J Neuroimmunol 57:143–153

Gladson CL, Cheresh DA (1991) Glioblastoma expression of vitronectin and the alpha v beta 3 integrin. Adhesion mechanism for transformed glial cells. J Clin Invest 88:1924–1932. doi:10. 1172/JCI115516

Golubovskaya VM, Huang G, Ho B et al (2013) Pharmacologic blockade of FAK autophospho-rylation decreases human glioblastoma tumor growth and synergizes with temozolomide. Mol Cancer Ther 12:162–172. doi:10.1158/1535-7163.MCT-12-0701

Goodman SL, Picard M (2012) Integrins as therapeutic targets. Trends Pharmacol Sci 33:405–412. doi:10.1016/j.tips.2012.04.002

Gui GP, Wells CA, Yeomans P et al (1996) Integrin expression in breast cancer cytology: a novel predictor of axillary metastasis. Eur J Surg Oncol 22:254–258

Guo W, Giancotti FG (2004) Integrin signalling during tumour progression. Nat Rev Mol Cell Biol 5:816–826. doi:10.1038/nrm1490

Gutheil JC (2000) Novel immunologic and biologic therapies for breast cancer. Curr Oncol Rep 2:582–586

Hall PA, Coates P, Lemoine NR, Horton MA (1991) Characterization of integrin chains in normal and neoplastic human pancreas. J Pathol 165:33–41. doi:10.1002/path.1711650107

Hanahan D, Weinberg RA (2011) Hallmarks of cancer: the next generation. Cell 144:646–674. doi:10.1016/j.cell.2011.02.013

Harburger DS, Calderwood DA (2009) Integrin signalling at a glance. J Cell Sci 122:1472. doi:10. 1242/jcs.052910

Hazlehurst LA, Damiano JS, Buyuksal I et al (2000) Adhesion to fibronectin via beta1 integrins regulates p27kip1 levels and contributes to cell adhesion mediated drug resistance (CAM-DR). Oncogene 19:4319–4327. doi:10.1038/sj.onc.1203782

Hazlehurst LA, Argilagos RF, Emmons M et al (2006) Cell adhesion to fibronectin (CAM-DR) influences acquired mitoxantrone resistance in U937 cells. Cancer Res 66:2338–2345. doi:10. 1158/0008-5472.CAN-05-3256

Hehlgans S, Haase M, Cordes N (2007) Signalling via integrins: implications for cell survival and anticancer strategies. Biochim Biophys Acta 1775:163–180. doi:10.1016/j.bbcan.2006.09.001

Hehlgans S, Eke I, Deuse Y, Cordes N (2008) Integrin-linked kinase: dispensable for radiation survival of three-dimensionally cultured fibroblasts. Radiother Oncol 86:329–335. doi:10. 1016/j.radonc.2007.09.007

Hehlgans S, Lange I, Eke I, Cordes N (2009) 3D cell cultures of human head and neck squamous cell carcinoma cells are radiosensitized by the focal adhesion kinase inhibitor TAE226. Radiother Oncol 92:371–378. doi:10.1016/j.radonc.2009.08.001

Hehlgans S, Eke I, Cordes N (2012) Targeting FAK radiosensitizes 3-dimensional grown human HNSCC cells through reduced Akt1 and MEK1/2 signaling. Int J Radiat Oncol Biol Phys 83: e669–e676. doi:10.1016/j.ijrobp.2012.01.065

Heng DYC, Kollmannsberger C, Chi KN (2010) Targeted therapy for metastatic renal cell carcinoma: current treatment and future directions. Ther Adv Med Oncol 2:39–49. doi:10. 1177/1758834009352498

Hersey P, Sosman J, O'Day S et al (2010) A randomized phase 2 study of etaracizumab, a monoclonal antibody against integrin alpha(v)beta(3), + or − dacarbazine in patients with stage IV metastatic melanoma. Cancer 116:1526–1534. doi:10.1002/cncr.24821

Higgins GS, O'Cathail SM, Muschel RJ, McKenna WG (2015) Drug radiotherapy combinations: review of previous failures and reasons for future optimism. Cancer Treat Rev 41:105–113. doi:10.1016/j.ctrv.2014.12.012

Hochwald SN, Nyberg C, Zheng M et al (2009) A novel small molecule inhibitor of FAK decreases growth of human pancreatic cancer. Cell Cycle 8:2435–2443

Horsley W, Nayar V, Auddy G (2015) Natalizumab use in multiple sclerosis: a real world evidence (Rwe) analysis of its impact on Nhs resources in England. Value Health 18:A764. doi:10.1016/ j.jval.2015.09.2506

Humphries JD, Byron A, Humphries MJ (2006) Integrin ligands at a glance. J Cell Sci 119:3901–3903. doi:10.1242/jcs.03098

Hynes RO (2002) Integrins: bidirectional, allosteric signaling machines. Cell 110:673–687. doi:10. 1016/S0092-8674(02)00971-6

Infante JR, Camidge DR, Mileshkin LR et al (2012) Safety, pharmacokinetic, and pharmacody-namic phase I dose-escalation trial of PF-00562271, an inhibitor of focal adhesion kinase, in advanced solid tumors. J Clin Oncol 30:1527–1533. doi:10.1200/JCO.2011.38.9346

Iwamoto DV, Calderwood DA (2015) Regulation of integrin-mediated adhesions. Curr Opin Cell Biol 36:41–47. doi:10.1016/j.ceb.2015.06.009

Jain RK (2013) Normalizing tumor microenvironment to treat cancer: bench to bedside to biomarkers. J Clin Oncol 31:2205–2218. doi:10.1200/JCO.2012.46.3653

Janes SM, Watt FM (2006) New roles for integrins in squamous-cell carcinoma. Nat Rev Cancer 6:175–183. doi:10.1038/nrc1817

Jones J, Sugiyama M, Watt FM, Speight PM (1993) Integrin expression in normal, hyperplastic, dysplastic, and malignant oral epithelium. J Pathol 169:235–243. doi:10.1002/path. 1711690210

Junttila MR, de Sauvage FJ (2013) Influence of tumour micro-environment heterogeneity on therapeutic response. Nature 501:346–354. doi:10.1038/nature12626

Kalluri R, Zeisberg M (2006) Fibroblasts in cancer. Nat Rev Cancer 6:392–401. doi:10.1038/nrc1877

Kessenbrock K, Plaks V, Werb Z (2010) Matrix metalloproteinases: regulators of the tumor microenvironment. Cell 141:52–67. doi:10.1016/j.cell.2010.03.015

Klemm F, Joyce JA (2014) Microenvironmental regulation of therapeutic response in cancer. Trends Cell Biol 25:198–213. doi:10.1016/j.tcb.2014.11.006

Koretz K, Schlag P, Boumsell L, Möller P (1991) Expression of VLA-alpha 2, VLA-alpha 6, and VLA-beta 1 chains in normal mucosa and adenomas of the colon, and in colon carcinomas and their liver metastases. Am J Pathol 138:741–750

Koukoulis GK, Virtanen I, Korhonen M et al (1991) Immunohistochemical localization of integrins in the normal, hyperplastic, and neoplastic breast. Correlations with their functions as receptors and cell adhesion molecules. Am J Pathol 139:787–799

Kumar S, Weaver VM (2009) Mechanics, malignancy, and metastasis: the force journey of a tumor cell. Cancer Metastasis Rev 28:113–127. doi:10.1007/s10555-008-9173-4

Kurokawa A, Nagata M, Kitamura N et al (2008) Diagnostic value of integrin alpha3, beta4, and beta5 gene expression levels for the clinical outcome of tongue squamous cell carcinoma. Cancer 112:1272–1281. doi:10.1002/cncr.23295

Lark AL, Livasy CA, Dressler L et al (2005) High focal adhesion kinase expression in invasive breast carcinomas is associated with an aggressive phenotype. Mod Pathol 18:1289–1294. doi:10.1038/modpathol.3800424

Legate KR, Montañez E, Kudlacek O, Füssler R (2006) ILK, PINCH and parvin: the tIPP of integrin signalling. Nat Rev Mol Cell Biol 7:20–31. doi:10.1038/nrm1789

Legate KR, Wickström S a, Fässler R et al (2009) Genetic and cell biological analysis of integrin outside-in signaling Genetic and cell biological analysis of integrin outside-in signaling. 23:397–418. doi:10.1101/gad.1758709

Levental KR, Yu H, Kass L et al (2009) Matrix crosslinking forces tumor progression by enhancing integrin signaling. Cell 139:891–906. doi:10.1016/j.cell.2009.10.027

Liu W, Bloom DA, Cance WG et al (2008) FAK and IGF-IR interact to provide survival signals in human pancreatic adenocarcinoma cells. Carcinogenesis 29:1096–1107. doi:10.1093/carcin/bgn026

Maurer GD, Tritschler I, Adams B et al (2009) Cilengitide modulates attachment and viability of human glioma cells, but not sensitivity to irradiation or temozolomide in vitro. Neuro Oncol 11:747–756. doi:10.1215/15228517-2009-012

McNeel DG (2005) Prostate cancer antigens and vaccines, preclinical developments. Cancer Chemother Biol Response Modif 22:247–261

Meads MB, Gatenby RA, Dalton WS (2009) Environment-mediated drug resistance: a major contributor to minimal residual disease. Nat Rev Cancer 9:665–674. doi:10.1038/nrc2714

Meineke V, Gilbertz K-P, Schilperoort K et al (2002) Ionizing radiation modulates cell surface integrin expression and adhesion of COLO-320 cells to collagen and fibronectin in vitro. Strahlentherapie und Onkol 178:709–714. doi:10.1007/s00066-002-0993-9

Micke P, Ostman A (2005) Exploring the tumour environment: cancer-associated fibroblasts as targets in cancer therapy. Expert Opin Ther Targets 9:1217–1233. doi:10.1517/14728222.9.6.1217

Mikkelsen T, Brodie C, Finniss S et al (2009) Radiation sensitization of glioblastoma by cilengitide has unanticipated schedule-dependency. Int J Cancer 124:2719–2727. doi:10.1002/ijc.24240

Miyazaki T, Kato H, Nakajima M et al (2003) FAK overexpression is correlated with tumour invasiveness and lymph node metastasis in oesophageal squamous cell carcinoma. Br J Cancer 89:140–145. doi:10.1038/sj.bjc.6601050

Monferran S, Skuli N, Delmas C et al (2008) Alphavbeta3 and alphavbeta5 integrins control glioma cell response to ionising radiation through ILK and RhoB. Int J Cancer 123:357–364. doi:10.1002/ijc.23498

Morse EM, Brahme NN, Calderwood DA (2014) Integrin cytoplasmic tail interactions. Biochemistry 53:810–820. doi:10.1021/bi401596q

Nagata M, Noman AA, Suzuki K et al (2013) ITGA3 and ITGB4 expression biomarkers estimate the risks of locoregional and hematogenous dissemination of oral squamous cell carcinoma. BMC Cancer 13:410. doi:10.1186/1471-2407-13-410

Nakasone ES, Askautrud HA, Kees T et al (2012) Imaging tumor-stroma interactions during chemotherapy reveals contributions of the microenvironment to resistance. Cancer Cell 21:488–503. doi:10.1016/j.ccr.2012.02.017

Nam J-M, Onodera Y, Bissell MJ, Park CC (2010) Breast cancer cells in three-dimensional culture display an enhanced radioresponse after coordinate targeting of integrin alpha5beta1 and fibronectin. Cancer Res 70:5238–5248. doi:10.1158/0008-5472.CAN-09-2319

Niyazi M, Maihoefer C, Krause M et al (2011) Radiotherapy and "new" drugs-new side effects? Radiat Oncol 6:177. doi:10.1186/1748-717X-6-177

O'Day S, Pavlick A, Loquai C et al (2011) A randomised, phase II study of intetumumab, an anti-αv-integrin mAb, alone and with dacarbazine in stage IV melanoma. Br J Cancer 105:346–352. doi:10.1038/bjc.2011.183

Oliveira-Ferrer L, Hauschild J, Fiedler W et al (2008) Cilengitide induces cellular detachment and apoptosis in endothelial and glioma cells mediated by inhibition of FAK/src/AKT pathway. J Exp Clin Cancer Res 27:86. doi:10.1186/1756-9966-27-86

Park CC, Henshall-Powell RL, Erickson AC et al (2003) Ionizing radiation induces heritable disruption of epithelial cell interactions. Proc Natl Acad Sci USA 100:10728–10733. doi:10.1073/pnas.1832185100

Park CC, Zhang H, Pallavicini M et al (2006) Beta1 integrin inhibitory antibody induces apoptosis of breast cancer cells, inhibits growth, and distinguishes malignant from normal phenotype in three dimensional cultures and in vivo. Cancer Res 66:1526–1535. doi:10.1158/0008-5472.CAN-05-3071

Park CC, Zhang HJ, Yao ES et al (2008) Beta1 integrin inhibition dramatically enhances radiotherapy efficacy in human breast cancer xenografts. Cancer Res 68:4398–4405. doi:10.1158/0008-5472.CAN-07-6390

Paulsson J, Micke P (2014) Prognostic relevance of cancer-associated fibroblasts in human cancer. Semin Cancer Biol 25:61–68. doi:10.1016/j.semcancer.2014.02.006

Paulus W, Baur I, Schuppan D, Roggendorf W (1993) Characterization of integrin receptors in normal and neoplastic human brain. Am J Pathol 143:154–163

Peng C-H, Liao C-T, Peng S-C et al (2011) A novel molecular signature identified by systems genetics approach predicts prognosis in oral squamous cell carcinoma. PLoS ONE 6:e23452. doi:10.1371/journal.pone.0023452

Plodinec M, Loparic M, Monnier CA et al (2012) The nanomechanical signature of breast cancer. Nat Nanotechnol 7:757–765. doi:10.1038/nnano.2012.167

Polte TR, Hanks SK (1995) Interaction between focal adhesion kinase and Crk-associated tyrosine kinase substrate p130Cas. Proc Natl Acad Sci USA 92:10678–10682

Previtali S, Quattrini A, Nemni R et al (1996) Alpha6 beta4 and alpha6 beta1 integrins in astrocytomas and other CNS tumors. J Neuropathol Exp Neurol 55:456–465

Qin J, Wu C (2012) ILK: a pseudokinase in the center stage of cell-matrix adhesion and signaling. Curr Opin Cell Biol 24:607–613. doi:10.1016/j.ceb.2012.06.003

Reardon DA, Fink KL, Mikkelsen T et al (2008) Randomized phase II study of cilengitide, an integrin-targeting arginine-glycine-aspartic acid peptide, in recurrent glioblastoma multiforme. J Clin Oncol 26:5610–5617. doi:10.1200/JCO.2008.16.7510

Ricart AD, Tolcher AW, Liu G et al (2008) Volociximab, a chimeric monoclonal antibody that specifically binds alpha5beta1 integrin: a phase I, pharmacokinetic, and biological correlative study. Clin Cancer Res 14:7924–7929. doi:10.1158/1078-0432.CCR-08-0378

Rieken S, Habermehl D, Mohr A et al (2011) Targeting $\alpha v \beta 3$ and $\alpha v \beta 5$ inhibits photon-induced hypermigration of malignant glioma cells. Radiat Oncol 6:132. doi:10.1186/1748-717X-6-132

Ritchie CK, Giordano A, Khalili K (2000) Integrin involvement in glioblastoma multiforme: possible regulation by NF-kappaB. J Cell Physiol 184:214–221. doi:10.1002/1097-4652 (200008)184:2<214:AID-JCP9>3.0.CO;2-Z

Roberts WG, Ung E, Whalen P et al (2008) Antitumor activity and pharmacology of a selective focal adhesion kinase inhibitor, PF-562,271. Cancer Res 68:1935–1944. doi:10.1158/0008-5472.CAN-07-5155

Rønnov-Jessen L, Petersen OW, Bissell MJ (1996) Cellular changes involved in conversion of normal to malignant breast: importance of the stromal reaction. Physiol Rev 76:69–125

Rossow L, Eke I, Dickreuter E, Cordes N (2015) Targeting of the EGFR/$\beta 1$ integrin connecting proteins PINCH1 and Nck2 radiosensitizes three-dimensional SCC cell cultures. Oncol Rep 34:469–476

Salzler GG, Graham A, Connolly PH et al (2015) Safety and effectiveness of adjunctive intra-arterial abciximab in the management of acute limb ischemia. Ann Vasc Surg. doi:10.1016/j.avsg.2015.09.004

Sanchez-Lopez E, Flashner-Abramson E, Shalapour S et al (2015) Targeting colorectal cancer via its microenvironment by inhibiting IGF-1 receptor-insulin receptor substrate and STAT3 signaling. Oncogene. doi:10.1038/onc.2015.326

Sandfort V, Koch U, Cordes N (2007) Cell adhesion-mediated radioresistance revisited. Int J Radiat Biol 83:727–732. doi:10.1080/09553000701694335

Sandfort V, Eke I, Cordes N (2010) The role of the focal adhesion protein PINCH1 for the radiosensitivity of adhesion and suspension cell cultures. PLoS ONE. doi:10.1371/journal.pone.0013056

Schnell O, Krebs B, Wagner E et al (2008) Expression of integrin alphavbeta3 in gliomas correlates with tumor grade and is not restricted to tumor vasculature. Brain Pathol 18:378–386. doi:10.1111/j.1750-3639.2008.00137.x

Searle EJ, Illidge TM, Stratford IJ (2014) Emerging opportunities for the combination of molecularly targeted drugs with radiotherapy. Clin Oncol 26:266–276. doi:10.1016/j.clon.2014.02.006

Shi X, Meng X, Sun X et al (2014) PET/CT imaging-guided dose painting in radiation therapy. Cancer Lett 355:169–175. doi:10.1016/j.canlet.2014.07.042

Shimoyama S, Gansauge F, Gansauge S et al (1995) Altered expression of extracellular matrix molecules and their receptors in chronic pancreatitis and pancreatic adenocarcinoma in comparison with normal pancreas. Int J Pancreatol 18:227–234

Shirakihara T, Kawasaki T, Fukagawa A et al (2013) Identification of integrin $\alpha 3$ as a molecular marker of cells undergoing epithelial-mesenchymal transition and of cancer cells with aggressive phenotypes. Cancer Sci 104:1189–1197. doi:10.1111/cas.12220

Shishido S, Bönig H, Kim Y-M (2014) Role of integrin alpha4 in drug resistance of leukemia. Front Oncol 4:1–10. doi:10.3389/fonc.2014.00099

Stallmach A, von Lampe B, Matthes H et al (1992) Diminished expression of integrin adhesion molecules on human colonic epithelial cells during the benign to malign tumour transformation. Gut 33:342–346. doi:10.1136/gut.33.3.342

Steglich A, Vehlow A, Eke I, Cordes N (2015) α integrin targeting for radiosensitization of three-dimensionally grown human head and neck squamous cell carcinoma cells. Cancer Lett 357:542–548. doi:10.1016/j.canlet.2014.12.009

Storch K, Cordes N (2012) Focal adhesion-chromatin linkage controls tumor cell resistance to radio- and chemotherapy. Chemother Res Pract 2012:319287. doi:10.1155/2012/319287

Stupp R, Hegi ME, Gorlia T et al (2014) Cilengitide combined with standard treatment for patients with newly diagnosed glioblastoma with methylated MGMT promoter (CENTRIC EORTC 26071-22072 study): a multicentre, randomised, open-label, phase 3 trial. Lancet Oncol 15:1100–1108. doi:10.1016/S1470-2045(14)70379-1

Tavora B, Reynolds LE, Batista S et al (2014) Endothelial-cell FAK targeting sensitizes tumours to DNA-damaging therapy. Nature 514:112–116. doi:10.1038/nature13541

Thundimadathil J (2012) Cancer treatment using peptides: current therapies and future prospects. J Amino Acids 2012:967347. doi:10.1155/2012/967347

Tilghman RW, Parsons JT (2008) Focal adhesion kinase as a regulator of cell tension in the progression of cancer. Semin Cancer Biol 18:45–52. doi:10.1016/j.semcancer.2007.08.002

Vehlow A, Cordes N (2013) Invasion as target for therapy of glioblastoma multiforme. Biochim Biophys Acta—Rev Cancer 1836:236–244. doi:10.1016/j.bbcan.2013.07.001

Vogetseder A, Thies S, Ingold B et al (2013) αv-Integrin isoform expression in primary human tumors and brain metastases. Int J Cancer 133:2362–2371. doi:10.1002/ijc.28267

Wei SC, Yang J (2015) Forcing through tumor metastasis : the interplay between tissue rigidity and epithelial—mesenchymal transition. Trends Cell Biol xx:1–10. doi:10.1016/j.tcb.2015.09.009

Weis SM, Cheresh DA (2011) αv integrins in angiogenesis and cancer. Cold Spring Harb Perspect Med 1:1–14. doi:10.1101/cshperspect.a006478

Wick W, Wick A, Schulz B et al (2002) Prevention of irradiation-induced glioma cell invasion by temozolomide involves caspase 3 activity and cleavage of focal adhesion kinase. Cancer Res 62:1915–1919

Wickström SA, Lange A, Hess MW et al (2010) Integrin-linked kinase controls microtubule dynamics required for plasma membrane targeting of caveolae. Dev Cell 19:574–588. doi:10.1016/j.devcel.2010.09.007

Wild-bode C, Weller M, Rimner A et al (2001) Sublethal irradiation promotes migration and invasiveness of glioma cells : implications for radiotherapy of human glioblastoma sublethal irradiation promotes migration and invasiveness of glioma cells : implications for radiotherapy of human glioblastoma. Cancer Res 61:2744–2750

Yamada KM, Even-Ram S (2002) Integrin regulation of growth factor receptors. Nat Cell Biol 4: E75–E76. doi:10.1038/ncb0402-e75

Zaidel-Bar R, Itzkovitz S, Ma'ayan A et al (2007) Functional atlas of the integrin adhesome. Nat Cell Biol 9:858–867. doi:10.1038/ncb0807-858

Zhou B, Gibson-Corley KN, Herndon ME et al (2014) Integrin alpha3beta1 can function to promote spontaneous metastasis and lung colonization of invasive breast carcinoma. Mol Cancer Res 12:143–154. doi:10.1158/1541-7786.mcr-13-0184

Zutter MM, Krigman HR, Santoro SA (1993) Altered integrin expression in adenocarcinoma of the breast. Analysis by in situ hybridization. Am J Pathol 142:1439–1448

Personalized Radiation Oncology: Epidermal Growth Factor Receptor and Other Receptor Tyrosine Kinase Inhibitors

Geoff S. Higgins, Mechthild Krause, W. Gillies McKenna and Michael Baumann

Abstract

Molecular biomarkers are currently evaluated in preclinical and clinical studies in order to establish predictors for treatment decisions in radiation oncology. The receptor tyrosine kinases (RTK) are described in the following text. Among them, the most data are available for the epidermal growth factor receptor (EGFR) that plays a major role for prognosis of patients after radiotherapy, but seems also to be involved in mechanisms of radioresistance, specifically in repopulation of tumour cells between radiotherapy fractions. Monoclonal

G.S. Higgins, M. Krause: Equal contribution

G.S. Higgins · W.G. McKenna
Gray Laboratories, Department of Oncology, Cancer Research UK/MRC Oxford
Institute for Radiation Oncology, University of Oxford, Old Road Campus
Research Building, Oxford, UK

M. Krause (✉) · M. Baumann
OncoRay - National Center for Radiation Research in Oncology (NCRO),
Carl Gustav Carus Faculty of Medicine, University Hospital, Technische Universität
Dresden and Helmholtz-Zentrum Dresden—Rossendorf, Dresden, Germany
e-mail: mechthild.krause@uniklinikum-dresden.de

M. Baumann
e-mail: michael.baumann@uniklinikum-dresden.de

M. Krause · M. Baumann
German Cancer Consortium (DKTK) Dresden, German Cancer Research
Center (DKFZ), Heidelberg, Germany

M. Krause · M. Baumann
Helmholtz-Zentrum Dresden—Rossendorf, Insititute of Radiooncology, Dresden, Germany

M. Krause · M. Baumann
Department of Radiation Oncology, Carl Gustav Carus Faculty of Medicine,
University Hospital, Technische Universität Dresden, Dresden, Germany

© Springer-Verlag Berlin Heidelberg 2016
M. Baumann et al. (eds.), *Molecular Radio-Oncology*, Recent Results
in Cancer Research 198, DOI 10.1007/978-3-662-49651-0_5

antibodies against the EGFR improve locoregional tumour control and survival when applied during radiotherapy, however, the effects are heterogeneous and biomarkers for patient selection are warranted. Also other RTK´s such as c-Met and IGF-1R seem to play important roles in tumour radioresistance. Beside the potential to select patients for molecular targeting approaches combined with radiotherapy, studies are also needed to evluate radiotherapy adaptation approaches for selected patients, i.e. adaptation of radiation dose, or, more sophisticated, of target volumes.

Keywords

EGFR, Biomarker, Radiotherapy, HER-2, Receptor tyrosine kinases

1   Introduction

Treatment decisions in clinical radiation oncology are today based on general predictive biomarkers such as tumour histology or tumour mass (macroscopic tumour vs. postoperative residuals). Beside indications for radio- or radiochemotherapy or total radiation dose, also decisions on fractionation schedules can be based on such factors. Examples are squamous cell carcinoma of the head and neck (HNSCC) that express a considerable time factor, i.e. improvement of local tumour control at shorter overall treatment time by repopulating cancer stem cells during treatment, and are thus better treated using accelerated radiation treatment schedules. Recent data showed that also tumour size can impact the outcome after different fractionation schedules with a larger time factor for larger compared to smaller non-small-cell lung cancer (Soliman et al. 2013). Beyond these "classical" biomarkers, there are currently no molecular biomarkers in clinical use as a basis for treatment decisions in radiation oncology. However, a number of promising candidate biomarkers are currently being tested in preclinical and clinical studies. Notably, such biomarkers need to be evaluated separately for radio-oncological combined treatment approaches as compared to drug treatments alone. The reasons are the different endpoints (mostly curative for combined treatment, palliative for systemic treatment alone in solid tumours) and the potential interactions between both treatment modalities when combination schedules are used.

2   Epidermal Growth Factor Receptor and Other Receptor Tyrosine Kinases

2.1   Importance of EGFR for Radiotherapy Outcome

The ErbB receptor family presents one of about 20 known subfamilies of the receptor tyrosine kinase (RTK) receptors. It includes four receptor subtypes (EGFR/HER1/ErbB1, HER2/neu/ErbB2, HER3/ErbB3 and HER4/ErbB4), of which the epidermal growth factor receptor (EGFR) is the best-evaluated receptor. Compared to the normal tissues of the tumour's origin, the EGFR is the most frequently overexpressed receptor in human tumours. A prominent example is squamous cell carcinoma of the skin and head and neck, where 80–100 % of the tumours were found to show a high EGFR expression, but also carcinoma of the cervix uteri (80 %), endometrial cancer (90 %), non-small-cell lung cancer (40–80 %) and glioblastoma (40–50 %) belong to the high EGFR-expressing tumours [reviewed in Salomon et al. (1995)]. A high EGFR expression has been reported to be associated with lower tumour control rates after radiotherapy for several tumour entities (Nicholson et al. 2001; Baumann et al. 2007); however, there are also contradictory results showing no or only weak or even reverse associations between both parameters (Chakravarti et al. 2005a; Chakravarti et al. 2005b; Lee et al. 2005; Marioni et al. 2011). It needs to be mentioned that an association of the EGFR expression with survival or tumour control has also been shown for other oncologic treatment modalities, supporting a prognostic rather than predictive value of the protein expression: in addition to retrospective data on patient outcome after surgery or chemotherapy of different tumour entities, a recent analysis of head and neck squamous cell cancer (HNSCC) patients treated within two different prospective clinical trials either with surgery without an EGFR-targeted agent or with radiochemotherapy in combination with the anti-EGFR antibody cetuximab has shown that a high EGFR protein expression and elevated phosphorylation of the tyrosine kinase at Y1068 correlated with lower survival, supporting a prognostic value independent on the kind of treatment (Wheeler et al. 2012). Interestingly, evaluation of HNSCC patients enrolled in a randomized RTOG trial revealed an independent prognostic value of EGFR protein expression for overall survival, disease-free survival and local tumour control, but not for metastases-free survival (Ang et al. 2002), suggesting that the reason for the different response is indeed local tumour resistance and not metastatic potential. These data support strategies on local treatment intensification to overcome this resistance.

The EGFR seems to be involved also in mechanisms of radiation resistance, specifically in repopulation of cancer stem cells between radiation fractions. Repopulation determines an increase of the number of cancer stem cells between irradiation fractions by accelerated proliferation and/or by decreased cell loss. It causes the so-called time factor of radiotherapy that is the decrease of tumour cure probability with increasing overall treatment time. Although heterogeneity exists between different tumour models, a coincidence between onset of repopulation and increase of membranous EGFR protein expression has been shown experimentally in FaDu xenografts (Eicheler et al. 2005; Petersen et al. 2003). The causal relationship of EGFR expression and repopulation is supported by post hoc analyses of clinical randomized trials. Both in the CHARTWEL-bronchus as well as in DAHANCA trials, non-small-cell lung cancer or HNSCC has been treated in different overall treatment times. Both post hoc analyses showed that specifically tumours with high EGFR expression have significantly lower local tumour control probabilities when overall treatment times are prolonged and that this disadvantage can be partly or completely dissolved with shortening overall treatment time (Bentzen et al. 2005; Eriksen et al. 2005). This mechanism is schematically shown

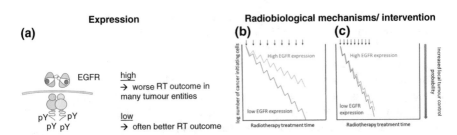

Fig. 1 EGFR protein expression is often associated with radiotherapy outcome, i.e. locoregional tumour control or survival **a** The EGFR seems to be involved in biological mechanisms of radiation resistance, specifically repopulation of cancer stem cells **b**, **c**. After each radiation fraction ($\downarrow$), a percentage of the cancer (stem) cells are inactivated, but the surviving cancer stem cells repopulate within the time interval to the next fraction, thus again increasing their number. This repopulation is obviously more distinct in high EGFR-expressing tumours, leading to lower tumour control probabilities in this subgroup (**b**). Applying the radiotherapy treatment schedule within a shorter overall treatment time (**c**) reduces the amount of repopulation and outweights this disadvantage for high EGFR-expressing tumours

in Fig. 1. Thus, promising experimental interventions include not only local treatment modifications by radiation dose, but also modifications of the radiotherapy fractionation schedule, i.e. the application of accelerated radiotherapy specifically in high EGFR-expressing tumours.

EGFR expression has been shown to be associated also with expression of other RTKs, and consideration of both may help to refine different prognostic groups of patients. Retrospective data on non-small-cell lung cancer suggest that a genetic amplification of the EGFR measured by fluorescence in situ hybridization (FISH) is more frequent in squamous cell carcinoma and is associated with an amplification of the insulin-like growth factor 1 receptor (IGF-1R, see below), and the amplification of both receptors or a protein overexpression defines a patient group with lower disease-free survival (DFS) (Ludovini et al. 2013; Gately et al. 2014).

2.2 Importance of Other ErbB Receptors for Radiotherapy Outcome

ErbB2 (HER2) is frequently overexpressed in breast cancer but also in a variety of other cancers. In clinical data sets, ErbB2 seems to be associated with higher tumour stage and aggressiveness in different tumour entities (Salomon et al. 1995); however, it is not clear whether this phenomenon has any association to resistance to specific treatments or is just a feature of these tumours. Overexpression of ErbB2 together with the putative cancer stem cell marker CD44 has been shown to be more frequent in breast cancer recurrences compared to primary breast cancer (Duru et al. 2012). In vitro, HER2+/CD44+/CD24−/low MCF7/C6 cells showed elevated aldehyde dehydrogenase (ALDH) activity, invasion and sphere formation as well as faster tumour formation after cell inoculation in vivo. After irradiation in vitro, clonogenic cell survival was lower in HER2 siRNA knock-down cells compared to HER2 positive cells, indicating a higher radioresistance in HER2 positive cells (Duru et al. 2012). These data suggest a potential value of ErbB2 as a marker of tumour aggressiveness and radioresistance that needs to be validated in clinical data sets.

For ErbB3, there are some clinical data suggesting a prognostic role of a high expression with clinical outcome in colorectal cancer (Ledel et al. 2014). In ErbB2 positive breast cancer, low ErbB3 expression has been shown to be associated with better progression-free survival compared to high ErbB3-expressing tumours (Lipton et al. 2013). Also here, there is currently no evidence for specific interaction with cancer treatments. However, preclinical data suggest that compensatory ErbB3 can be activated when EGFR signalling is blocked and that this activation, via src signalling, increases radioresistance by preventing apoptosis in breast cancer cells in vitro (Contessa et al. 2006).

Little is known about the importance of ErbB4 for cancer prognosis and specifically for radiation resistance. While few mostly preclinical data sets suggest an importance of specific mutations for tumour aggressiveness, there are no valid data on a potential value of the receptor expression or mutations for treatment resistance.

2.3 Importance of EGFR and Its Downstream Signal Transduction for the Outcome of Combined Radiotherapy and EGFR-Targeted Agents

For EGFR targeting, specifically for the application of EGFR tyrosine kinase inhibitors outside the context of radiotherapy, some biomarkers have been established that can predict tumour response to treatment [reviewed in Krause and Baumann (2008)]. One example are specific mutations of the EGFR tyrosine kinase that are mostly in-frame deletions in exon 19 (codon 746–750), missense mutations in exon 21 (codon 858) or missense or insertion mutations in exon 18–21 [reviewed in Johnson and Janne (2005)]. EGFR gene amplification measured by FISH can be shown in about 30 % of non-small-cell lung cancer (NSCLC). While NSCC with EGFR amplification seems to have a generally worse prognosis (Hirsch et al. 2003; Jeon et al. 2006), this can be counteracted by the application of EGFR-TK inhibitors (Hirsch et al. 2006; Tsao et al. 2005; Temam et al. 2007), supporting a predictive value of high EGFR gene copy numbers for EGFR-TK inhibition alone. The EGFR downstream signal transduction molecule RAS plays a role in mediating radio- and chemotherapy resistance (Bernhard et al. 2000; Chakravarti et al. 2002). In contrast to KRAS wildtype tumours, antiproliferative effects of EGFR-TK inhibitors are not evident in tumours harbouring activating KRAS mutations. Beyond several retrospective data sets, this is supported by results from clinical randomized phase III trial on patients with NSCLC and colorectal cancer, where a correlation of activating KRAS mutations with shorter survival time and time to progression after EGFR-TK inhibition or application of anti-EGFR antibodies has been established (Eberhard et al. 2005; Bokemeyer et al. 2009; Karapetis et al. 2008).

In the context of combined EGFR inhibition with radiotherapy, so far no specific molecular biomarker has been established for clinical use. This is in parts caused by the fact that the group of EGFR-TK inhibitors have not shown any improvement in the curative effect of radiotherapy when both treatments are applied simultaneously or sequentially. Thus, biomarkers are currently only needed for combined radiotherapy and anti-EGFR antibodies, i.e. for simultaneous radiotherapy and cetuximab as the currently only approved treatment combination. Here, the combined treatment improves local tumour control and survival in patients with HNSCC when compared to radiotherapy alone (Bonner et al. 2006; Bonner et al. 2010). However, the average effect seems to be not superior to standard radiochemotherapy (Caudell et al. 2008). In the light of sometimes impressive responses of individual tumours to the combination of radiatio therapy and cetuximab, predictive markers that help to stratify patients for the treatment with radiotherapy plus cetuximab versus radiochemotherapy are urgently needed, because stratification alone would be expected to increase local tumour control rates and survival in this situation. Post hoc analyses of the above-mentioned trial are ongoing with so far no promising biomarkers reported. Preclinical analyses showed a correlation of genetic EGFR amplification measured by FISH with the improvement of local tumour control by cetuximab applied simultaneously to irradiation, whereas tumours without amplification show very heterogeneous response (Gurtner et al. 2011). Also tumour micromilieu parameters like perfusion appear to be potential candidate biomarkers (Gurtner et al. 2013). Using a theragnostic approach in preclinical experiments, i.e. radiollabelled ([(86)Y] Y-(CHX-A''-DTPA)$_4$-cetuximab for positron emission tomography (PET) and ([(90) Y]Y-(CHX-A''-DTPA)$_4$-cetuximb for radioimmunotherapy applied in combination with external beam radiotherapy, improvement of radiation response by radioimmunotherapy could be shown in tumours with higher expression of the EGFR and with high perfusion (Koi et al. 2014). These data support an important role of two simple factors, the target expression and the reachability of the target by the (in this case relatively large) molecules of the drug.

2.4   Non-EGFR family tyrosine kinases as therapeutic targets

Although the EGFR family of receptor tyrosine kinases (RTKs) have been the most widely studied as potential targets for tumour radiosensitization, the development of inhibitors against RTKs such as c-Met and IGF-1R has resulted in growing interest in the potential role of other RTKs. As discussed below, there is significant data showing that the overexpression of some of these RTKs is associated with adverse clinical outcomes following radiotherapy treatment and therefore representing prognostic biomarkers. It is currently unclear whether expression levels may also prove to be predictive markers of response to novel inhibitors of these RTKs when combined with RT.

3   c-Met

c-Met is a transmembrane RTK that is activated by the extracellular binding of its ligand, hepatocyte growth factor (HGF), leading to receptor dimerization and phosphorylation of internal tyrosine kinase domains (Ponzetto et al. 1994). Activation of the HGF/c-Met pathway has been linked to numerous biological changes including tumourigenesis, resistance to apoptosis and increased cell proliferation and motility (Maulik et al. 2002). The pathway can be aberrantly upregulated by multiple mechanisms including autocrine HGF/c-Met signalling and overexpression of c-Met and by activating mutations (Yi and Tsao 2000; Ma et al. 2008; Ma et al. 2003). Downstream signalling of c-Met involves both the PI3K/Akt and MAPK pathways and therefore shows significant crosstalk with EGFR activation (Organ and Tsao 2011).

Ionising radiation has been shown to induce c-Met expression and activation of tumour cells, resulting in a more aggressive phenotype such as increased cell invasiveness. De Bacco et al. have shown that c-Met inhibitors cause pronounced tumour radiosensitization both in vitro and in vivo (De Bacco et al. 2011) and several other groups have reported similar findings using different c-Met inhibitors (Welsh et al. 2009; Bhardwaj et al. 2012). The exact mechanism by which c-Met inhibition causes radiosensitization is currently unclear, but there is significant evidence linking c-Met inhibition to decreased DNA damage repair (Welsh et al. 2009; Fan et al. 1998; Fan et al. 2000).

There is growing evidence that c-Met activation is associated with an adverse prognosis in many different tumour types. c-Met overexpression has been shown to be associated with worse progression-free and overall survival when compared with patients with little or no c-Met expression in glioblastoma patients treated with surgical resection, followed by adjuvant radiotherapy or chemoradiotherapy (Kong et al. 2009). Increased c-Met copy number has also been associated with worse survival in surgically resected NSCLC (Cappuzzo et al. 2009). Recent data have shown that high c-MET gene expression significantly correlates also with locoregional tumour control after postoperative radiochemotherapy in HNSCC, where patients with high c-MET gene expression show a substantially lower tumour control rate compared to patients with low expression (Linge et al. 2016)

Since c-Met signalling is frequently upregulated in many cancers which are often treated with radical radiotherapy such as HNSCC and lung cancer, there is significant interest in combining c-Met inhibitors with radiotherapy treatment. c-Met is overexpressed in over 80 % of HNSCCs (Burtness et al. 2013). High expression of c-Met has been shown to be associated with reduced response rates, and worse local failure-free and overall survival rates in oropharyngeal cancer following radical radiotherapy (Aebersold et al. 2001).

Several inhibitors against c-met have been described. Since the side effect profiles of leading clinical candidates such as crizotinib (which also targets ALK) and tivantinib are becoming familiar, there will be significant interest in combining these agents with radiotherapy treatment (Ou 2011; Scagliotti et al. 2013). Once the toxicity associated with such combinations has been established, attempts can be made to identify biomarkers of response to these treatments including expression levels of c-Met.

4   Insulin-Like Growth Factor 1 Receptor

The insulin-like growth factor 1 receptor (IGF-1R) is a cell membrane receptor that belongs to the IGF/insulin family of receptors which play important roles in tissue growth and development as well as overall metabolism. However, IGF-IR signalling also appears to play an important role in the transformation of cells, and cancer cell proliferation and metastasis (Arcaro 2013).

The IGF-1 receptor functions as a homodimer with two α extracellular subunits containing a ligand-binding domain as well as two β transmembrane subunits which contain an intracellular tyrosine kinase component (Adams et al. 2000). IGF-1, IGF-2 and insulin interact with IGF-1R, although there is particularly high affinity between IGF-1 and IGF-1R. Ligand binding of IGF-1R results in autophosphorylation of tyrosine residues in the kinase domain and phosphorylation of the juxtamembrane tyrosines which act as a docking site for adaptor molecules such as Src-homology collagen protein (Shc) and the insulin receptor substrate (IRS) 1 and 2. This results in the activation of a complex downstream signalling cascade that includes the MAPK and PI3K/Akt pathways (Fig. 2) similar to EGFR activation (Favelyukis et al. 2001; Shelton et al. 2004; Zha and Lackner 2010).

Fig. 2 Principal components of the IGF-1R pathway. IGF-1 and IGF-2 ligands bind to the extracellular domain of IGF-1R resulting in receptor cross-linking and autophosphorylation. Docking proteins such as IRS and Shc trigger activation of the PI3K-AKT and Ras-RAF pathways, respectively, leading to increased cell proliferation and resistance to cell death

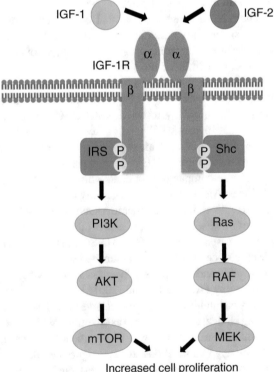

The ultimate effects of IGF-1R activation include increased cell proliferation and resistance to chemotherapy- and radiotherapy-induced cell death (Arnaldez and Helman 2012).

Although no cancer-specific mutations of IGF-1R have been described, multiple studies have reported dysregulated IGF-1 signalling in many different malignancies. These include overexpression of the IGF-1 receptor in breast and colorectal cancer and the presence of elevated IGF-1 levels in many different tumour types including prostate, gastric, breast and colorectal cancer (Arcaro 2013).

There is an abundance of evidence linking aberrant IGR-1R signalling to radioresistance. Fibroblasts overexpressing IGF-1R have been shown to have increased radioresistance, while IGF-1R silencing has been shown to increase tumour radiosensitivity (Turner et al. 1997; Yavari et al. 2010; Rochester et al. 2005). In addition, the use of anti-IGF-1R antibodies has been shown to cause tumour radiosensitiziation both in vitro and in vivo (Riesterer et al. 2011; Iwasa et al. 2009).

Alterations in cell proliferation and DNA repair are the primary mechanisms by which disruption of IGF-1R signalling causes radiosensitization. IGF-1R is involved in regulating the DNA damage response pathway by its interaction with ataxia-telangiectasia-mutated (ATM) protein with IGF-1R silencing decreasing the activity of ATM and inducing tumour radiosensitization (Peretz et al. 2001; Macaulay et al. 2001). IGF-1R has been particularly implicated in DNA double-strand break (DSB) repair with inhibition of the IGF-1 receptor reducing DSB repair post-radiation as measured by the presence of Rad51 and γH2AX (Iwasa et al. 2009). Although much work has been focused on the effects of IGF-1R on non-homologous end joining (NHEJ) by regulating Ku70/80, it has additionally recently been suggested that inhibition of IGF-1R also attenuates homologous recombination (Valenciano et al. 2012; Chitnis 2013).

The clinical effects of aberrant IGF1 signalling on patients treated with radio-therapy have been shown to be associated with adverse outcomes in many different tumours including breast (Turner et al. 1997); cervical (Lloret et al. 2008), and head and neck cancer (Lara et al. 2011). Data from a prospective head and neck cancer study showed that IGF-1R expression was associated with a 28.6-fold increased risk of treatment failure and supports the potential role of IGF-1R expression as a prognostic biomarker following radiotherapy (Moreno-Acosta et al. 2012).

Multiple monoclonal antibodies and small molecule inhibitors targeting IGF-1R have been described and have entered clinical trials (Arnaldez and Helman 2012). Figitumumab, a monoclonal antibody against IGF-IR, showed significant promise in a phase II study, but subsequent phase III studies in NSCLC with concurrent chemotherapy failed to demonstrate any benefit. Although it is possible that biomarkers could be developed and validated to identify subgroups of patients with metastatic disease who benefit from IGF1-R inhibition, the failure of these large phase III studies caused the development of several inhibitors to be discontinued (Yee 2012).

Disappointingly, even though the preclinical and clinical rationale for combining IGF-1R inhibitors with radiotherapy is compelling, there is a paucity of clinical studies in this area. Since there is ongoing interest in combining IGF-1R inhibitors in the metastatic setting with additional inhibitors against such targets as EGFR and mTOR (Fidler et al. 2012), it seems justifiable to initiate clinical studies combining IGF-IR inhibitors with radiotherapy in patients with IGF-1R overexpression.

5   Vascular Endothelial Growth Factor Receptor/Platelet-derived Growth Factor Receptor

As the vascular endothelial growth factor (VEGF) receptors and platelet-derived growth factor (PDGF) receptors have overlapping biological functions such as angiogenesis and are both inhibited by tyrosine kinase inhibitors such as sorafenib and sunitinib, which are already in clinical use, they will be considered together in this section (Homsi and Daud 2007).

The VEGF family is comprised of VEGF-A, -B, -C and -D and placental growth factor which can bind to three receptor tyrosine kinases (VEGFR-1, -2 and -3) (Olsson et al. 2006). The central role of VEGF-A binding to VEGFR-1 and VEGFR-2 to enable tumour angiogenesis has led to the development of several anti-VEGF treatments, of which the VEGF monoclonal antibody bevacizumab has been most widely used (Ferrara et al. 2004).

The PDGF family consists of PDFG-A, -B, -C and -D and exerts their effects by binding to the structurally similar PDGF transmembrane receptors (PDGFR-α and PDGFR-β). Ligand binding results in receptor dimerization and autophosphorylation of the PDGFR tyrosine kinase (Andrae et al. 2008). This propagates downstream signalling which, in common with EGFR, c-Met and IGF-1R, includes the MAPK and PI3K/Akt pathways known to be associated with increased cell proliferation and resistance to cell death.

PDGF has been implicated as a mediator of both acute and chronic inflammation and, in particular, has been associated with the development of pulmonary, hepatic, cardiac and renal fibrosis (Andrae et al. 2008). Preclinically, the expression levels of PDGF and PDGFR have been shown to be elevated in rats with radiation-induced pulmonary fibrosis (Tada et al. 2003). In vivo experiments have shown that three different drugs targeting the PDGF receptor tyrosine kinase reduced radiation-induced pulmonary fibrosis in irradiated mice on the basis of physiological, radiological and histological endpoints (Abdollahi et al. 2005). Since pulmonary pneumonitis and fibrosis are key dose-limiting factors in radiotherapy treatment for lung cancer, there is therefore potential interest in using PDGFR inhibitors as antifibrotic treatments to protect normal lung tissue from the side effects of radiotherapy (Gross 1977; Li et al. 2007).

PDGF is also known to contribute to tumour angiogenesis primarily through actions on pericytes and vascular smooth muscle cells (Battegay et al. 1994; Risau et al. 1992; Xue et al. 2012; Abramsson et al. 2003). Although it may seem surprising that disrupting tumour angiogenesis should augment the effects of radiotherapy, since disrupting the tumour vasculature could lead to reduced perfusion and therefore increased hypoxia, there is significant preclinical evidence that antiangiogenesis treatments cause tumour radiosensitization. This has resulted in the development of over forty clinical studies combining radiation and angiogenesis inhibition. Although many of these studies are with bevacizumab, several studies are combining radiotherapy with the tyrosine kinase inhibitors, sorafenib and sunitinib, which both inhibit PDGFR as well as VEGFR (Kleibeuker et al. 2012).

It has been suggested that the mechanism by which bevacizumab augments radiotherapy treatment may be due to "vascular normalization" in which the normal structure and function of the tumour vessels are restored, thereby reducing tumour hypoxia, rather than by true inhibition of angiogenesis (Goel et al. 2011). Bevacizumab has been shown to cause such changes in murine xenograft experiments, but even in these murine models, the effects appear to be transient, and treatment beyond five days may potentially increase tumour hypoxia (Dings et al. 2007). The transient nature of this normalization may account for the disappointing results seen in two phase III trials showing that the addition of bevacizumab to chemoradiotherapy treatment for glioblastoma multiforme (GBM) failed to improve overall survival (Chinot et al. 2014; Gilbert et al. 2014)

6   Conclusions

Although data are heterogeneous, EGFR expression itself plays a major role for prognosis of patients after radiotherapy. There is good evidence that the EGFR is involved in repopulation of tumour cells during fractionated radiotherapy, leading to worse locoregional tumour control rates for high EGFR-expressing head and neck squamous cell carcinoma as compared to lower EGFR-expressing tumours. Inhibition of the EGFR during radiotherapy leads to improvement of local tumour control in head and neck squamous cell carcinoma, when anti-EGFR antibodies (cetuximab) are used. However, the effects are heterogeneous and warrant the establishment of biomarkers to identify individuals likely to respond to combined cetuximab/RT treatment. For other ErbB inhibitors, similar functions may exist, but data are sparse and conclusions currently not justified.

The realization that non-EGFR receptor tyrosine kinases such as c-Met and IGF-1R may play important roles in tumour radioresistance, combined with the development of effective compounds against these targets, has prompted significant interest from within the radiation oncology community. There is clearly the potential for these RTKs to be used as biomarkers to predict response to radiotherapy treatment. In addition, future studies may ascertain whether patients with the activation of these pathways benefit from treatment adaptations such as radiation dose escalation. A potentially even more exciting approach is to combine radiotherapy with inhibitors against these RTKs, and this may significantly increase the effectiveness of radiotherapy.

Importantly, RTKs such as c-Met, IGF-1R and PDGFR all involve a degree of crosstalk with EGFR by signalling through the MAPK and PI3K/Akt pathways. Effective inhibitors against several downstream components of these pathways have been shown to cause tumour radiosensitization preclinically. These include MEK inhibitors such as AZD6244 (Astrazeneca) (Chung et al. 2009) which is now being used in phase I studies with concurrent radiotherapy in NSCLC and chemoradiotherapy in rectal carcinoma, and PI3K inhibitors such as BKM120 (Novartis) (Fokas et al. 2012) which is in early phase trials with radiotherapy in NSCLC and chemoradiotherapy in GBM. It remains to be seen whether inhibiting these downstream components of several different classes of RTK may be the most effective and pragmatic approach to radiosensitizing tumours clinically rather than by inhibiting the RTKs directly.

References

Abdollahi A et al (2005) Inhibition of platelet-derived growth factor signaling attenuates pulmonary fibrosis. J Exp Med 201(6):925–935

Abramsson A, Lindblom P, Betsholtz C (2003) Endothelial and nonendothelial sources of PDGF-B regulate pericyte recruitment and influence vascular pattern formation in tumors. J Clin Invest 112(8):1142–1151

Adams TE et al (2000) Structure and function of the type 1 insulin-like growth factor receptor. Cell Mol Life Sci 57(7):1050–1093

Aebersold DM et al (2001) Involvement of the hepatocyte growth factor/scatter factor receptor c-met and of Bcl-xL in the resistance of oropharyngeal cancer to ionizing. Int J Cancer 96 (1):41–54

Andrae J, Gallini R, Betsholtz C (2008) Role of platelet-derived growth factors in physiology and medicine. Genes Dev 22(10):1276–1312

Ang KK et al (2002) Impact of epidermal growth factor receptor expression on survival and pattern of relapse in patients with advanced head and neck carcinoma. Cancer Res 62 (24):7350–7356

Arcaro A (2013) Targeting the insulin-like growth factor-1 receptor in human cancer. Front Pharmacol 4:30

Arnaldez FI, Helman LJ (2012) Targeting the insulin growth factor receptor 1. Hematol Oncol Clin North Am 26(3):527–542

Battegay EJ et al (1994) PDGF-BB modulates endothelial proliferation and angiogenesis in vitro via PDGF beta-receptors. J Cell Biol 125(4):917–928

Baumann M et al (2007) EGFR-targeted anti-cancer drugs in radiotherapy: preclinical evaluation of mechanisms. Radiother Oncol 83(3):238–248

Bentzen SM et al (2005) Epidermal growth factor receptor expression in pretreatment biopsies from head and neck squamous cell carcinoma as a predictive factor for a benefit from accelerated radiation therapy in a randomized controlled trial. J Clin Oncol 23(24):5560–5567

Bernhard EJ et al (2000) Direct evidence for the contribution of activated N-ras and K-ras oncogenes to increased intrinsic radiation resistance in human tumor cell lines. Cancer Res 60 (23):6597–6600

Bhardwaj V et al (2012) C-Met inhibitor MK-8003 radiosensitizes c-Met-expressing non-small-cell lung cancer cells with radiation-induced c-Met-expression. J Thorac Oncol 7 (8):1211–1217

Bokemeyer C et al (2009) Fluorouracil, leucovorin, and oxaliplatin with and without cetuximab in the first-line treatment of metastatic colorectal cancer. J Clin Oncol 27(5):663–671

Bonner JA et al (2006) Radiotherapy plus cetuximab for squamous-cell carcinoma of the head and neck. N Engl J Med 354(6):567–578

Bonner JA et al (2010) Radiotherapy plus cetuximab for locoregionally advanced head and neck cancer: 5-year survival data from a phase 3 randomised trial, and relation between cetuximab-induced rash and survival. Lancet Oncol 11(1):21–28

Burtness B, Bauman JE, Galloway T (2013) Novel targets in HPV-negative head and neck cancer: overcoming resistance to EGFR inhibition. Lancet Oncol 14(8):e302–e309

Cappuzzo F et al (2009) Increased MET gene copy number negatively affects survival of surgically resected non-small-cell lung cancer patients. J Clin Oncol 27(10):1667–1674

Caudell JJ et al (2008) Locoregionally advanced head and neck cancer treated with primary radiotherapy: a comparison of the addition of cetuximab or chemotherapy and the impact of protocol treatment. Int J Radiat Oncol Biol Phys 71(3):676–681

Chakravarti A et al (2002) The epidermal growth factor receptor pathway mediates resistance to sequential administration of radiation and chemotherapy in primary human glioblastoma cells in a RAS-dependent manner. Cancer Res 62(15):4307–4315

Chakravarti A et al. (2005a) Expression of the epidermal growth factor receptor and HER-2 are predictors of favorable outcome and reduced complete response rates, respectively, in patients with muscle-invading bladder cancers treated by concurrent radiation and cisplatin-based chemotherapy: a report from the radiation therapy oncology group. Int J Radiat Oncol Biol Phys 62(2):309–317

Chakravarti A et al. (2005b) Immunohistochemically determined total epidermal growth factor receptor levels not of prognostic value in newly diagnosed glioblastoma multiforme: report from the radiation therapy oncology group. Int J Radiat Oncol Biol Phys 62(2)318–327

Chinot OL et al (2014) Bevacizumab plus radiotherapy-temozolomide for newly diagnosed glioblastoma. N Engl J Med 370(8):709–722

Chitnis MM et al. (2013) IGF-1R inhibition enhances radiosensitivity and delays double-strand break repair by both non-homologous end-joining and homologous recombination. Oncogene

Chung EJ et al (2009) In vitro and in vivo radiosensitization with AZD6244 (ARRY-142886), an inhibitor of mitogen-activated protein kinase/extracellular signal-regulated kinase 1/2 kinase. Clin Cancer Res 15(9):3050–3057

Contessa JN et al (2006) Compensatory ErbB3/c-Src signaling enhances carcinoma cell survival to ionizing radiation. Breast Cancer Res Treat 95(1):17–27

De Bacco F et al (2011) Induction of MET by ionizing radiation and its role in radioresistance and invasive growth of cancer. J Natl Cancer Inst 103(8):645–661

Dings RP et al (2007) Scheduling of radiation with angiogenesis inhibitors anginex and Avastin improves therapeutic outcome via vessel normalization. Clin Cancer Res 13(11):3395–3402

Duru N et al (2012) HER2-associated radioresistance of breast cancer stem cells isolated from HER2-negative breast cancer cells. Clin Cancer Res 18(24):6634–6647

Eberhard DA et al (2005) Mutations in the epidermal growth factor receptor and in KRAS are predictive and prognostic indicators in patients with non-small-cell lung cancer treated with chemotherapy alone and in combination with erlotinib. J Clin Oncol 23(25):5900–5909

Eicheler W et al (2005) Kinetics of EGFR expression during fractionated irradiation varies between different human squamous cell carcinoma lines in nude mice. Radiother Oncol 76(2):151–156

Eriksen JG, Steiniche T, Overgaard J et al (2005) The influence of epidermal growth factor receptor and tumor differentiation on the response to accelerated radiotherapy of squamous cell carcinomas of the head and neck in the randomized DAHANCA 6 and 7 study. Radiother Oncol 74(2):93–100

Fan S et al (1998) Scatter factor protects epithelial and carcinoma cells against apoptosis induced by DNA-damaging agents. Oncogene 17(2):131–141

Fan S et al (2000) The cytokine hepatocyte growth factor/scatter factor inhibits apoptosis and enhances DNA repair by a common mechanism involving signaling through phosphatidyl inositol 3' kinase. Oncogene 19(18):2212–2223

Favelyukis S et al (2001) Structure and autoregulation of the insulin-like growth factor 1 receptor kinase. Nat Struct Biol 8(12):1058–1063

Ferrara N et al (2004) Discovery and development of bevacizumab, an anti-VEGF antibody for treating cancer. Nat Rev Drug Discov 3(5):391–400

Fidler MJ et al (2012) Targeting the insulin-like growth factor receptor pathway in lung cancer: problems and pitfalls. Ther Adv Med Oncol 4(2):51–60

Fokas E et al (2012) Dual inhibition of the PI3K/mTOR pathway increases tumor radiosensitivity by normalizing tumor vasculature. Cancer Res 72(1):239–248

Gately K et al (2014) High coexpression of both EGFR and IGF1R correlates with poor patient prognosis in resected non-small-cell lung cancer. Clin Lung Cancer 15(1):58–66

Gilbert MR et al (2014) A randomized trial of bevacizumab for newly diagnosed glioblastoma. N Engl J Med 370(8):699–708

Goel S et al (2011) Normalization of the vasculature for treatment of cancer and other diseases. Physiol Rev 91(3):1071–1121

Gross NJ (1977) Pulmonary effects of radiation therapy. Ann Intern Med 86(1):81–92

Gurtner K et al (2011) Diverse effects of combined radiotherapy and EGFR inhibition with antibodies or TK inhibitors on local tumour control and correlation with EGFR gene expression. Radiother Oncol 99:323–330

Gurtner K et al. (2013) EGFR-amplification correlates with response to combined treatment of fractionated irradiation and EGFR-inhibition in HNSCC tumour xenografts. In: 17th European Cancer conference (ECCO), Amsterdam, p 51

Hirsch FR et al (2003) Epidermal growth factor receptor in non-small-cell lung carcinomas: correlation between gene copy number and protein expression and impact on prognosis. J Clin Oncol 21(20):3798–3807

Hirsch FR et al (2006) Molecular predictors of outcome with gefitinib in a phase III placebo-controlled study in advanced non-small-cell lung cancer. J Clin Oncol 24(31):5034–5042

Homsi J, Daud AI (2007) Spectrum of activity and mechanism of action of VEGF/PDGF inhibitors. Cancer Control 14(3):285–294

Iwasa T et al (2009) Inhibition of insulin-like growth factor 1 receptor by CP-751,871 radiosensitizes non-small cell lung cancer cells. Clin Cancer Res 15(16):5117–5125

Jeon YK et al (2006) Clinicopathologic features and prognostic implications of epidermal growth factor receptor (EGFR) gene copy number and protein expression in non-small cell lung cancer. Lung Cancer 54(3):387–398

Johnson BE, Janne PA (2005) Epidermal growth factor receptor mutations in patients with non-small cell lung cancer. Cancer Res 65(17):7525–7529

Karapetis CS et al (2008) K-ras mutations and benefit from cetuximab in advanced colorectal cancer. N Engl J Med 359(17):1757–1765

Kleibeuker EA et al (2012) Combining angiogenesis inhibition and radiotherapy: a double-edged sword. Drug Resist Updat 15(3):173–182

Koi L et al (2014) Radiolabeled anti-EGFR-antibody improves local tumor control after external beam radiotherapy and offers theragnostic potential. Radiother Oncol 110(2):362–369

Kong DS et al (2009) Prognostic significance of c-Met expression in glioblastomas. Cancer 115 (1):140–148

Krause M, Baumann M (2008) Clinical biomarkers of kinase activity: examples from EGFR inhibition trials. Cancer Metastasis Rev 27(3):387–402

Lara PC et al (2011) IGF-1R expression predicts clinical outcome in patients with locally advanced oral squamous cell carcinoma. Oral Oncol 47(7):615–619

Ledel F et al (2014) HER3 expression in patients with primary colorectal cancer and corresponding lymph node metastases related to clinical outcome. Eur J Cancer 50(3):656–662

Lee CM et al (2005) Correlation between human epidermal growth factor receptor family (EGFR, HER2, HER3, HER4), phosphorylated Akt (P-Akt), and clinical outcomes after radiation therapy in carcinoma of the cervix. Gynecol Oncol 99(2):415–421

Li M, Jendrossek V, Belka C (2007) The role of PDGF in radiation oncology. Radiat Oncol 2:5

Linge et al (2016) Clin Cancer Res, epub doi: 10.1158/1078-0432.CCR-15-1990

Lipton A et al (2013) HER3, p95HER2, and HER2 protein expression levels define multiple subtypes of HER2-positive metastatic breast cancer. Breast Cancer Res Treat 141(1):43–53

Lloret M et al (2008) MVP expression is related to IGF1-R in cervical carcinoma patients treated by radiochemotherapy. Gynecol Oncol 110(3):304–307

Ludovini V et al (2013) Concomitant high gene copy number and protein overexpression of IGF1R and EGFR negatively affect disease-free survival of surgically resected non-small-cell-lung cancer patients. Cancer Chemother Pharmacol 71(3):671–680

Ma PC et al (2003) c-MET mutational analysis in small cell lung cancer: novel juxtamembrane domain mutations regulating cytoskeletal functions. Cancer Res 63(19):6272–6281

Ma PC et al (2008) Expression and mutational analysis of MET in human solid cancers. Genes Chromosomes Cancer 47(12):1025–1037

Macaulay VM et al (2001) Downregulation of the type 1 insulin-like growth factor receptor in mouse melanoma cells is associated with enhanced radiosensitivity and impaired activation of Atm kinase. Oncogene 20(30):4029–4040

Marioni G et al (2011) Laryngeal carcinoma prognosis after postoperative radiotherapy correlates with CD105 expression, but not with angiogenin or EGFR expression. Eur Arch Otorhinolaryngol 268(12):1779–1787

Maulik G et al (2002) Role of the hepatocyte growth factor receptor, c-Met, in oncogenesis and potential for therapeutic inhibition. Cytokine Growth Factor Rev 13(1):41–59

Moreno-Acosta P et al (2012) IGF1R gene expression as a predictive marker of response to ionizing radiation for patients with locally advanced HPV16-positive cervical cancer. Anticancer Res 32(10):4319–4325

Nicholson RI, Gee JM, Harper ME (2001) EGFR and cancer prognosis. Eur J Cancer 37(Suppl 4):9–15

Olsson AK et al (2006) VEGF receptor signalling—in control of vascular function. Nat Rev Mol Cell Biol 7(5):359–371

Organ SL, Tsao MS (2011) An overview of the c-MET signaling pathway. Ther Adv Med Oncol 3(1 Suppl):S7–S19

Ou SH (2011) Crizotinib: a novel and first-in-class multitargeted tyrosine kinase inhibitor for the treatment of anaplastic lymphoma kinase rearranged non-small cell lung cancer and beyond. Drug Des Devel Ther 5:471–485

Peretz S et al (2001) ATM-dependent expression of the insulin-like growth factor-I receptor in a pathway regulating radiation response. Proc Natl Acad Sci U.S.A. 98(4):1676–1681

Petersen C et al (2003) Proliferation and micromilieu during fractionated irradiation of human FaDu squamous cell carcinoma in nude mice. Int J Radiat Biol 79(7):469–477

Ponzetto C et al (1994) A multifunctional docking site mediates signaling and transformation by the hepatocyte growth factor/scatter factor receptor family. Cell 77(2):261–271

Riesterer O et al (2011) Combination of anti-IGF-1R antibody A12 and ionizing radiation in upper respiratory tract cancers. Int J Radiat Oncol Biol Phys 79(4):1179–1187

Risau W et al (1992) Platelet-derived growth factor is angiogenic in vivo. Growth Factors 7(4):261–266

Rochester MA et al (2005) Silencing of the IGF1R gene enhances sensitivity to DNA-damaging agents in both PTEN wild-type and mutant human prostate cancer. Cancer Gene Ther 12(1):90–100

Salomon DS et al (1995) Epidermal growth factor-related peptides and their receptors in human malignancies. Crit Rev Oncol Hematol 19(3):183–232

Scagliotti GV, Novello S, von Pawel J (2013) The emerging role of MET/HGF inhibitors in oncology. Cancer Treat Rev 39(7):793–801

Shelton JG et al (2004) Synergy between PI3K/Akt and Raf/MEK/ERK pathways in IGF-1R mediated cell cycle progression and prevention of apoptosis in hematopoietic cells. Cell Cycle 3(3):372–379

Soliman M et al (2013) GTV differentially impacts locoregional control of non-small cell lung cancer (NSCLC) after different fractionation schedules: subgroup analysis of the prospective randomized CHARTWEL trial. Radiother Oncol 106(3):299–304

Tada H et al (2003) Increased binding and chemotactic capacities of PDGF-BB on fibroblasts in radiation pneumonitis. Radiat Res 159(6):805–811

Temam S et al (2007) Epidermal growth factor receptor copy number alterations correlate with poor clinical outcome in patients with head and neck squamous cancer. J Clin Oncol 25(16):2164–2170

Tsao MS et al (2005) Erlotinib in lung cancer—molecular and clinical predictors of outcome. N Engl J Med 353(2):133–144

Turner BC et al (1997) Insulin-like growth factor-I receptor overexpression mediates cellular radioresistance and local breast cancer recurrence after lumpectomy and radiation. Cancer Res 57(15):3079–3083

Valenciano A et al (2012) Role of IGF-1 receptor in radiation response. Transl Oncol 5(1):1–9

Welsh JW et al (2009) The c-Met receptor tyrosine kinase inhibitor MP470 radiosensitizes glioblastoma cells. Radiat Oncol 4:69

Wheeler S et al (2012) Tumor epidermal growth factor receptor and EGFR PY1068 are independent prognostic indicators for head and neck squamous cell carcinoma. Clin Cancer Res 18(8):2278–2289

Xue Y et al (2012) PDGF-BB modulates hematopoiesis and tumor angiogenesis by inducing erythropoietin production in stromal cells. Nat 18(1):100–110

Yavari K et al (2010) SiRNA-mediated IGF-1R inhibition sensitizes human colon cancer SW480 cells to radiation. Acta Oncol 49(1):70–75

Yee D (2012) Insulin-like growth factor receptor inhibitors: baby or the bathwater? J Natl Cancer Inst 104(13):975–981

Yi S, Tsao MS (2000) Activation of hepatocyte growth factor-met autocrine loop enhances tumorigenicity in a human lung adenocarcinoma cell line. Neoplasia 2(3):226–234

Zha J, Lackner MR (2010) Targeting the insulin-like growth factor receptor-1R pathway for cancer therapy. Clin Cancer Res 16(9):2512–2517

Hypoxia as a Biomarker and for Personalized Radiation Oncology

Dirk Vordermark and Michael R. Horsman

Abstract

Tumor hypoxia is a clinically relevant cause of radiation resistance. Direct measurements of tumor oxygenation have been performed predominantly with the Eppendorf histograph and these have defined the reduced prognosis after radiotherapy in poorly oxygenated tumors, especially head-and-neck cancer, cervix cancer and sarcoma. Exogenous markers have been used for immunohistochemical detection of hypoxic tumor areas (pimonidazole) or for positron-emission tomography (PET) imaging (misonidazole). Overexpression of hypoxia-related proteins such as hypoxia-inducible factor-1α (HIF-1α) has also been linked to poor prognosis after radiotherapy and such proteins are considered as potential endogenous hypoxia markers.

Keywords

Tumor hypoxia · Tumor oxygenation · Pimonidazole · Hypoxia-inducible factor-1α

1 Introduction

Intratumoural hypoxia is a clinically relevant condition causing radiation resistance of tumour cells. The insufficient supply of fast-growing tumours with blood vessels and the pathologic structure of intratumoural vessels, respectively, have been

D. Vordermark (✉)
Universitätsklinik und Poliklinik für Strahlentherapie, Martin-Luther-Universität
Halle-Wittenberg, Halle/Saale, Germany
e-mail: dirk.vordermark@medizin.uni-halle.de

M.R. Horsman
Department of Experimental Clinical Oncology, Aarhus University Hospital,
Aarhus, Denmark
e-mail: mike@oncology.au.dk

© Springer-Verlag Berlin Heidelberg 2016
M. Baumann et al. (eds.), *Molecular Radio-Oncology*, Recent Results
in Cancer Research 198, DOI 10.1007/978-3-662-49651-0_6

123

associated with two mechanisms of tumour hypoxia. Specifically, these are diffusion-limited hypoxia caused by long distances of individual tumour cells from the nearest blood vessel versus perfusion-limited tumour hypoxia which can also occur close to (non-perfused) blood vessels due to the presence of vascular leaks, thrombosis or shunts. These two types have also been referred to as "chronic" and "acute" hypoxia, respectively. However, oxygenation of a tumour is considered a dynamic process, and in many tissues, intermittent changes of oxygen concentration are observed ("cyclic hypoxia").

The classic explanation of hypoxia-associated radioresistance in tumour cells is the interference of molecular oxygen with DNA repair. Oxygen has been shown to bind to sites of radiation-induced DNA damage, thereby causing fixation of DNA lesions and preventing repair. In in vitro experiments, an oxygen-enhancement ratio (OER) of 2–3 has been determined, meaning that compared to a reference dose of ionizing radiation under normoxic conditions, 2–3 times this dose has to be given to achieve equivalent cell kill under anoxic (0 % oxygen) conditions.

In vivo, an additional mechanism causing treatment resistance of hypoxic tumours is the selection of tumour cells with increased anti-apoptotic, proliferative and metastatic characteristics by conditions of hypoxia (Graeber et al. 1996). This chapter will discuss currently available methods to detect intratumoural hypoxia and their clinical applicability.

2 Direct Measurements of Tumour Oxygenation

Probably, the most direct method for identifying hypoxia in tumours involves inserting electrodes into the tissue and monitoring the actual oxygenation status. This approach was first applied to human tumours in the 1960s using "home-made" glass electrodes. These early polarographic electrodes were, however, generally cumbersome and fragile, and only a few pO_2 values 3–4 mm below the surface of the tumour were possible. Nevertheless, clinical data were obtained in cervix (Kolstad 1968) and head-and-neck (Gatenby et al. 1988) cancer patients that clearly demonstrated a relationship between the oxygenation measurements and outcome to radiation therapy, in that those patients with tumours that were better oxygenated had a significantly superior local response to irradiation.

This whole area was revolutionized with the development of the Eppendorf histograph, which had two distinct improvements. The first was having a more robust electrode with the oxygen sensor protected inside a metal needle. A second improvement was the attachment of this needle to a stepping motor that allowed for multiple measurements along the needle track through the tumour; thus, detailed oxygen partial pressure (pO_2) distributions were possible. Numerous clinical studies were thus undertaken in a variety of human tumour types. The results clearly showed that hypoxia was a characteristic feature of virtually all human tumours investigated, although the degree of hypoxia could be variable (Vaupel et al. 1989). Probably, the most significant finding from these studies was the confirmation that hypoxia influenced outcome to therapy. This has been reported for head and neck

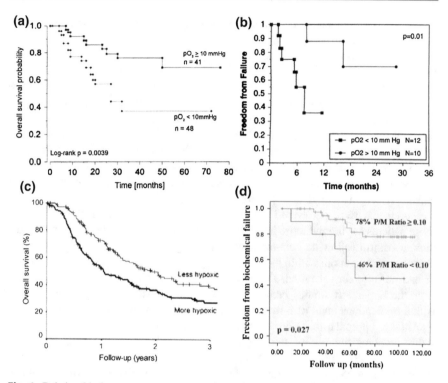

Fig. 1 Relationship between tumour oxygenation estimated prior to therapy using the Eppendorf histograph and eventual outcome to that therapy. **a** Overall survival for 89 cervix patients given surgery or radiotherapy with curative intent in which the median pO_2 values were above or below 10 mmHg. **b** Freedom from distant failure in 22 patients with soft tissue sarcomas receiving preoperative irradiation and hyperthermia in which the tumour median pO_2 values were above or below 10 mmHg. **c** Overall survival for 397 head-and-neck cancer patients after primary radiation therapy in which the percentage of pO_2 values less than or equal to 2.5 mmHg was above (more hypoxic) or below (less hypoxic) the median value of 19 %. **d** Freedom from biochemical failure for 57 prostate patients treated with brachytherapy in which the prostate/muscle (P/M) mean pO_2 ratio was above or below 0.10. Composite figure derived from Hoeckel et al. (1996) (**a**); Brizel et al. (1996) (**b**); Nordsmark et al. (2005) (**c**); and Turaka et al. (2011) (**d**)

(Nordsmark et al. 1996, 2005; Brizel et al. 1997; Stadler et al. 1999; Rudat et al. 2001), cervix (Hoeckel et al. 1993, 1996; Knocke et al. 1999; Fyles et al. 1998, 2006; Lyng et al. 2000), soft tissue sarcomas (Brizel et al. 1996; Nordsmark et al. 2001), and prostate (Turaka et al. 2011). Examples of the typical results obtained in each of these clinical sites are illustrated in Fig. 1 and clearly show that patients with more hypoxic tumours had a poorer outcome to therapy. Perhaps the most striking results were those made in cervix and sarcomas that showed hypoxia to influence outcome in patients in which surgery was the primary or only treatment (Hoeckel et al. 1996; Nordsmark et al. 2001), suggesting that hypoxia could also influence malignant progression, especially metastatic spread. In fact, one other study in cervix was able to show that the primary tumours of patients with metastases were indeed more poorly oxygenated than those of patients without metastases (Sundfør et al. 1998).

Today, the Eppendorf electrode is no longer commercially available, and there are a number of reasons for this. Without using concurrent imaging during the oxygen measurements, it was impossible to state whether the values obtained were from viable tissue, and even where this was done one could not state whether the cells in the hypoxic regions were clonogenic; the tumours themselves had generally to be easily accessible; and the technique was invasive. Furthermore, despite the positive findings between the Eppendorf measurements and treatment outcome, the machine was never predictive of response on a patient-to-patient basis. This was clearly illustrated in one of the first clinical studies using head-and-neck cancer patients (Nordsmark et al. 1996). Here, the 35 patients in which tumour oxygenation measurements were performed could be separated into two distinct groups with those patients having the more hypoxic tumours showing a significantly lower local tumour control following conventional radiation therapy. However, some 40 % of the patients did not fall within the correct category; they were hypoxic but controlled or had no hypoxia yet failed. Despite the various limitations, the results obtained from the Eppendorf studies must still be considered positive in that it supplied us with a tremendous level of information about tumour hypoxia and its importance.

Another approach that may have the potential to measure tumour oxygenation status involves the use of fibre optic probes. Unlike the Eppendorf histogram electrode, these do not consume oxygen with each measurement; thus; continuous observations of oxygenation status in the same tumour region is possible (Griffiths and Robinson 1999). Preclinical studies comparing the commercially available Oxford-Optronix OxyLite sensor with the polarographic techniques (Collingridge et al. 1997; Braun et al. 2001; Seddon et al. 2001; Wen et al. 2008), or classical paired survival curve estimates of radiobiological hypoxia (Urano et al. 2002), reported similarities and differences depending on the tissue type, tumour size or the changes observed using various modifiers of tumour hypoxia. Although fibre optic probes have the potential to not only measure the pretreatment level of tumour hypoxia, but also to monitor tumour oxygenation status continuously during and after treatment, there has as yet been no clinical application in cancer.

Other less invasive attempts to directly measure tumour oxygenation have involved phosphorescence tomography- or magnetic resonance (MR)-based approaches. The former requires the infusion of water-soluble phosphor probes into the vasculature (Vikram et al. 2007) and has been used to map oxygen concentration in preclinical tumour models (Wilson and Cerniglia 1992; Fukumura et al. 2001), but again has not been used in patients. The MR approaches include monitoring oxygen-sensitive reporter molecules (^{19}F-oximetry). Several such molecules have been developed including perfluorochemical emulsions and hexafluorobenzene (Pacheco-Torres et al. 2011). The latter approach allowed for actual quantification of the MR signals and conversion into oxygen concentrations at the pixel level (Zhao et al. 2005). However, systemic toxicity required the imaging agent to be injected directly into tumours limiting its potential clinical application. An alternative MR method is electron paramagnetic resonance (EPR), which detects paramagnetic materials that have been injected into tissues (Krishna et al. 2012). It can provide quantitative and repeated 3D estimates of oxygenation and has been extensively used in preclinical studies and even in patients for a range of different clinical problems (Swartz et al. 2004). Although many of the preclinical studies have focused on tumour hypoxia, the clinical application of EPR in cancer has, however, been somewhat limited (Krishna et al. 2012).

3 Exogenous Markers of Hypoxia

The oxygen mapping techniques described above involve injecting exogenous agents to directly ascertain oxygen values that are low and equivalent to hypoxia. A more widely studied method for indirectly detecting tumour hypoxia involves the administration of exogenous compounds that under hypoxic conditions undergoes a chemical change from a non-reactive species to a highly reactive product that then binds to macromolecules within the cell. Subsequent application of techniques that can identify this bound product will allow us to demonstrate the presence of hypoxia. The most popular agents used in this context have been 2-nitroimidazole-based markers. These nitroimidazole compounds were originally developed as hypoxic cell radiosensitizers, with the 2-nitroimidazoles being the most effective agents for enhancing radiation response in preclinical models (Adams and Cooke 1969). Such compounds are characterized by having an NO_2 grouping attached to the imidazole ring structure. This NO_2 group can undergo a 6-electron intracellular reduction to produce NH_2, and although the NO_2 and NH_2 moieties are generally inactive, one of the formed intermediates is highly reactive and can bind to any macromolecule within the cell (Horsman et al. 2012). In the presence of oxygen, typically above 10 mmHg, the first electron reduction species formed reacts with oxygen and returns to the NO_2 moiety with the subsequent production of oxygen radicals that ultimately form hydrogen peroxide, and it is this lack of further reduction that gives rise to the hypoxia specificity. The bound product formed under hypoxia can be identified either using an antibody to the product or by labelling the original compound with a radioactive tracer such as ^1H or ^{14}C. The most commonly used nitroimidazole is pimonidazole, the binding of which in preclinical studies was found to correlate with radiobiological hypoxia (Raleigh et al. 1999). Additional clinical studies showed that the degree of pimonidazole binding was related to radiation-induced local tumour control in head-and-neck cancer (Kaanders et al. 2002), but not cervix (Nordsmark et al. 2006). Similar positive findings for head-and-neck cancer patients were reported between radiotherapy outcome and the degree of hypoxia estimated using another nitroimidazole marker, EF5 (Evans et al. 2007).

By labelling the nitroimidazole compound with ^{18}F will allow for the hypoxia produced bound product to be identified using positron emission tomography (PET). The first tracer developed for hypoxia PET imaging was a $[^{18}F]$-fluorinated version of the radiosensitizer misonidazole (FMISO) and was found to be capable of identifying hypoxia in a range of human tumours (Rasey et al. 1996). It was followed by a group of compounds based on another radiosensitizer, etanidazole (i.e. EF3/5). These markers have a relatively high lipophilicity which allows for easy penetration of cell membranes and diffusion into tumour tissue, but simultaneously limited the clearance of unbound tracer, thus leading to relatively low tumour-to-reference tissue ratios. Other fluorinated nitroimidazole compounds have been developed which are more water soluble than FMISO and therefore easier to clear from non-hypoxic tissue. These have included fluoroetanidazole (FETA), fluoroerythronitroimidazole (FETNIM), fluoroazomycinarabinofuranoside (FAZA) and HX4, of which the latter two are currently in clinical evaluation (Schuetz et al. 2010; van Loon et al. 2010). It is difficult to say whether one tracer is superior to another in identifying tumour hypoxia, since there has never been any systematic examination of all the 2-nitroimidazoles tracers in the same tumour model or patient population. The ideal tracer would be one in which clearance of unbound tracer is complete at the time of imaging; thus, only bound material indicative of hypoxia is measured. This can take many hours and even days to achieve, but such measurements have to take into account decay of the radioactive marker and normal clinical schedules. As a result, static scans are typically made 2–4 h after tracer administration, which results in low inter-tissue and intratumour contrast. An alternative approach involves labelling the nitroimidazoles with long-lived radionuclides, for example $[^{124}I]$-iodoazomycin arabinoside (^{124}I-AZA) and $[^{124}I]$-iodoazomycin galactoside (^{124}I-AZG), allowing for delayed scans up to 24 and 48 h after tracer administration. Unfortunately, the results have been disappointing with no improvement in image contrast and poor counting statistics (Rischin et al. 2006; Reischi et al. 2007), and it is unlikely that the problems inherent to hypoxia PET can be solved exclusively by better tracers. One small study in head-and-neck cancer patients (Thorwarth et al. 2005) demonstrated that pharmacokinetic analysis of the shape of tumour time activity curves (TACs) obtained from dynamic PET scans increased prognostic accuracy compared to traditional analysis of static PET images. However, dynamic scans are cumbersome and expensive, and cause inconvenience to patients; the analysis is complex; and different estimates of hypoxia can be obtained depending on the kinetic model and tumour type used.

Regardless of whether static or dynamic assessment is applied, one of the major issues with PET markers is that the cells must be hypoxic for significant time periods to be detected, which means that such markers are more likely to identify diffusion-limited chronic hypoxia rather than acute hypoxia resulting from transient fluctuations in blood flow (Horsman et al. 2012). Another significant problem facing the application of PET hypoxia markers is one of resolution in which the voxel sizes identified in the PET scans are much larger than most of the hypoxic structures (Horsman et al. 2012). Thus, the actual PET image does not accurately reflect the true hypoxia heterogeneity at the microregional level.

Several of the nitroimidazole-based PET markers have undergone clinical evaluation with respect to correlating the hypoxia estimates with outcome to radiation therapy. The majority of studies involved FMISO measurements in head-and-neck cancer patients (Rajendran et al. 2006; Rischin et al. 2006; Thorwarth et al. 2006; Eschmann et al. 2007; Dirix et al. 2009; Lee et al. 2009; Kikuchi et al. 2011;

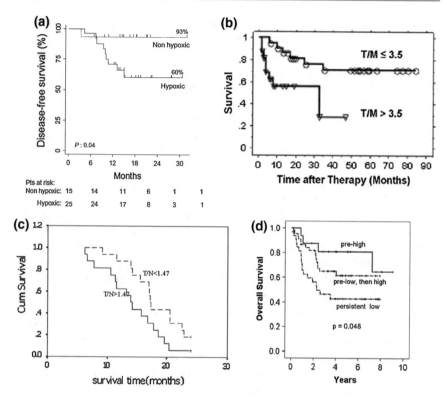

Fig. 2 Results from four different clinical trials showing the relationship between hypoxia imaging and outcome to therapy. **a** Disease-free survival in 40 head-and-neck cancer patients based on the preradiation therapy estimate of hypoxia as determined by a tumour-to-muscle ratio of ≥ 1.4 from [^{18}F] FAZA PET measurements. **b** Progression-free survival in 38 cervical cancer patients receiving radiotherapy and chemoradiotherapy in which the tumour/muscle (T/M) levels of ^{60}Cu-ATSM were above or below the threshold dose of 3.5. **c** Overall survival for 32 non-small-cell lung cancer patients in which the tumour-to-normal tissue (T/N) ratio measured with ^{99m}Tc-HL91 SPECT before radiation therapy was above/below 1.47. **d** Disease-specific survival in 98 cancer patients based on the level of perfusion measured with DCE-MRI either before or before and during radiation treatment. Composite figure derived from Mortensen et al. (2012) (**a**); Dehdashti et al. (2008) (**b**); Li et al. (2006) (**c**); and Mayr et al. (2010) (**d**)

Zips et al. 2012). Two other studies in head and neck used either FETNIM (Lehtio et al. 2004) or FAZA (Mortensen et al. 2012). Results from the latter study using FAZA as the imaging agent are illustrated in Fig. 2 and clearly show that like all the other head-and-neck studies, patients with hypoxic tumours had a significantly poorer outcome. Similar findings were found using FETNIM in lung (Li et al. 2010) and oesophagus (Yue et al. 2012), FAZA in sarcomas (Khamly et al. 2008) and cervix (Scheutz et al. 2010) and FMISO in central nervous system tumours (Spence et al. 2008). Despite the positive findings obtained with all these nitroimidazole-based hypoxia PET markers, the situation remains the same as seen with the oxygen electrode methods in that although we can verify the presence of hypoxia in human tumours and demonstrate that it influences outcome to therapy, we still cannot use the results to select those patients that are hypoxic on an individual basis.

A chemically different group of putative PET markers that may have the potential to identify tumour hypoxia includes Cu-ATSM [Cu(II)-diacetyl-*bis*(N^4-methyl-thiosemicarbazone)], which can be labelled with a variety of positron-emitting isotopes of copper. Cu-ATSM has been shown to have high membrane permeability and fast tumour uptake, thus allowing for rapid imaging after injection (Dearling et al. 1998), but its exact retention mechanism is still not completely understood. The hypoxia specificity is believed to occur because while the Cu^{2+} moiety can easily pass across cell membranes, under low oxygen conditions the Cu^{2+} is converted to Cu^{1+} which is then trapped within cells (Vävere and lewis 2007). A good correlation between Cu-ATSM and pO_2 measurements (Lewis and Welch 2001; O'Donoghue et al. 2005) and nitroimidazole-based hypoxia markers (O'Donoghue et al. 2005; Dence et al. 2008) have been shown in preclinical studies, although these effects are time- and tumour-dependent (O'Donoghue et al. 2005). Measurements in patients with lung (Dehdashti et al. 2003), cervix (Dehdashti et al. 2008), rectal (Dietz et al. 2008) or head-and-neck (Minagawa et al. 2011) cancer support the possibility of using Cu-ATSM as a marker of outcome to radiotherapy. The results from the cervix trial (Dehdashti et al. 2008) are shown in Fig. 2 and clearly demonstrate that those patients with a higher tumour uptake of Cu-ATSM, and presumably more hypoxic, had a lower progression-free survival. However, additional studies have shown Cu-ATSM to be affected by mechanisms other than hypoxia and that it is also insensitive to treatments that modify tumour oxygenation (Yuan et al. 2006); thus, its potential to be used as a specific marker for tumour hypoxia remains unclear.

The use of alternative radioactive labels allows for the possibility to use other non-invasive imaging techniques to identify hypoxia in tumours. Such an approach has been achieved with a number of [^{123}I/^{125}I]-iodoazomycin derivatives which can be detected using single-photon emission computer tomography (SPECT). Of these, only [^{123}I]-iodoazomycin arabinoside (IAZA) has undergone clinical evaluation (Urtasun et al. 1996), and it was found that head-and-neck cancer patients with positive IAZA scans had a poorer outcome to radiotherapy than those patients with negative scans. Other potential SPECT markers for hypoxia that have been developed include ^{99m}Technetium-labelled compounds, such as BMS 181321 and BRU59-21, and complex ligands, specifically HL91. BRU59-21 was investigated in a phase I study in patients with head-and-neck cancer, and a significant correlation was found with pimonidazole binding (Hoebers et al. 2002). HL91 uptake was studied in non-small-cell lung cancer patients prior to radiation therapy, and the results, as shown in Fig. 2, demonstrated that those patients with the highest uptake had a significantly poorer response (Li et al. 2006). Various [^{19}F]-labelled nitorimidazole compounds have also been developed which can be detected using MR. To-date, two [^{19}F]-labelled nitroimidazoles have been developed, namely [^{19}F]-EF5 and [^{19}F]-SR 4554. Of these, only [^{19}F]-SR 4554 underwent some clinical evaluations (Seddon et al. 2003), but there has not been any real follow-up.

An alternative MR approach that utilizes measurements made after injecting an exogenous marker is dynamic contrast-enhanced magnetic resonance imaging (DCE-MRI). This involves intravenously injecting a contrast agent and then monitoring its extravasation over several minutes from a region of interest (Nielsen et al. 2012). The focus with these estimates is actually on tumour perfusion, but this may still be an excellent method for identifying tumour hypoxia; oxygen delivery occurs via the vascular supply so the measurements could reflect chronic hypoxia, and changes in perfusion are clearly responsible for fluctuating hypoxia (Horsman et al. 2012). Clinical studies have been performed with DCE-MRI and reported that the parameters obtained actually correlated with oxygen electrode measurements in cervix (Cooper et al. 2000; Lyng et al. 2001), pimonidazole binding in head and neck (Newbold et al. 2009; Donaldson et al. 2011) and [^{18}F]-FMISO uptake in glioblastoma multiforme (Swanson et al. 2009) and head-and-neck nodal metastases (Jansen et al. 2010). Several studies have also attempted to correlate the DCE-MRI measurements with radiotherapy outcome in patients with cervical cancer (Loncaster et al. 2002; Mayr et al. 2010; Andersen et al. 2012) and reported that those patients with supposedly more hypoxic tumours had a poorer response to radiotherapy, as illustrated in Fig. 2. Tumour perfusion can also be estimated with PET following administration of [^{15}O]-labelled water. However, the clinical studies that used this method in head-and-neck cancer have produced conflicting results. One study reported that the [^{15}O]-labelled water perfusion estimates correlated reasonably well with [^{18}F]-EF5 measurements of hypoxia (Komar et al. 2008), but another study found that poor local tumour control and survival after radiation therapy were associated with high blood perfusion rather than the low perfusion one would expect to be indicative of hypoxia (Lehtio et al. 2004).

4 Endogenous Markers of Hypoxia

As an alternative to invasive electrode measurements or exogenously applied hypoxia markers, molecules expressed under (patho)physiological conditions of low oxygenation have been studied as potential "endogenous" or "intrinsic" hypoxia markers. Most of these studies are related to hypoxia-inducible factor-1α (HIF-1α), a transcription factor subunit considered to be the main regulator of the hypoxia response in mammalian cells. HIF-1α protein accumulates in the nucleus under hypoxic conditions and binds to hypoxia-responsive elements in the promoter regions of hypoxia-regulated genes, including erythropoietin (EPO), carbonic anhydrase IX (CA IX), glucose transporter 1 (GLUT1) and vascular endothelial growth factor (VEGF). Therefore, both HIF-1α protein itself and mRNA or protein of HIF-1-regulated genes could serve as indicators of tumour hypoxia.

An appropriate marker of hypoxic radioresistance should become overexpressed or accumulate at a level of hypoxia which is relevant for cellular radiosensitivity. The half-maximal oxygen effect on radiosensitivity is observed at about 0.5 % O_2 (Hall 1988). HIF-1α protein has been shown to be detectable in HeLa cells after 4 h at 20 % O_2 with a moderate increase between 20 and 6 %, a strong increase below

6 % and a maximum expression at 0.5 % (Jiang et al. 1996). In U87 MG human glioma cells, a constant increase in HIF-1α protein could be shown between 2 and <0.02 % O_2, for *in vitro* hypoxia durations between 1 and 18 h (Vordermark and Brown 2003).

The temporal response of HIF-1α protein response to hypoxia (and reoxygenation) has been described as rather rapid: in HeLa cells, induction of HIF-1α protein was observed after 2 min of hypoxia, a maximum expression was seen after 1 h, and after 32 min of reoxygenation, the protein was again undetectable (Jewell et al. 2001). These data indicate that HIF-1α protein expression in tissue can occur already at higher oxygen concentrations where radiosensitivity of cells is not yet compromised and that care must be taken in processing of surgical/biopsy tissue to account for the immediate response to changes in oxygenation. Colocalization studies of HIF-1α and injectable hypoxia markers in xenograft tumours have supported the assumption that HIF-1-related hypoxia markers accumulate at higher O_2 concentrations (i.e. closer to perfused blood vessels) than exogenous markers such as EF5 (Vukovic et al. 2001).

Among the HIF-1-regulated genes, the membrane enzyme carbonic anhydrase IX (CA IX) has received the most attention as a potential endogenous hypoxia marker for use in radiotherapy. In vitro, a continuous increase of CA IX protein expression has been described in A-549 lung carcinoma cells exposed to decreasing O_2 concentrations from 5 to 0.1 % (Wykoff et al. 2000). Long-term hypoxia (24 h at 1.5 % O_2) was found to result in higher CA IX levels than exposure for up to 10 h, suggesting that CA IX indicates predominantly prolonged exposure of cells to hypoxia (Lal et al. 2001). In FaDu head-and-neck squamous cell carcinoma, expression of CA IX increased over a radiosensitivity-relevant range of oxygen concentrations, resulting in a correlation of CA IX protein and cellular radioresistance (Vordermark et al. 2005).

The possibility to detect HIF-1α protein and related proteins such as CA IX in archival tumour material from patients with an already known clinical course of disease has motivated researchers to analyse the relationship of marker expression on immunohistochemistry and clinical outcome (e.g. survival and local control) after cancer treatment, especially radiotherapy. In early histopathological series investigating a number of different tumour types, HIF-1α has been detected in 40–82 % of prostate cancers, 80–100 % of colon adenocarcinomas and 29–83 % of breast adenocarcinomas (Zhong et al. 1999; Talks et al. 2000), with respective corresponding numbers for CA IX protein of 0, 100 and 26 % (Ivanov et al. 2001).

The HIF-1α immunohistochemical staining pattern observed in sections of human tumour material is not consistent across tumour types and individual studies. In oropharyngeal carcinoma, a typical staining pattern of "diffusion-limited hypoxia" (i.e. positive cells in ring shape at a distance from a central blood vessel) was described in 65 % of positive tumours, with more diffuse patterns in the remainder (Aebersold et al. 2001). Other authors characterized the area of HIF-1α-positive cells as close to a blood vessel (compatible with perfusion-related or "acute" hypoxia) versus distant from a vessel versus unspecific pattern (Haugland et al. 2002). A so-called perinecrotic staining pattern (i.e. accumulation of the marker in the zone most distant from a blood vessel, near regions of necrosis) was also reported in studies of CA IX expression in cervical carcinoma, head-and-neck cancer and non-small-cell lung cancer (Beasley et al. 2001; Giatromanolaki et al. 2001; Loncaster et al. 2001). The use of the term "endogenous hypoxia marker" has been criticized, since immunohistochemical studies of pO_2 electrode measurement tracks in cervix cancer tumour tissue have shown no direct correlation of overexpression of the proteins HIF-1α, CA IX or GLUT1 with the corresponding pO_2 reading (Mayer et al. 2006). This suggests that in vivo additional mechanisms other than the mere oxygenation level modulate expression of the putative endogenous hypoxia markers and that their expression is at least not hypoxia-specific.

However, a vast body of clinical literature suggests that a high level of expression of HIF-1-related proteins is related to poor outcome after cancer treatment. In head-and-neck cancer, several groups reported an association of HIF-1α overexpression and reduced overall survival or disease-specific survival following surgery or radiotherapy or combination treatment (Aebersold et al. 2001; Beasley et al. 2002; Winter et al. 2006). The association of high CA IX expression with poor prognosis in head-and-neck cancer was seen to a lesser extent in comparable studies, and some groups found this marker to be prognostic only in combination with other potential hypoxia markers (Hui et al. 2002; De Schutter et al. 2005) or not at all (Eriksen and Overgaard 2007; Nordsmark et al. 2007).

Cervix cancer, the other tumour entity with strong evidence from oxygen electrode studies of a relationship between tumour oxygenation and clinical response to radiotherapy, has been studied extensively regarding endogenous hypoxia marker expression. In three of the largest series treated with radiotherapy and/or surgery, HIF-1α expression was also significantly associated with overall survival or disease-specific survival on multivariate analysis (Birner et al. 2000; Bachtiary et al. 2003; Burri et al. 2003). Similar associations were found in some, but not all studies of CA IX expression in cervix cancer (Loncaster et al. 2001; Lee et al. 2007).

Other cancer types have been studied extensively regarding endogenous hypoxia marker expression, but with a stronger therapeutic focus on surgery and less impact of radiotherapy, among them breast cancer and lung cancer. Predominant associations of high marker expression and poor survival were observed here as well (review in Bache et al. 2008).

5 Plasma Hypoxia Markers

In theory, the measurement of a hypoxia-related protein secreted from hypoxic tumour cells into the plasma could permit an integrated assessment of both the total tumour burden ("number of cells") and their oxygenation level ("percentage of hypoxic tumour cells"). The best-studied secreted hypoxia-related protein is osteopontin (OPN), a tumour-associated glycoprotein secreted into bodily fluids and in the plasma of tumour patients. Plasma OPN level was shown by Le et al. (2003) to correspond with Eppendorf electrode measurements of tumour oxygenation in patients with head-and-neck cancer, suggesting a role for OPN as an endogenous marker of tumour hypoxia. In a landmark study, Overgaard et al. (2005) showed that only patients with high plasma levels of OPN (upper tertile) significantly benefitted from the addition of nimorazole, a hypoxic radiosensitizer, compared to standard radiotherapy in patients with head-and-neck cancer. OPN may therefore serve as a marker by which to select head-and-neck cancer patients for intensified, hypoxia-specific, treatment. A molecular mechanism for the intracellular accumulation of OPN under hypoxia has been described (Sorensen et al. 2005; Zhu et al. 2005), although secretion of OPN may require additional steps (Said et al. 2005; Lukacova et al. 2006).

Elevated plasma or serum levels of OPN have been reported for several human cancer types including pancreatic, hepatocellular, colon, breast, prostate and lung cancer (Fedarko et al. 2001; Koopmann et al. 2004; Zhang et al. 2006). An association of high OPN plasma levels with poor prognosis has been established for different clinical situations. For instance, Isa et al. (2009) demonstrated that low plasma OPN measured before treatment correlated with improved overall survival and progression-free interval after chemotherapy for non-small-cell lung cancer. Mack et al. (2008) reported an association of elevated OPN plasma levels and inferior overall survival after carboplatin-/paclitaxel-based chemotherapy for advanced non-small-cell lung cancer. Blasberg et al. (2010) could show that OPN plasma levels significantly decreased after resection of early stage lung cancer and increased with later relapse, supporting the potential value of OPN as a biomarker for monitoring the treatment response in lung cancer. Recently, a pilot study of plasma hypoxia markers has also suggested a prognostic role of osteopontin response to radiotherapy of locally advanced non-small-cell lung cancer (Ostheimer et al. 2013)

Given the strong association with both electrode-measured oxygenation (Le et al. 2006) and response of tumour to surgery or chemotherapy in non-small-cell lung cancer, the prognostic potential of plasma OPN in radiotherapy of non-small-cell lung cancer was recently studied. Ostheimer et al. (2013) found in a pilot study of 55 patients with locoregionally advanced non-small-cell lung cancer that a panel of plasma biomarkers (OPN, CA IX and VEGF) in combination was an independent prognostic factor for overall survival in multivariate analysis. Early data on repeated measurements of OPN suggest a prognostic value of increasing plasma OPN over time in patients undergoing radiotherapy. In malignant glioma patients, OPN plasma levels did not decrease after surgical resection which may in part be explained by the fact that resection of such tumours is microscopically incomplete by nature, but also suggests that tumour-unrelated factors, such as wound healing, may contribute to total plasma osteopontin levels (Güttler et al. 2013). Nevertheless, a low plasma level of osteopontin at the end of postoperative radiotherapy identified patients with significantly improved overall survival in this pilot study. In patients with head-and-neck cancer, pretreatment OPN plasma levels were evaluated for outcome after surgery, radiotherapy, combined chemoradiation or sequential combinations. An adverse effect of high pretreatment OPN levels on survival and tumour control was confirmed for the different treatment arms (Petrik et al. 2006). In a separate series, lower pretreatment OPN levels were in favour of better tumour response and superior survival in head-and-neck cancer patients after radiotherapy alone (Snitcovsky et al. 2009).

6 Conclusions and Future Perspectives

Hypoxia is a characteristic feature of human tumours that has a major negative influence on determining tumour response to conventional therapy and is also an important factor in influencing malignant progression, both in terms of the aggressive growth of the primary tumour and its ability for metastatic spread. What is now needed is a method that allows us to identify those individual patients that have tumours containing significant levels of hypoxia, so that we can predict their outcome to therapy and where necessary select alternative treatments to eliminate that hypoxia.

Of course, one of the problems here is that hypoxia is often considered as a single entity when in fact we know that the degree and type of hypoxia found in tumours are very heterogenous (Horsman et al. 2012). At the very least, we have chronic and acute hypoxia, and it is not known whether both types respond equally well to therapy. Even if we could identify regions of both chronic and acute hypoxia within tumours, it is often difficult to state whether the cells in those hostile environments are actually viable and clonogenic. The situation becomes even more complicated because we also know that other microenvironmental factors such as intermediate hypoxia, low pH and glucose deprivation can influence malignant progression and thus outcome. The ideal imaging method must be able to identify all the critical factors. Furthermore, it must also give accurate, reliable and repro-ducible measurements, be easy to use on a routine basis and be applicable to any tumour type regardless of location. A non-invasive method would also be prefer-able. Clearly, no one technique that is currently available can achieve all these criteria. We must, therefore, either rely on measurements made with the best method there is or begin to combine modalities that can give us a better indication of the relevant parameters.

Once we have decided on the most relevant technique for imaging hypoxia, then there is the question of how do we deal with that hypoxia? Numerous preclinical studies have demonstrated a variety of methods that can be applied to eliminate hypoxia (Horsman et al. 2011), and many of these have been successfully applied in the clinic (Horsman and Overgaard 2007; Overgaard 2007), but none is currently in routine clinical use. It has also been suggested that in situations where we can actually image the distribution of hypoxia in tumours, we can then use that infor-mation to increase the radiation dose delivered to the tumour (Ling et al. 2000; Søvik et al. 2009; Bentzen and Gregoire 2011). But, whether that should be an increase to the gross tumour volume in which a substantial hypoxic volume has been identified or simply increase the dose to the biological target volume defined by the hypoxic area is not clear.

At present, we have a wealth of information about tumour hypoxia from a variety of clinically relevant techniques. Although we are not yet in a position to use that data to help us predict outcome on an individual patient basis or decide what we should do to tackle the hypoxia problem, the amount of effort being applied to this area would suggest that it is only a matter of time before we achieve those goals and the hypoxia problem eventually becomes obsolete.

Acknowledgements The authors would like to thank the following organizations for financial support: the Danish Agency for Science Technology and Innovation; the Danish Cancer Society; the EC FP7 project METOXIA (project no. 222741); the German Research Foundation (Deutsche Forschungsgemeinschaft); the Wilhelm Sander Foundation and CIRRO—the Lundbeck Foundation Center for Interventional Research in Radiation Oncology and the Danish Council for Strategic Research.

References

Adams GE, Cooke MS (1969) Electron–affinic sensitization. I. A structural basis for chemical radiosensitizers in bacteria. Int J Radiat Biol 15:457–471

Aebersold DM, Burri P, Beer KT et al (2001) Expression of hypoxia-inducible factor-1alpha: a novel predictive and prognostic parameter in the radiotherapy of oropharyngeal cancer. Cancer Res 61:2911–2916

Andersen EKF, Hole KH, Lund KV et al (2012) Dynamic contrast-enhanced MRI of cervical cancers: temporal percentile screening of contrast enhancement identifies parameters for prediction of chemoradioresistance. Int J Radiat Oncol Biol Phys 82:485–492

Bache M, Kappler M, Said HM et al (2008) Detection and specific targeting of hypoxic regions within solid tumors: current preclinical and clinical strategies. Curr Med Chem 15:322–338

Bachtiary B, Schindl M, Potter R et al (2003) Overexpression of hypoxia-inducible factor 1alpha indicates diminished response to radiotherapy and unfavorable prognosis in patients receiving radical radiotherapy for cervical cancer. Clin Cancer Res 9:2234–2240

Beasley NJ, Wykoff CC, Watson PH et al (2001) Carbonic anhydrase IX, an endogenous hypoxia marker, expression in head and neck squamous cell carcinoma and its relationship to hypoxia, necrosis, and microvessel density. Cancer Res 61:5262–5267

Beasley NJ, Leek R, Alam M et al (2002) Hypoxia-inducible factors HIF-1alpha and HIF-2alpha in head and neck cancer: relationship to tumor biology and treatment outcome in surgically resected patients. Cancer Res 62:2493–2497

Bentzen SM, Gregoire V (2011) Molecular imaging-based dose painting: a novel paradigm for radiation therapy prescription. Sem Radiat Oncol 21:101–110

Birner P, Schindl M, Obermair A et al (2000) Overexpression of hypoxia-inducible factor 1alpha is a marker for an unfavorable prognosis in early-stage invasive cervical cancer. Cancer Res 60:4693–4696

Blasberg JD, Pass HI, Goparaju CM et al (2010) Reduction of elevated plasma osteopontin levels with resection of non-small-cell lung cancer. J Clin Oncol 28:936–941

Braun RD, Lanzen JL, Snyder SA, Dewhirst MW (2001) Comparison of tumor and normal tissue oxygen tension measurements using Oxylite or microelectrodes in rodents. Am J Physiol Heart Circ Physiol 280:H2533–H2544

Brizel DM, Scully SP, Harrelson JM et al (1996) Tumor oxygenation predicts for the likelihood of distant metastases in human soft tissue sarcoma. Cancer Res 56:941–943

Brizel DM, Sibley GS, Prosnitz LR, Scher RL, Dewhirst MW (1997) Tumor hypoxia adversely affects the prognosis of carcinoma of the head and neck. Int J Radiat Oncol Biol Phys 38:285–289

Burri P, Djonov V, Aebersold DM et al (2003) Significant correlation of hypoxia-inducible factor-1alpha with treatment outcome in cervical cancer treated with radical radiotherapy. Int J Radiat Oncol Biol Phys 56:494–501

Collingridge DR, Young WK, Vojnovic B et al (1997) Measurement of tumor oxygenation: a comparison between polarographic needle electrodes and a time-resolved luminescence-based optical sensor. Radiat Res 147:329–334

Cooper RA, Carrington BM, Loncaster JA et al (2000) Tumour oxygenation levels correlate with dynamic contrast-enhanced magnetic resonance imaging parameters in carcinoma of the cervix. Radiother Oncol 57:53–59

De Schutter H, Landuyt W, Verbeken E et al (2005) The prognostic value of the hypoxia markers CA IX and GLUT 1 and the cytokines VEGF and IL 6 in head and neck squamous cell carcinoma treated by radiotherapy ± chemotherapy. BMC Cancer 5:42

Dearling JL, Lewis JS, Mullen GE, Rae MT, Zweit J, Blower PJ (1998) Design of hypoxia-targeting radiopharmaceuticals: selective uptake of copper-64 complexes in hypoxic cells in vitro. Eur J Nucl Med 25:788–792

Dehdashti F, Mintun MA, Lewis JS et al (2003) In vivo assessment of tumor hypoxia in lung cancer with ^{60}Cu-ATSM. Eur J Nucl Med Mol Imaging 30:844–850

Dehdashti F, Grigsby PW, Lewis JS, Laforest R, Siegel BA, Welch MJ et al (2008) Assessing tumor hypoxia in cervical cancer by PET with 60Cu-labeled diacetyl-bis (N4-methylthiosemicarbazone). J Nucl Med 49:201–205

Dence CS, Ponde DE, Welch MJ, Lewis JS (2008) Autoradiographic and small-animal PET comparisons between (18)F-FMISO, (18)F-FDG, (18)F-FLT and the hypoxic selective (64) Cu-ATSM in a rodent model of cancer. Nucl Med Biol 35:713–720

Dietz DW, Dehdashti F, Grigsby PW et al (2008) Tumor hypoxia detected by positron emission tomography with 60Cu-ATSM as a predictor of response and survival in patients undergoing neoadjuvant chemoradiotherapy for rectal carcinoma: a pilot study. Dis Colon Rectum 51:1641–1648

Dirix P, Vandecaveye V, De Keyzer F, Stroobants S, Hermans R, Nuyts S (2009) Dose painting in radiotherapy for head and neck squamous cell carcinoma: value of repeated functional imaging with (18)F-FDG PET, (18)F-fluoromisonidazole PET, diffusion-weighted MRI, and dynamic contrast-enhanced MRI. J Nucl Med 50:1020–1027

Donaldson SB, Betts G, Bonington SC et al (2011) Perfusion estimated with rapid dynamic contrast-enhanced magnetic resonance imaging correlates inversely with vascular endothelial growth factor expression and pimonidazole staining in head-and-neck cancer: a pilot study. Int J Radiat Oncol Biol Phys 81:1176–1183

Eriksen JG, Overgaard J (2007) Lack of prognostic and predictive value of CA IX in radiotherapy of squamous cell carcinoma of the head and neck with known modifiable hypoxia: an evaluation of the DAHANCA 5 study. Radiother Oncol 83:383–388

Eschmann SM, Paulsen F, Bedeshem C et al (2007) Hypoxia-imaging with (18)F-Misonidazole and PET: changes of kinetics during radiotherapy of head-and-neck cancer. Radiother Oncol 83:406–410

Evans SM, Du KL, Chalian AA et al (2007) Patterns and levels of hypoxia in head and neck squamous cell carcinomas and their relationship to patient outcome. Int J Radiat Oncol Biol Phys 69:1024–1031

Fedarko NS, Jain A, Karadag A et al (2001) Elevated serum bone sialoprotein and osteopontin in colon, breast, prostate, and lung cancer. Clin Cancer Res 7:4060–4066

Fukumura D, Xu L, Chen Y, Gohongi T, Seed B, Jain RK (2001) Hypoxia and acidosis independently up-regulate vascular endothelial growth factor transcription in brain tumors in vivo. Cancer Res 61:6020–6024

Fyles AW, Milosevic M, Wong R et al (1998) Oxygenation predicts radiation response and survival in patients with cervix cancer. Radiother Oncol 48:149–156

Fyles A, Milosevic M, Pintilie M et al (2006) Long-term performance of interstitial fluid pressure and hypoxia as prognostic factors in cervix cancer. Radiother Oncol 80:132–137

Gatenby RA, Kessler HB, Rosenblum JS et al (1988) Oxygen distribution in squamous cell carcinoma metastases and its relationship to outcome of radiation therapy. Int J Radiat Oncol Biol Phys 14:831–838

Giatromanolaki A, Koukourakis MI, Sivridis E et al (2001) Expression of hypoxia-inducible carbonic anhydrase-9 relates to angiogenic pathways and independently to poor outcome in non-small cell lung cancer. Cancer Res 61:7992–7998

Graeber T, Osmanian C, Jacks T et al (1996) Hypoxia-mediated selection of cells with diminished apoptotic potential in solid tumors. Nature 379(6560):88–91

Griffiths JR, Robinson SP (1999) The oxylite: a fibre-optic oxygen sensor. Br J Radiol 72:627–630

Güttler A, Giebler M, Cuno P et al (2013) Osteopontin and splice variant expression level in human malignant glioma: radiobiologic effects and prognosis after radiotherapy. Radiother Oncol 108:535–540

Hall EJ (1988) Radiobiology for the radiologist. Lippincott, Philadelphia

Haugland HK, Vukovic V, Pintilie M et al (2002) Expression of hypoxia-inducible factor-1alpha in cervical carcinomas: correlation with tumor oxygenation. Int J Radiat Oncol Biol Phys 53:854–861

Hoebers FJP, Janssen HLK, Valdés Olmos RA et al (2002) Phase 1 study to identify tumour hypoxia in patients with head and neck cancer using technetium-99 m BRU 59-21. Eur J Nucl Med 29:1206–1211

Hoeckel M, Knoop C, Schlenger K et al (1993) Intratumoral pO_2 predicts survival in advanced cancer of the uterine cervix. Radiother Oncol 26:45–50

Hoeckel M, Schlenger K, Aral B, Mitze M, Schaffer U, Vaupel P (1996) Association between tumor hypoxia and malignant progression in advanced cancer of the uterine cervix. Cancer Res 56:4509–4515

Horsman MR, Overgaard J (2007) Hyperthermia: a potent enhancer of radiotherapy. Clin Oncol 19:418–426

Horsman MR, Overgaard J, Siemann DW (2011) Impact on radiotherapy. In: Siemann DW (ed) Tumor Microenvironment. Wiley, Chichester

Horsman MR, Mortensen LS, Petersen JB, Busk M, Overgaard J (2012) Imaging hypoxia to improve radiotherapy outcome. Nat Rev Clin Oncol 9:674–687

Hui EP, Chan AT, Pezzella F et al (2002) Coexpression of hypoxia-inducible factors 1alpha and 2alpha, carbonic anhydrase IX, and vascular endothelial growth factor in nasopharyngeal carcinoma and relationship to survival. Clin Cancer Res 8:2595–2604

Isa S, Kawaguchi T, Teramukai S et al (2009) Serum osteopontin levels are highly prognostic for survival in advanced non-small cell lung cancer: results from JMTO LC 0004. J Thorac Oncol 4:1104–1110

Ivanov S, Liao SY, Ivanova A et al (2001) Expression of hypoxia-inducible cell-surface transmembrane carbonic anhydrases in human cancer. Am J Pathol 158:905–919

Jansen JFA, Schöder H, Lee NY et al (2010) Noninvasive assessment of tumor microenvironment using dynamic contrast-enhanced magnetic resonance imaging and 18F-fluoromisonidazole positron emission tomography imaging in neck nodal metastases. Int J Radiat Oncol Biol Phys 77:1403–1410

Jewell UR, Kvietikova I, Scheid A et al (2001) Induction of HIF-1alpha in response to hypoxia is instantaneous. FASEB J 15:1312–1314

Jiang BH, Semenza GL, Bauer C et al (1996) Hypoxia-inducible factor 1 levels vary exponentially over a physiologically relevant range of O_2 tension. Am J Physiol 271:C1172–C1180

Kaanders JH, Wijffels KI, Marres HA et al (2002) Pimonidazole binding and tumor vascularity predict for treatment outcome in head and neck cancer. Cancer Res 62:7066–7074

Khamly K, Choong P, Ngan S et al (2008) Hypoxia in soft-tissue sarcomas on [18F]-fluoroazomycin arabinoside positron emission tomography (FAZA-PET) powerfully predicts response to radiotherapy and early relapse (abstract 35029). Presented at the 14th Connective Tissue Oncology Society Annual Meeting, November 13–15 (London)

Kikuchi M, Yamane T, Shinoharas S et al (2011) 18F-fluoromisonidazole positron emission tomography before treatment is a predictor of radiotherapy outcome and survival prognosis in patients with head and neck squamous cell carcinoma. Ann Nucl Med 25:625–633

Knocke TH, Weitmann HD, Feldmann HJ, Selzer E, Pötter R (1999) Intratumoral pO_2-measurements as predictive assay in the treatment of carcinoma of the uterine cervix. Radiother Oncol 53:99–104

Kolstad P (1968) Intercapillary distance, oxygen tension and local recurrence in cervix cancer. Scand J Clin Lab Invest Suppl 106:145–157

Komar G, Seppänen M, Eskola O et al (2008) 18F-EF5: a new PET tracer for imaging hypoxia in head and neck cancer. J Nucl Med 49:1944–1951

Koopmann J, Fedarko NS, Jain A et al (2004) Evaluation of osteopontin as biomarker for pancreatic adenocarcinoma. Cancer Epidemiol Biomarkers Prev 13:487–491

Krishna MC, Matsumoto S, Yasui H et al (2012) Electron paramagnetic resonance imaging of tumor pO_2. Radiat Res 177:376–386

Lal A, Peters H, St Croix B et al (2001) Transcriptional response to hypoxia in human tumors. J Natl Cancer Inst 93:1337–1343

Le QT, Sutphin PD, Raychaudhuri S et al (2003) Identification of osteopontin as a prognostic plasma marker for head and neck squamous cell carcinomas. Clin Cancer Res 9:59–67

Le QT, Chen E, Salim A et al (2006) Evaluation of tumor oxygenation and gene expression in patients with early stage non-small cell lung cancers. Clin Cancer Res 12:1507–1514

Lee S, Shin HJ, Han IO et al (2007) Tumor carbonic anhydrase 9 expression is associated with the presence of lymph node metastases in uterine cervical cancer. Cancer Sci 98:329–333

Lee N, Nehmeh S, Schöder H et al (2009) Prospective trial incorporating pre-/mid-treatment [^{18}F]-misonidazole positron emission tomography for head-and-neck cancer patients undergoing concurrent chemoradiotherapy. Int J Radiat Oncol Biol Phys 75:101–108

Lehtio K, Eskola O, Vijanen T et al (2004) Imaging perfusion and hypoxia with PET to predict radiotherapy response in head-and-neck cancer. Int J Radiat Oncol Biol Phys 59:971–982

Lewis JS, Welch MJ (2001) PET imaging of hypoxia. Quant J Nucl Med 45:183–188

Li L, Yu J, Xing L et al (2006) Serial hypoxia imaging with ^{99m}Tc-HL91 SPECT to predict radiotherapy response in non small cell lung cancer. Amer J Clin Oncol 29:628–633

Li L, Hu M, Zhu H, Zhao W, Yang G, Yu J (2010) Comparison of 18F-Fluoroerythronitroimidazole and 18F-fluorodeoxyglucose positron emission tomography and prognostic value in locally advanced non-small-cell lung cancer. Clin Lung Cancer 11:335–340

Ling CC, Humm J, Larson S et al (2000) Towards multidimensional radiotherapy (MD-CRT): biological imaging and biological conformality. Int J Radiat Oncol Biol Phys 47:551–560

Loncaster JA, Harris AL, Davidson SE et al (2001) Carbonic anhydrase (CA IX) expression, a potential new intrinsic marker of hypoxia: correlations with tumor oxygen measurements and prognosis in locally advanced carcinoma of the cervix. Cancer Res 61:6394–6399

Loncaster JA, Carrington BM, Sykes JR et al (2002) Prediction of radiotherapy outcome using dynamic contrast enhanced MRI of carcinoma of the cervix. Int J Radiat Oncol Biol Phys 54:759–767

Lukacova S, Khalil AA, Overgaard J et al (2006) Relationship between radiobiological hypoxia in a C3H mouse mammary carcinoma and osteopontin levels in mouse serum. Int J Radiat Biol 81:937–944

Lyng H, Sundfør K, Tropé C, Rofstad EK (2000) Disease control of uterine cervical cancer: relationships to tumor oxygen tension, vascular density, cell density, and frequency of mitosis and apoptosis measured before treatment and during radiotherapy. Clin Cancer Res 6:1104–1112

Lyng H, Vorren AO, Sundfør K et al (2001) Assessment of tumor oxygenation in human cervical carcinoma by use of dynamic Gd-DTPA-enhanced MR imaging. J Magn Reson Imaging 14:750–756

Mack PC, Redman MW, Chansky K et al (2008) Lower osteopontin plasma levels are associated with superior outcomes in advanced non-small-cell lung cancer patients receiving platinum-based chemotherapy: SWOG Study S0003. J Clin Oncol 26:4771–4776

Mayer A, Hockel M, Vaupel P (2006) Endogenous hypoxia markers in locally advanced cancers of the uterine cervix: reality or wishful thinking? Strahlenther Onkol 182:501–510

Mayr NA, Wang JZ, Zhang D et al (2010) Longitudinal changes in tumor perfusion pattern during the radiation therapy course and its clinical impact in cervical cancer. Int J Radiat Oncol Biol Phys 77:502–508

Minagawa Y, Shizukuishi K, Koike I et al (2011) Assessment of tumor hypoxia by 62Cu-ATSM PET/CT as a predictor of response in head and neck cancer: a pilot study. Ann Nucl Med 25:339–345

Mortensen LS, Johansen J, Kallehauge J et al (2012) FAZA PET/CT hypoxia imaging in patients with squamous cell carcinoma of the head and neck treated with radiotherapy: results from the DAHANCA 24 trial. Radiother Oncol 105:14–20

Newbold K, Castellano I, Charles-Edwards E et al (2009) An exploratory study into the role of dynamic contrast-enhanced magnetic resonance imaging or perfusion computed tomography for detection of intratumoral hypoxia in head-and-neck cancer. Int J Radiat Oncol Biol Phys 74:29–37

Nielsen T, Wittenborn T, Horsman MR (2012) Dynamic contrast-enhanced magnetic resonance imaging (DCE-MRI) in preclinical studies of antivascular treatments. Pharmaceutics 4:563–589

Nordsmark M, Overgaard M, Overgaard J (1996) Pretreatment oxygenation predicts radiation response in advanced squamous cell carcinoma of the head and neck. Radiother Oncol 41:31–39

Nordsmark M, Alsner J, Keller J et al (2001) Hypoxia in human soft tissue sarcomas: adverse impact on survival and no association with p53 mutations. Br J Cancer 84:1070–1075

Nordsmark M, Bentzen SM, Rudat V et al (2005) Prognostic value of tumor oxygenation in 397 head and neck tumors after primary radiation therapy. An international multi-center study. Radiother Oncol 77:18–24

Nordsmark M, Loncaster J, Aquino-Parsons C et al (2006) The prognostic value of pimonidazole and tumour pO_2 in human cervix carcinomas after radiation therapy: a prospective international multi-center study. Radiother Oncol 80:123–131

Nordsmark M, Eriksen JG, Gebski V et al (2007) Differential risk assessments from five hypoxia specific assays: the basis for biologically adapted individualized radiotherapy in advanced head and neck cancer patients. Radiother Oncol 83:389–397

O'Donoghue JA, Zanzonico P, Pugachev A et al (2005) Assessment of regional tumor hypoxia using 18F-fluoromisonidazole and 64Cu(II)-diacetyl-bis(N4-methylthiosemicarbazone) positron emission tomography: Comparative study featuring microPET imaging, Po2 probe measurement, autoradiography, and fluorescent microscopy in the R3327-AT and FaDu rat tumor models. Int J Radiat Oncol Biol Phys 61:1493–1502

Ostheimer C, Bache M, Güttler A et al (2013) Osteopontin, carbonic anhydrase 9 and vascular endothelial growth factor. A pilot study on potential plasma hypoxia markers in the radiotherapy o non-small-cell lung cancer. Strahlenther Onkol 190:276–282

Overgaard J (2007) Hypoxic radiosensitization: adored and ignored. J Clin Oncol 25:4066–4074

Overgaard J, Eriksen JG, Nordsmark M et al (2005) Plasma osteopontin, hypoxia, and response to the hypoxia sensitiser nimorazole in radiotherapy of head and neck cancer: results from the DAHANCA 5 randomised double-blind placebo-controlled trial. Lancet Oncol 6:757–764

Pacheco-Torres J, López-Larrubia P, Ballesteros P, Cerdán S (2011) Imaging tumor hypoxia by magnetic resonance methods. NMR Biomed 24:1–16

Petrik D, Lavori PW, Cao H et al (2006) Plasma osteopontin is an independent prognostic marker for head and neck cancers. J Clin Oncol 24:5291–5297

Rajendran JG, Schwartz DL, O'Sullivan J et al (2006) Tumor hypoxia imaging with [F-18] fluoromisonidazole positron emission tomography in head and neck cancer. Clin Cancer Res 12:5435–5441

Raleigh JA, Chou SC, Arteel GE, Horsman MR (1999) Comparisons among pimonidazole binding, oxygen electrode measurements and radiation response in C3H mouse tumors. Radiat Res 151:580–589

Rasey JS, Koh WJ, Evans ML et al (1996) Quantifying regional hypoxia in human tumors with positron emission tomography of [^{18}F]fluoromisonidazole: a pretherapy study of 37 patients. Int J Radiat Oncol Biol Phys 36:417–428

Reischl G, Dorow DS, Cullinane C et al (2007) Imaging of tumor hypoxia with [124I]IAZA in comparison with [18F]FMISO and [18F]FAZA–first small animal PET results. J Pharm Pharm Sci 10:203–211

Rischin D, Hicks RJ, Fischer R et al (2006) Prognostic significance of [18F]-misonidazole positron emission tomography-detected tumor hypoxia in patients with advanced head and neck cancer randomly assigned to chemoradiation with or without tirapazamine: a substudy of Trans-Tasman Radiation Oncology Group study 98.02. J Clin Oncol 24:2098–2104

Rudat V, Stadler P, Becker A et al (2001) Predictive value of the tumor oxygenation by means of pO_2 histography in patients with advanced head and neck cancer. Strahlenther Onkol 177:462–468

Said HM, Katzer A, Flentje M, Vordermark D (2005) Response of the plasma hypoxia marker osteopontin to in vitro hypoxia in human tumor cells. Radiother Oncol 76:200–205

Schuetz M, Schmid MP, Pötter R et al (2010) Evaluating repetitive 18F-fluoroazomycin-arabinoside (18FAZA) PET in the setting of MRI guided adaptive radiotherapy in cervical cancer. Acta Oncol 49:941–947

Seddon BM, Honess DJ, Vojnovic B, Tozer GM, Workman P (2001) Measurement of tumor oxygenation: in vivo comparison of a luminescence fiber-optic sensor and a polarographic electrode in the p22 tumor. Radiat Res 155:837–846

Seddon BM, Payne GS, Simmons L et al (2003) A phase I study of SR-4554 via intravenous administration for noninvasive investigation of tumor hypoxia by magnetic resonance spectroscopy in patients with malignancy. Clin Cancer Res 9:5101–5112

Snitcovsky I, Leitao GM, Pasini FS et al (2009) Plasma osteopontin levels in patients with head and neck cancer undergoing chemoradiotherapy. Arch Otolaryngol Head Neck Surg 135:807–811

Sorensen BS, Hao J, Overgaard J et al (2005) Influence of oxygen concentration and pH on expression of hypoxia induced genes. Radiother Oncol 76:187–193

Søvik Å, Malinen E, Olsen DR (2009) Strategies for biologic image-guided dose escalation: a review. Int J Radiat Oncol Biol Phys 73:650–658

Spence AM, Muzi M, Swanson KR et al (2008) Regional hypoxia in glioblastoma multiforme quantified with [18F]fluoromisonidazole positron emission tomography before radiotherapy: correlation with time to progression and survival. Clin Cancer Res 14:2623–2630

Stadler P, Becker A, Feldmann HJ et al (1999) Influence of the hypoxic subvolume on the survival of patients with head and neck cancer. Int J Radiat Oncol Biol Phys 44:749–754

Sundfør K, Lyng H, Rofstad EK (1998) Tumour hypoxia and vascular density as predictors of metastasis in squamous cell carcinoma of the uterine cervix. Br J Cancer 78:822–827

Swanson KR, Chakraborty G, Wang CH et al (2009) Complementary but distinct roles for MRI and ^{18}F-fluoromisonidazole PET in the assessment of human glioblastomas. J Nucl Med 50:36–44

Swartz HM, Khan N, Buckey J et al (2004) Clinical applications of EPR: overview and perspectives. NMR Biomed 17:335–351

Talks KL, Turley H, Gatter KC et al (2000) The expression and distribution of the hypoxia-inducible factors HIF-1alpha and HIF-2alpha in normal human tissues, cancers, and tumor-associated macrophages. Am J Pathol 157:411–421

Thorwarth D, Eschmann SM, Scheiderbauer J, Paulsen F, Alber M (2005) Kinetic analysis of dynamic 18F-fluoromisonidazole PET correlates with radiation treatment outcome in head-and-neck cancer. BMC Cancer 5:152

Thorwarth D, Eschmann SM, Holzner F, Paulsen F, Alber M (2006) Combined uptake of [18F] FDG and [18F]FMISO correlates with radiation therapy outcome in head-and-neck cancer patients. Radiother Oncol 80:151–156

Turaka A, Buyyounouski MK, Hanlon AL, Horwitz EM, Greenberg RE, Movsas B (2011) Hypoxic prostate/muscle Po2 ratio predicts for outcome in patients with localized prostate cancer: long-term results. Int J Radiat Oncol Biol Phys 82:e433–e439

Urano M, Chen Y, Humm J, Koutcher JA, Zanzonico P, Ling C (2002) Measurements of tumor tissue oxygen tension using a time-resolved luminescence-based optical oxylite probe: comparison with a paired survival assay. Radiat Res 158:167–173

Urtasun RC, Parliament MB, McEwan AJ et al (1996) Measurement of hypoxia in human tumours by non-invasive spect imaging of iodoazomycin arabinoside. Br J Cancer 74(Suppl.): S209–S212

van Loon J, Janssen MHM, Öllers M et al (2010) PET imaging of hypoxia using [^{18}F] HX4: a phase I trial. Eur J Nucl Med Mol Imaging 37:1663–1668

Vaupel P, Kallinowski F, Okunieff P (1989) Blood flow, oxygen and nutrient supply, and metabolic micro-environment of human tumors: a review. Cancer Res 49:6449–6465

Vävere AL, Lewis JS (2007) Cu-ATSM: a radiopharmaceutical for the PET imaging of hypoxia. Dalton Trans 21:4893–4902

Vikram DS, Zweier JL, Kuppusamy P (2007) Methods for noninvasive imaging of tissue hypoxia. Antioxid Redox Signal 9:1745–1756

Vordermark D, Brown JM (2003) Evaluation of hypoxia-inducible factor-1α (HIF-1α) as an intrinsic marker of tumor hypoxia in U87 MG human glioblastoma: in-vitro and xenograft studies. Int J Radiat Oncol Biol Phys 56:1184–1193

Vordermark D, Kaffer A, Riedl S et al (2005) Characterization of carbonic anhydrase IX (CA IX) as an endogenous marker of chronic hypoxia in live human tumor cells. Int J Radiat Oncol Biol Phys 61:1197–1207

Vukovic V, Haugland HK, Nicklee T et al (2001) Hypoxia-inducible factor-1alpha is an intrinsic marker for hypoxia in cervical cancer xenografts. Cancer Res 61:7394–7398

Wen B, Urano M, Humm JL, Seshan VE, Li GC, Ling CC (2008) Comparison of helzel and oxylite systems in the measurement of tumor partial pressure (pO$_2$). Radiat Res 169:67–75

Wilson DF, Cerniglia GJ (1992) Localization of tumors and evaluation of their state of oxygenation by phosphorescence imaging. Cancer Res 52:3988–3993

Winter SC, Shah KA, Han C et al (2006) The relation between hypoxia-inducible factor (HIF)-1alpha and HIF-2alpha expression with anemia and outcome in surgically treated head and neck cancer. Cancer 107:757–766

Wykoff CC, Beasley NJ, Watson PH et al (2000) Hypoxia-inducible expression of tumor-associated carbonic anhydrases. Cancer Res 60:7075–7083

Yuan H, Schroeder T, Bowsher JE, Hedlund LW, Wong T, Dewhirst MW (2006) Intertumoral differences in hypoxia selectivity of the PET imaging agent 64Cu(II)-diacetyl-bis (N4-methylthiosemicarbazone). J Nucl Med 47:989–998

Yue J, Yang Y, Cabrera AR et al (2012) Measuring tumor hypoxia with ^{18}F-FETNIM PET in esophageal squamous cell carcinoma: a pilot clinical study. Dis Esophagus 25:54–61

Zhang H, Ye QH, Ren N et al (2006) The prognostic significance of preoperative plasma levels of osteopontin in patients with hepatocellular carcinoma. J Cancer Res Clin Oncol 132:709–717

Zhao D, Jiang L, Hahn EW, Mason RP (2005) Tumor physiologic response to combretastatin A4 phosphate assessed by MRI. Int J Radiat Oncol Biol Phys 62:872–880

Zhong H, De Marzo AM, Laughner E et al (1999) Overexpression of hypoxia-inducible factor 1alpha in common human cancers and their metastases. Cancer Res 59:5830–5935

Zhu Y, Denhardt DT, Cao H et al (2005) Hypoxia upregulates osteopontin expression in NIH-3T3 cells via a Ras-activated enhancer. Oncogene 24:6555–6563

Zips D, Zöphel K, Abolmaali N et al (2012) Exploratory prospective trial of hypoxia imaging during radiochemotherapy in patients with locally advanced head-and-neck cancer. Radiother Oncol 105:21–28

Human Papilloma Virus as a Biomarker for Personalized Head and Neck Cancer Radiotherapy

Jesper Grau Eriksen and Pernille Lassen

Abstract

A dramatic increase in the incidence of HPV-related oropharyngeal cancer has been reported in some parts of the western world over the past 30 years. They constitute a clinically distinct subgroup of cancers in terms of molecular biology, patient characteristics, and treatment outcome. This chapter describes the molecular characteristics, epidemiology, and demographics of the HPV-related head and neck cancers and discuss available methods to detect HPV-related tumours. The impact of HPV-related biomarkers in clinical studies on radiotherapy only, altered fractionation, modulation of hypoxia, and concurrent chemo- or bio-radiotherapy are reviewed as well as the perspectives of de-escalation and immune-modulation are discussed.

Keywords

Head and neck cancer · Radiotherapy · HPV · P16 · Hypoxia · De-intensification

J.G. Eriksen (✉)
Department of Oncology, Odense University Hospital, Odense, Denmark
e-mail: jesper.grau.eriksen@rsyd.dk

P. Lassen
Department of Oncology, Department of Clinical Experimental Oncology, Aarhus University Hospital, 8000 Aarhus C, Denmark
e-mail: pernille@oncology.dk

© Springer-Verlag Berlin Heidelberg 2016
M. Baumann et al. (eds.), *Molecular Radio-Oncology*, Recent Results in Cancer Research 198, DOI 10.1007/978-3-662-49651-0_7

1   Introduction

A causal relationship between human papillomavirus (HPV) and cervical cancer
was established almost 40 years ago (Zur Hausen 1994) and HPV is necessary for
the development of cervical cancers. Tobacco and alcohol were, until recently,
considered to be the major risk factors in carcinogenesis of head and neck squamous cell carcinoma (HNSCC), but the putative role of HPV in HNSCC has been
investigated since the 1980s, and at present sufficient molecular and pathological
evidence exists to etiologically link HPV to a subset of HNSCCs, especially
tumours arising in the oropharynx (OPSCC) (Gillison et al. 2000, 2012; Sudhoff
et al. 2011). During the past 30 years, a rapid increase in the incidence of
HPV-associated OPSCC has been reported in several Western countries while the
incidence of HNSCC overall has declined (Chaturvedi et al. 2008; Hammarstedt
et al. 2007; Lassen 2010; Mehanna et al. 2013). HPV DNA has been found in
HNSCC from all sites (Kreimer et al. 2005) with a significantly higher prevalence
in OPSCC compared to tumours arising in non-oropharyngeal sites. Moreover,
HPV 16 is the dominant type in HNSCC, accounting for about 90 % of HPV
DNA-positive HNSCCs, whereas HPV 18, 31, 33, and 35 are found in most of the
remaining cases.

   HPV-related HNSCC constitutes a clinically distinct subgroup of cancers in
terms of molecular biology, patient characteristics (demographic and risk factor
profile) and treatment outcome, and this on the whole differentiates it markedly
from HPV-negative tumours, that typically have a strong association with tobacco.
Tumour HPV status has proven to be the single strongest prognostic factor for
outcome in radiotherapy of HNSCC, and separate therapeutic treatment strategies
based on tumour HPV status are in the pipeline. The aim of this chapter is to
summarize the current knowledge and understanding of HPV in HNSCC, with
specific focus on the influence of HPV on radiotherapy outcome, including an
assessment of the radiobiological modifications of head and neck cancer
radiotherapy.

2   HPV-Induced Oncogenesis

HPVs are strictly epitheliotropic and depend on epithelial differentiation for com-
pletion of their life cycle. Infection is established when the virus gains access to the
basal cells of the skin or mucosal epithelium through micro-abrasions on the sur-
faces. Viral particles are then formed progressively as the basal cells differentiate
and are eventually released when the cells reach the outer layer of the epithelium
(Doorbar 1979; Doorbar 2005; Zur Hausen 2002). Currently, almost 150 different
HPV types are isolated of which 120 types are fully sequenced. Based on their
malignant potential, the HPVs are further subdivided into high-risk and low-risk
types. HPVs are small double-stranded, circular DNA viruses with a genome of
approximately 8,000 base pairs. The coding sequences have been classified as early

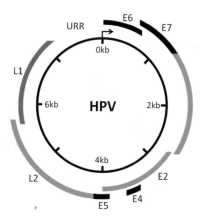

Fig. 1 The HPV genome

(E) containing the early genes E1, E2, E4, E5, E6 and E7 and late (L) containing the late genes encoding the major (L1) and minor (L2) capsid proteins (Fig. 1). The presence of E3 and E8 has been recently described in only a few HPV types, but their function is yet unknown. Viral integration into the host cell genome occurs downstream the E6 and E7, often in the E1 or E2 region. However, in HNSCCs that can be attributed to HPV the viral genome is not exclusively integrated into the host genome but can also be found in episomal (extrachromosomal) form or a mixture of both similar to what is observed in cervical cancer samples. The E5 protein seems to be important in the early phase of infection, but in case of viral integration into host cell DNA the coding sequence of E5 is often deleted (Doorbar 2005). The molecular pathways in HPV-induced oncogenesis have been well described and the E6 and E7 oncoproteins play a key role in malignant transformation and mainte-nance, abrogating p53 and pRb tumour suppressor functions, respectively. The E6 oncoprotein disrupts the p53 pathway by ubiquitination and subsequent degradation of the p53 protein, which leads to uncontrolled cell cycle progression caused by lack of control at the G1/S and G2/M checkpoints (Nevins 2001). As a consequence of feedback loops, the functional inactivation of Rb by the E7 oncoprotein results in upregulation of the p16-protein. p16, encoded by the CDKN2A tumour suppressor gene, regulates the activity of CyclinD-CDK4/6 complexes (CDKs). When not inhibited by p16, these CDKs phosphorylate Rb leading to the release of the transcription factor E2F, which initiates cell cycle progression (Khleif 1996). In contrast, the bound Rb-E2F protein acts as a negative regulator, inhibiting tran-scription of several genes including CDKN2A. The functional inactivation of Rb by E7 therefore results in the release of the p16 gene from its transcriptional inhibition, by loss of negative feedback, and high expression levels of p16 is a characteristic feature of HPV-positive tumours (Khleif 1996; Chung and Gillison 2009; Smeets et al. 2007) (Fig. 2).

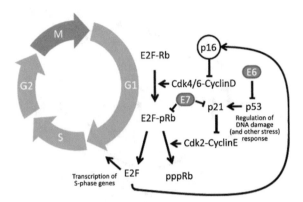

Fig. 2 HPV E6 and E7 oncoproteins disrupt p53 and pRb regulatory pathways that govern the cell division cycle. The functional inactivation of pRb by E7 leads to upregulation of p16 as a consequence of feedback loops. With permission from Lassen P.

Genetic alterations caused by the actions of HPV oncoproteins E6 and E7 differ from the molecular profiles observed in HPV E6/E7 mRNA-negative HNSCC besides the upregulation of p16. Based on the current evidence, apparently HPV-induced carcinogenesis involves significantly fewer genomic alterations/ accumulation of mutations than oncogenesis independent of HPV (Braakhuis et al. 2004; Slebos et al. 2006; Stransky et al. 2011). Particularly mutations in the tumour suppressor gene TP53 are less common in HPV-positive HNSCC compared to HPV-negative tumours (Gillison et al. 2000; Braakhuis et al. 2004) and also chromosomal aberrations of 3p, 9p and 17p are less frequent in HPV-related HNSCC (Braakhuis et al. 2004; Smeets et al. 2006). Thus, as a consequence of the specific HPV-induced carcinogenesis, primarily exerted by the E6 and E7 onco-proteins, HPV-positive tumours are characterized by a unique genotype and a molecular biological profile that distinguishes them from their virus-negative counterparts.

3   Epidemiology

A dramatic increase in the incidence of oropharyngeal cancer has been reported in several Western countries over the past 30 years (Chaturvedi et al. 2008; Ham-marstedt et al. 2007; Lassen 2010; Marur et al. 2010; Blomberg et al. 2011). Based on the observations that, simultaneously, there has been an increase in the fre-quency of HPV-positivity among OPSCCs infection with HPV seems to be the dominant cause of this development. Moreover, in the same time period a decrease in tobacco-smoking seems to be responsible for a reduction in the incidence of HNSCC outside the oropharynx at least in Western countries. As a result, these opposite incidence trends are presently changing the traditional epidemiological pattern in HNSCC and will continue to do so in the near future, and it is estimated that in countries with well-established, efficient screening-programs against cervical cancer, the incidence of HPV-related OPSCC will exceed that of cervical cancer by the year 2020 (Chaturvedi et al. 2011).

In 2007, the International Agency of Research of Cancer (IARC) declared that there is sufficient molecular and pathological evidence to etiologically link HPV 16 to a subset of HNSCCs, especially OPSCC. However, the natural history of oral high-risk HPV infection still remains to be fully elucidated and this is complicated by the fact that dysplasia is almost never detected in this region. Consequently, no efficient screening method exists to detect precancerous lesions in the oropharyngeal region. Although the exact mechanism is not known, oral–genital contact is assumed to be the primary mode by which HPV is transmitted to the oral mucosa, and several case control studies have shown an association between HPV-related HNSCC and sexual behaviour, most consistently the lifetime number of genital and oral sexual partners (Gillison et al. 2012).

4   Demography and Clinical Profile of HPV-Related HNSCC

HPV-related HNSCCs frequently present with smaller primary tumours (T1–2), but more advanced nodal stage (Lassen et al. 2011; Rischin et al. 2010) resulting in the majority of patients with HPV-positive tumours being diagnosed at overall advanced clinical stages (American Joint Committee on Cancer, AACJ): Stage III–IV. The anatomical AJCC stage has traditionally been a reasonable prognostic indicator in HNSCC and is incorporated into treatment guidelines all over the world. However, based on the consistent findings from clinical trials that HPV-related disease has a favourable prognosis despite advanced stage at time of diagnosis, a revision of the AJCC stage and its prognostic implication is currently under debate.

Patients diagnosed with HPV-related HNSCC tend to be younger, have better performance status and less comorbidity and also a higher socioeconomic status compared with HPV-negative patients (Gillison et al. 2008; Smith et al. 2004; Worden et al. 2008). A history of heavy smoking (defined by >10 pack-years) is significantly less common among patients with HPV-related HNSCC than HPV-negative HNSCC although many patients with HPV-related disease do have a history of smoking (Chaturvedi et al. 2008; Gillison et al. 2008; Ang et al. 2010). Based on observations from the USA, there also seems to be quite a striking difference in the frequency of HPV-positivity between white and black patients with about 30 % of whites' tumours being HPV-positive compared with only 0–4 % of blacks' tumours (Settle et al. 2009). Moreover, the incidence of OPSCC has increased in whites but has decreased in blacks (Jemal et al. 2013) despite an apparent higher prevalence of oral HPV infections in blacks than whites (Gillison et al. 2012).

The characteristic microscopic appearance of HPV-related HNSCC, especially OPSCC, is another parameter separating this disease entity from the classical HNSCC, which has traditionally been grouped into poorly, moderately or highly differentiated squamous cell carcinomas. The apparent predilection for HPV to target the highly specialized lymphoepithelium lining the lingual or palatine tonsillar crypts leads to a morphological resemblance between the tumours and this unique crypt epithelium. Consequently, HPV-related HNSCC tends to demonstrate non-keratinizing or only partially keratinizing morphology, with characteristic secondary features consisting of central necrosis with cystic change, tumour infiltrating lymphocytes and basaloid features, and very often surface dysplasia and prominent stromal desmoplasia are absent (Westra 2012). Based on these characteristic histopathological features of HPV-related HNSCC, it has been recommended by head and neck pathologists that the historical nomenclature of poorly, moderately or highly differentiated squamous cell carcinomas should be avoided and instead replaced by "HPV-related squamous cell carcinoma". Moreover, incorporation of the typical microscopic appearance of an HPV-related tumour into the interpretation of various HPV detection assays (e.g. p16 immunohistochemical staining) is considered to be of significant importance and may ultimately lead to a more reliable and reproducible correlation with HPV status in HNSCC as described and recommended by El-Naggar and Westra (2012).

5   HPV Detection Methods

The reported prevalence rates of HPV DNA in head and neck cancer specimens show considerable variation (Kreimer et al. 2005; Braakhuis et al. 2004) which in part can be explained by tumour site differences, i.e. viral prevalence is relatively low in the oral cavity and high in the tonsil (Gillison et al. 2000; Kreimer et al. 2005; Isayeva et al. 2012; Lingen et al. 2013). Another important contributing factor to the observed differences in HPV prevalence can be ascribed to the use of different detection methods. The most widely applied detection methods are based on PCR amplification of viral DNA. Generally, these assays have a high sensitivity, enabling detection of very few DNA copies per sample. However, this might yield false-positive results, due to sample to sample contaminations or detection of transient infections in which the virus is transcriptionally inactive, and as such the specificity of the methods is reduced (Smeets et al. 2007). Measuring levels of E6 and E7 mRNA by quantitative real-time PCR (qRT-PCR) assays increase specificity (Smeets et al. 2007; D'Souza et al. 2007), but fresh frozen tissue material is required for this method (Braakhuis et al. 2004; Smeets et al. 2006) which limits the present clinical applicability. Another commonly used method is the type-specific HPV DNA detection by in situ hybridization (ISH) assays. These assays are capable of detecting multiple HPV subtypes, their sensitivity is somewhat lower than the PCR-based assays, but on the other hand, they allow for visual confirmation of HPV DNA within individual tumour cell nuclei (Chung and Gillison 2009; Begum et al. 2005). Immunohistochemical (IHC) staining of tumour p16 expression has gained broad acceptance as a biomarker of infection with HPV in HNSCC, and a high correlation between HPV and p16 expression in HNSCC, particularly oropharyngeal carcinomas, has consistently been reported (Smeets et al. 2007; Shi et al. 2009; Licitra et al. 2006; Lassen et al. 2009; Weinberger et al. 2006). The method is relatively standardized and easily applicable on formalin-fixed paraffin-embedded (FFPE) samples, which makes implementation of the method in the daily clinical routine feasible (Lewis 2012). Moreover, since transcription of E7 precedes upregulation of p16, it has been suggested that p16 positivity may identify specifically those HPV infections that are biologically relevant in carcinogenesis. Expression of p16 is not limited to HPV-positive tumours though, and using this marker alone as an indicator of biologically relevant HPV infections inevitably entails the risk of including some virally false-positive results.

There are limitations to all methods of HPV detection, and which method to choose ultimately depends on the purpose of viral detection and consequently the extent of acceptable uncertainty of the test. Combined assays may represent an alternative way to reliably detect biologically relevant HPV infections in FFPE head and neck specimens, as proposed by Smeets et al. (2007). In previous randomized trials (Ang et al. 2010), p16-IHC was found to be a stronger prognostic factor for outcome than detection of HPV DNA by ISH and presently the most widespread clinical testing for tumour HPV status incorporates p16-IHC and ISH, either as stand-alone test or in combination (Jordan et al. 2012).

6 Effect of HPV on Response to Single-Modality Radiotherapy of HNSCC

Although, at present, the use of conventional radiotherapy as single-modality treatment in locally advanced HNSCC has been replaced by altered fractionation and combined modality schedules, the influence of tumour HPV status on outcome has been investigated in a few original studies in which conventionally fractionated radiotherapy was the predominant treatment. Among the first to suggest HPV-positivity to be a favourable prognostic factor in HNSCC were Friesland et al. (2001), Mellin et al. (2005, 2000) and Lindel et al. (2001) based on their analyses of single-institution retrospective case series. Methodologically, the studies differed from each other in several aspects, including disparities between the endpoints, definitions of time to event and the reported estimates used to evaluate the prognostic impact of HPV, which complicates a direct comparison of the results. Nevertheless, although not unambiguous, their observations supported the hypothesis that HPV infection had a positive influence on radiotherapy outcome for patients with HNSCC. The studies were all included in a meta-analysis, predominantly based on retrospective case series (Ragin and Taioli 2007) which confirmed the favourable impact of HPV-positivity. The meta-analysis also demonstrated that apparently the beneficial prognosis was restricted to tumours of oropharyngeal origin. In a well-characterized and prospectively collected cohort of head and neck cancer patients treated homogeneously with conventional radiotherapy alone, evaluation of tumour HPV status, expressed by p16, demonstrated that p16 expression was the strongest independent determinant of loco-regional tumour control as well as disease-specific and overall survival (Fig. 3) (Lassen et al. 2009).

Fig. 3 The influence of
HPV-associated p16
expression on response to
conventionally fractionated
radiotherapy. Actuarial
estimated loco-regional
tumour control (**a**),
disease-specific (**b**) and
overall survival (**c**) rates in
patients with p16-positive and
p16-negative carcinomas of
the pharynx and supraglottic
larynx. With permission from
Lassen P.

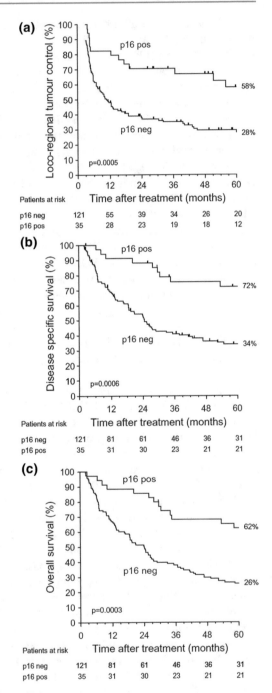

Thus, this study demonstrated a major impact of HPV-associated p16 expression on treatment response and survival in patients with head and neck cancers treated with conventionally fractionated radiotherapy alone.

The randomized DAHANCA 6 and 7 trials (Overgaard et al. 2003) compared the use of 5 fractions/week with 6 fractions/week, thereby shortening overall treatment time from 6½ weeks to 5½ weeks, while preserving the same total dose and fraction number. The study showed a significant benefit in favour of the 6 fractions/week schedule in terms of loco-regional control and disease-specific survival. Using p16 as retrospective stratification parameter within this prospective trial (Lassen et al. 2011) confirmed the strong independent prognostic impact of HPV-associated p16 expression on outcome after radiotherapy, both in terms of tumour control, disease-specific and overall survival. Moreover, the analysis suggested that HNSCC, regardless of tumour p16-status, reacts in a similar beneficial manner when treated with moderately accelerated fractionation compared to conventional fractionation as also shown in the updated meta-analysis of altered fractionation in HNSCC (Pignon et al. 2009). The cellular and molecular mechanisms underlying the favourable outcome for HPV-positive tumours treated with radiotherapy have recently been subject to further investigation. In preclinical investigation of HNSCC cell lines, Rieckmann et al. (Fig. 4) demonstrated a significantly higher radiosensitivity in HPV-positive cell lines compared to HPV-negative cells (Rieckmann et al. 2013). Furthermore, they found that, apparently, the increased radiosensitivity was due to accumulation of residual-DNA double-strand breaks (DSB) and associated with extensive G2 arrest in HPV-positive cells, indicating that the enhanced radio-responsiveness in HPV-positive tumours could reside in compromised DNA repair capacity of the cells.

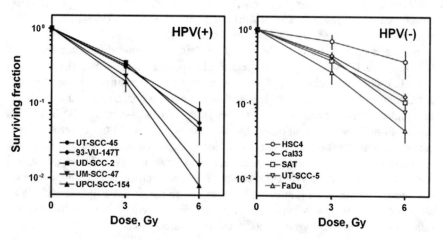

Fig. 4 Cellular radiosensitivity of HPV-positive and HPV-negative cell lines. Clonogenic survival of HPV-positive (*left*) and HPV-negative (*right*) cell lines after irradiation. With permission from Rieckmann T.

7   The Role of HPV in Hypoxic Modification During Radiotherapy

Hypoxia plays a pivotal element in radiotherapy of HNSCC and modification of hypoxia during radiotherapy improves loco-regional control, cancer-specific as well as overall survival (Overgaard 2011). In the DAHANCA 5 trial (Overgaard et al. 1998), patients were randomized to receive the hypoxic radiosensitizer nimorazole or placebo. A retrospective analysis of p16 status (Lassen et al. 2010) of 331 of the 414 patients in the original trial suggested that the response to hypoxic modification during radiotherapy differed by tumour p16 status. No significant benefit from nimorazole was observed in p16-positive tumours but only in the p16-negative tumours. In line with this are the observations from a retrospective analysis of another concept of hypoxic modification. In the TROG 02.02, "HeadSTART" (Rischin et al. 2010) trial from the Trans-Tasman Radiation Oncology Group, 853 patients with previously untreated locally advanced HNSCC of the oral cavity, pharynx, or larynx were randomized to conventional radiotherapy (70 Gy in seven weeks) concurrently with either high-dose cisplatin or cisplatin plus the hypoxia-selective cytotoxic drug tirapazamine. The original study failed its primary endpoint, but a later retrospective analysis in a small subset of these patients using HPV/p16 analysis suggested that only HPV-negative patients did benefit from treatment with tirapazamine (Rischin et al. 2010).

Toustrup et al. (2012) took another approach and tested a hypoxic gene expression classifier in the same patients from DAHANCA 5 as described above and found that nimorazole only improved loco-regional control in p16-negative, hypoxic tumours, although the hypoxic gene profile could also be found in a subset of the p16-positive tumours. The finding of hypoxic p16-positive tumours was confirmed, when estimating hypoxia using FAZA PET/CT imaging in HNSCC before curative radiotherapy (Mortensen et al. 2012) demonstrating that p16-positive and p16-negative tumours were equally hypoxic.

Sorensen et al. (2013) recently confirmed the pronounced radiosensitivity of HPV-positive HNSCC cells in a preclinical experiment. They also demonstrated that HPV-positive HNSCC cell lines display similar sensitivity under hypoxic conditions as the HPV-negative cell lines under normoxic conditions and moreover that under extreme hypoxia both HPV-positive and HPV-negative HNSCC cells benefit from hypoxic modification by nimorazole. Although, the experiment was performed under extreme hypoxic conditions, it is reasonable to suggest that the same results would be found under more moderate hypoxia. These preclinical findings suggest that HPV-positive tumour cells are hypoxic, but this hypoxia does not become of clinical significance because due to the extreme radiosensitivity of HPV-positive cells radiation doses of about 66 Gy will kill the cells anyhow, offsetting the effect of hypoxic modification by nimorazole.

8   The Role of HPV in Chemo–radiotherapy

HPV/p16 status has been estimated retrospectively in several studies involving chemo–radiotherapy (Attner et al. 2012; Fakhry and Gillison 2006; Lau et al. 2011). Ang and colleagues analysed the HPV/p16-status in 721 patients from the RTOG 0129 trial (Ang et al. 2010) randomizing between accelerated fractionation radio-therapy of 72 Gy/42 fractions in six weeks, with a concomitant boost of twice-daily irradiation for the last 12 treatment days versus 70 Gy/35 fractions over a seven-week period. Intravenous cisplatin was administered at a dose of 100 mg/m^2 of body surface on days one and 22 in the accelerated fractionation arm on days one, 22, and 43 in the standard fractionation group. The three-year rate of overall survival was similar in both arms, but when stratifying for HPV/p16 status, HPV-positive tumours did significantly better than the HPV-negative tumours using progression-free survival and overall survival as the endpoints. However, an analysis of whether the outcomes in the different chemo–radiotherapy arms differed by tumour HPV status is not available and an important purpose remains in exploring the optimal combination of radiotherapy and chemotherapy. The group from Princess Margaret Hospital in Toronto sought to elucidate this problem further in a non-randomized cohort of 505 oropharyngeal cancer patients treated with either chemo–radiotherapy (primarily high-dose cisplatin every third week) compared to primarily accelerated radiotherapy as single modality (O'Sullivan et al. 2013; O'Sullivan et al. 2012). They divided patients according to HPV status, stage and pack-years using the same algorithm as Ang and colleagues (Ang et al. 2010). Based on multivariate analyses using overall death and recurrence-free failure as endpoints as well as risk-profiling for having distant metastases, it seemed that HPV-positive oropharyngeal patients with T1-3 with N0-2b and less than 10 pack-years had minimal risk of distant recurrence irrespective of treatment with chemo–radiotherapy or radiation alone. Thus, these patients could be a possible target group for a prospective treatment de-intensification study. Nevertheless, one have to bear in mind that such studies are retrospective and conducted in an uncontrolled cohort consequently leading to a risk of introducing bias or confounders.

The use of a high-dose cisplatin schedule every third week or combination chemotherapy was the predominant treatment strategy in the above-mentioned studies. Recently, the first data from the registration protocol DAHANCA 18 were presented (Bentzen et al. 2015). In total, 227 patients with locally advanced HNSCC were treated with moderately accelerated radiotherapy, 66–68 Gy/33–34 fractions, six fractions per week and concomitant weekly low-dose cisplatin 40 mg/m^2. Pretreatment tumour p16 status was determined upfront. For p16-positive tumours, the five-year loco-regional control and overall survival were 89 and 93 %, respectively. These data indicate that the use of this less toxic regime might be sufficient for HPV-positive locally advanced HNSCC instead of high-dose cisplatin regimes. The hypothesis is also supported by the results of a recent small pairwise-matched analysis of weekly low-dose platinum versus high-dose cisplatin, showing no difference in survival between the two treatment schedules (Dobrosotskaya et al. 2014). However, since a non-inferiority randomized study of low-dose weekly cisplatin versus high-dose cisplatin every third week has never been (and probably never will be) conducted, no data exist to firmly address this question.

9   The Role of HPV in Bioradiation

Expectations to bioradiation have been high since the first results of the randomized phase lll trial of radiotherapy plus/minus cetuximab was presented in 2006 (Bonner et al. 2006) and updated in 2010 (Bonner et al. 2010). Based on the toxicity profile, it was suggested that bioradiation could be a reasonable alternative to concomitant chemotherapy in low-risk HPV-positive cancer. Supportive of this theory is the subgroup analysis performed along with the five-year update of the study, suggesting that the strongest benefit of additional EGFR-inhibition was found in younger patients with good performance and tumours with oropharyngeal origin, small T-stage, large nodal stage and consequently locally advanced disease (Bonner et al. 2010). This is exactly the characteristics of the patient with an HPV-positive tumour (Eriksen et al. 2010). One surprising piece of information from the five-year update is that it is primarily the tumours with a low expression of EGFR that seems to benefit from concomitant cetuximab. Moreover, low EGFR-expression seems to be a characteristic feature of HPV-positive tumours and might be explained by the deletion of E5 when the HPV genome is integrated in the host DNA during malignant progression (Burk et al. 2009). Tumour HPV/p16 status was never examined in the trial, but an influence of HPV on the results is likely. In a DAHANCA study cohort of 336 patients with oropharyngeal cancer, p16 and EGFR were examined according to previously described immunohistochemical methods (Lassen et al. 2009; Eriksen et al. 2004) and an inverse relation between the two markers was found: p16-positive tumours tended to express low levels of EGFR, $p = 0.0001$. This correlation was only present in the oropharynx (Lassen et al. 2013). Until now, no trial has upfront investigated the HPV/p16-status and balanced patients according to this in the treatment arms. In the DAHANCA 19 trial (clinicaltrials.gov NCT00496652) stratification according to site, stage and p16-status was done prior to randomization of patients to (chemotherapy) radiotherapy plus/minus the EGFR-inhibitor zalutumumab. The first data from this trial was presented recently and indicated that neither the p16-positive nor the p16-negative tumours did benefit from addition of zalutumumab to curatively intended (chemotherapy) radiotherapy. These findings were supported by retrospective data on 895 patients from the RTOG 0552 showing, that the effect of adding cetuximab to chemoradiation might result in competitive effects and the results presented at ASCO 2011 (Ang et al. 2011) indicated no benefit of adding an EGFR-inhibitor to chemoradiation. In contrast, in a recent study from Pajares et al. (Pajares et al. 2013), tumour blocks from 108 stage III/IV HNSCC patients treated with chemo–radiotherapy or radiotherapy plus EGFR-inhibitors were retrospectively analysed in a non-randomized setting. They showed that in this limited series, only the HPV-positive tumours did benefit from concomitant cetuximab when overall survival was used as endpoint. The design allowed for bias and confounding and data should be considered with caution. The RTOG 1016 is the first prospective trial to randomize between chemo–radiotherapy with high-dose cisplatin and bio-radiotherapy with cetuximab in HPV-positive oropharyngeal HNSCC only. The study that was launched in summer 2011 is rapidly accruing and aims at 706 randomized patients.

10 Perspectives for Future Treatment for HPV-Positive Tumours

In general, patients with HPV/p16-positive tumours have a very favourable prognosis and it is discussed how to reduce treatment burden without jeopardizing treatment outcome. To date, no prospective randomized data exist as guidance for treatment de-intensification of HPV/p16-positive HNSCC. Data suggest that loco-regional control and consequently disease-specific and overall survival are especially favourable in HPV/p16-positive non-smoking patients (Ang et al. 2010; O'Sullivan et al. 2013) and that they could be a candidate group for treatment de-intensification. However, as the risk of loco-regional recurrence becomes low, then the importance of distant recurrences might be of increasing importance (O'Sullivan et al. 2013) and HPV/p16-positive patients might even recur with an unusual metastasis pattern (Huang et al. 2010).

Based on the present evidence, data suggest that radiotherapy alone might be suitable for the low stages, HPV-positive HNSCC preferably with accelerated fractionation and presumably without hypoxic modification. The latter should ideally be estimated upfront by hypoxic profiling (Toustrup et al. 2012). For larger T-stages and higher nodal involvement (N2c/N3) chemo–radiotherapy still seems to be the choice, but the use of the less toxic weekly low-dose cisplatin schedule seems promising. Data on the replacement of chemotherapy with cetuximab is primarily driven by the idea that the latter is less toxic, but sufficient data do not exist at the moment. The RTOG 1016 study, mentioned above, will together with further exploration of the DAHANCA 19 trial hopefully provide the data needed. A third arm in the RTOG 1016 trial with accelerated fractionation radiotherapy only would have been optimal for answering these burning questions.

Other approaches are underway. Combination of radiotherapy with recombinant vaccines with inserted transgenes that code for E6 and E7 oncoproteins modified to remove their oncogenic potential and adjuvant human interleukin-2 (IL-2) are in progress and seems promising bearing the immunogenic potential of HPV in mind (Wansom et al. 2010). Testing of this vaccine in women with cervix HPV16 CIN grade 2/3 showed that seven out of eight patients were free of CIN 2/3 relapse and HPV 16 infection one year after treatment and therefore did not require conization (Brun et al. 2011). Another promising concept of immunotherapy would be blockade of the programmed death 1 protein (PD-1), an inhibitory receptor expressed by T cells, that can overcome immune resistance (ideally, as performed by the HPV) (Topalian et al. 2012). The experience in HNSCC is still very limited, but the biological basis is promising (Badoual et al. 2013).

In summary, the present data support the hypothesis that de-intensification of treatment might be possible in selected groups of HPV-positive HNSCC. However, all data so far are based on retrospective studies and cautiousness should be taken, when interpreting the suggested risk stratifications, since these low-risk groups might not have the same result with de-intensified treatment. So far the radiation oncology community has only limited experience in de-intensification of treatment schedules and therefore further investigation should be done within clinical randomized controlled trials. Finally, focus in these years has been very much on the HPV-positive tumours with a good prognosis, but still a substantial part of the patients are HPV-negative, smoking patients with comorbidities and a rather poor outcome. Optimization of treatment in these patients is much warranted as well.

References

Ang KK, Harris J, Wheeler R, Weber R, Rosenthal DI, Nguyen-Tan PF, Westra WH, Chung CH, Jordan RC, Lu C, Kim H, Axelrod R, Silverman CC, Redmond KP, Gillison ML (2010) Human papillomavirus and survival of patients with oropharyngeal cancer. N Engl J Med 363:24–35

Ang KK, Zhang Q, Rosenthal DI, Nguyen-Tan PF, Sherman E, Weber RS, Galvin JM, Schwartz DL, El-Naggar AK, Gillison ML, Jordan R, List MA, Konski AA, Thorstad A, Trotti A, Beitler JJ, Garden AS, Spanos WJ, Yom SS, Axelrod R (2011) A randomized phase III trial (RTOG 0522) of concurrent accelerated radiation plus cisplatin with or without cetuximab for stage III-IV head and neck squamous cell carcinomas (HNC). J Clin Oncol 29:5500 ASCO meeting abtracts

Attner P, Nasman A, Du J, Hammarstedt L, Ramqvist T, Lindholm J, Munck-Wikland E, Dalianis T, Marklund L (2012) Survival in patients with human papillomavirus positive tonsillar cancer in relation to treatment. Int J Cancer 131:1124–1130

Badoual C, Hans S, Merillon N, Van RC, Ravel P, Benhamouda N, Levionnois E, Nizard M, Si-Mohamed A, Besnier N, Gey A, Rotem-Yehudar R, Pere H, Tran T, Guerin CL, Chauvat A, Dransart E, Alanio C, Albert S, Barry B, Sandoval F, Quintin-Colonna F, Bruneval P, Fridman WH, Lemoine FM, Oudard S, Johannes L, Olive D, Brasnu D, Tartour E (2013) PD-1-expressing tumor-infiltrating T cells are a favorable prognostic biomarker in HPV-associated head and neck cancer. Cancer Res 73:128–138

Begum S, Cao D, Gillison ML, Zahurak M, Westra WH (2005) Tissue distribution of human papillomavirus 16 DNA integration in patients with tonsillar carcinoma. Clin Cancer Res 11:5694–5699

Bentzen J, Toustrup K, Eriksen JG, Primdahl H, Andersen LJ, Overgaard J (2015) Locally advanced head and neck cancer treated with accelerated radiotherapy, the hypoxic modifier nimorazole and weekly cisplatin. Results from the DAHANCA 18 phase II study. Acta Oncol 54:1001–1007

Blomberg M, Nielsen A, Munk C, Kjaer SK (2011) Trends in head and neck cancer incidence in Denmark, 1978–2007: focus on human papillomavirus associated sites. Int J Cancer 129:733–741

Bonner JA, Harari PM, Giralt J, Azarnia N, Shin DM, Cohen RB, Jones CU, Sur R, Raben D, Jassem J, Ove R, Kies MS, Baselga J, Youssoufian H, Amellal N, Rowinsky EK, Ang KK

(2006) Radiotherapy plus cetuximab for squamous-cell carcinoma of the head and neck. N Engl J Med 354:567–578

Bonner JA, Harari PM, Giralt J, Cohen RB, Jones CU, Sur RK, Raben D, Baselga J, Spencer SA, Zhu J, Youssoufian H, Rowinsky EK, Ang KK (2010) Radiotherapy plus cetuximab for locoregionally advanced head and neck cancer: 5-year survival data from a phase 3 randomised trial, and relation between cetuximab-induced rash and survival. Lancet Oncol 11:21–28

Braakhuis BJ, Snijders PJ, Keune JWH, Meijer CJ, Ruijter-Schippers HJ, Leemans R, Brakenhoff RH (2004) Genetic patterns in head and neck cancers that contain or lack transcriptionally active human papillomavirus. J Natl Cancer 96:998–1006

Brun JL, Dalstein V, Leveque J, Mathevet P, Raulic P, Baldauf JJ, Scholl S, Huynh B, Douvier S, Riethmuller D, Clavel C, Birembaut P, Calenda V, Baudin M, Bory JP (2011) Regression of high-grade cervical intraepithelial neoplasia with TG4001 targeted immunotherapy. Am J Obstet Gynecol 204:169.e1–169.e8

Burk RD, Chen Z, Van DK (2009) Human papillomaviruses: genetic basis of carcinogenicity. Pub Health Gen 12:281–290

Chaturvedi AK, Engels EA, Anderson WF, Gillison ML (2008) Incidence trends for human papillomavirus-related and -unrelated oral squamous cell carcinomas in the United States. J Clin Oncol 26:612–619

Chaturvedi AK, Engels EA, Pfeiffer RM, Hernandez BY, Xiao E, Kin E, Jiang B, Goodman MT, Siburg-Saber M, Cozen W, Liu L, Lynch CF, Wentzensen N, Jordan RC, Altekruse S, Anderson WF, Rosenberg PS, Gillison ML (2011) Human papillomavirus and rising oropharyngeal cancer incidence in the United States. J Clin Oncol 29:4294–4301

Chung CH, Gillison ML (2009) Human papillomavirus in head and neck cancer: its role in pathogenesis and clinical implications. Clin Cancer Res 15(22):6758–6762

Dobrosotskaya IY, Bellile E, Spector ME, Kumar B, Feng F, Eisbruch A, Wolf GT, Prince ME, Moyer JS, Teknos T, Chepeha DB, Walline HM, McHugh JB, Cordell KG, Ward PD, Byrd S, Maxwell JH, Urba S, Bradford CR, Carey TE, Worden FP (2014) Weekly chemotherapy with radiation versus high-dose cisplatin with radiation as organ preservation for patients with HPV positive and HPV negative locally advanced squamous cell carcinoma of the oropharynx (SCCOP). Head Neck 36:617–623

Doorbar J (1979) Molecular biology of human papillomavirus infection and cervical cancer. Clin Sci 2006(110):525–541

Doorbar J (2005) The papillomavirus life cycle. J Clin Virol 32(Suppl 1):S7–S15

D'Souza G, Kreimer AR, Viscidi R, Pawlita M, Fakhry C, Koch WM, Westra WH, Gillison ML (2007) Case-control study of human papillomavirus and oropharyngeal cancer. N Engl J Med 356:1944–1956

El-Naggar AK, Westra WH (2012) p16 expression as a surrogate marker for HPV-related oropharyngeal carcinoma: a guide for interpretative relevance and consistency. Head Neck 34:459–461

Eriksen JG, Steiniche T, Alsner J, Askaa J, Overgaard J (2004) The prognostic value of epidermal growth factor receptor is related to tumor differentiation and the overall treatment time of radiotherapy in squamous cell carcinomas of the head and neck. Int J Radiat Oncol Biol Phys 58:561–566

Eriksen JG, Lassen P, Overgaard J (2010) Do all patients with head and neck cancer benefit from radiotherapy and concurrent cetuximab? Lancet Oncol 11:312–313

Fakhry C, Gillison ML (2006) Clinical implications of human papillomavirus in head and neck cancers. J Clin Oncol 24:2606–2611

Friesland S, Mellin H, Munck-Wikland E, Nilsson A, Lindholm J, Dalianis T, Lewensohn R (2001) Human papilloma virus (HPV) and p53 immunostaining in advanced tonsillar carcinoma—relation to radiotherapy response and survival. Anticancer Res 21:529–534

Gillison ML, Koch WM, Capone RB, Spafford M, Westra WH, Wu L, Zahurak ML, Daniel RW, Viglione M, Symer DE, Shah KV, Sidransky D (2000) Evidence for a causal association between human papillomavirus and a subset of head and neck cancers. J Natl Cancer Inst 92:709–720

Gillison ML, D'Souza G, Westra W, Sugar E, Xiao W, Begum S, Viscidi R (2008) Distinct risk factor profiles for human papillomavirus type 16-positive and human papillomavirus type 16-negative head and neck cancers. J Natl Cancer Inst 100:407–420

Gillison ML, Snijders PJ, Chaturvedi AK, Steinberg BM, Schwartz S, Castellsague X (2012a) Human papillomavirus and diseases of the upper airway: head and neck cancer and respiratory papillomatosis. Vaccine 30(Suppl 5):F34–F54

Gillison ML, Broutian T, Pickard RK, Tong ZY, Xiao W, Kahle L, Graubard BI, Chaturvedi AK (2012b) Prevalence of oral HPV infection in the United States, 2009–2010. JAMA 307:693–703

Hammarstedt L, Dahlstrand H, Lindquist D, Onelöv L, Ryott M, Luo J, Dalianis T, Ye W, Munck-Wikland E (2007) The incidence of tonsillar cancer in Sweden is increasing. Acta oto-laryngol 127:988–992

Huang SH, Perez-Ordonez B, Liu FF, Waldron J, Ringash J, Irish J, Cummings B, Siu LL, Kim J, Weinreb I, Hope A, Gullane P, Brown D, Shi W, O'Sullivan B (2010) Atypical clinical behavior of p16-confirmed HPV-related oropharyngeal squamous cell carcinoma treated with radical radiotherapy. Int J Radiat Oncol Biol Phys 82:276–283

Isayeva T, Maswahu D, Brandwein-Gensler M (2012) Human papillomavirus in non-oropharyngeal head and neck cancers: a systematic literature review. Head Neck Pathol 6(Suppl 1):S104–S120

Jemal A, Simard EP, Dorell C, Noone AM, Markowitz LE, Kohler B, Eheman C, Saraiya M, Bandi P, Saslow D, Cronin KA, Watson M, Schiffmann M, Henley SJ, Schymura MJ, Anderson RN, Yankey D, Edwards BK (2013) Annual report to the nation on the status of cancer, 1975–2009, featuring the burden and trends in human papillomavirus (HPV)-associated cancers and HPV vaccination coverage levels. J Natl Cancer 105:175–201

Jordan RC, Lingen MW, Perez-Ordonez B, He X, Pickard R, Koluder M, Jiang B, Wakely P, Xiao W, Gillison ML (2012) Validation of methods for oropharyngeal cancer HPV status determination in US cooperative group trials. Am J Surg Pathol 36:945–954

Khleif SN (1996) Inhibition of cyclin D-CDK4/CDK6 activity is associated with an E2F-mediated induction of cyclin kinase inhibitor activity. PNAS 93:4350–4354

Kreimer AR, Clifford GM, Boyle P, Franceschi S (2005) Human papillomavirus types in head and neck squamous cell carcinomas worldwide: a systematic review. Cancer Epidemiol Biomark Prev 14:467–475

Lassen P (2010) The role of Human papillomavirus in head and neck cancer and the impact on radiotherapy outcome. Radiother Oncol 95:371–380

Lassen P, Eriksen JG, Hamilton-Dutoit S, Tramm T, Alsner J, Overgaard J (2009) Effect of HPV-associated p16INK4A expression on response to radiotherapy and survival in squamous cell carcinoma of the head and neck. J Clin Oncol 27:1992–1998

Lassen P, Eriksen JG, Hamilton-Dutoit S, Tramm T, Alsner J, Overgaard J (2010) HPV-associated p16-expression and response to hypoxic modification of radiotherapy in head and neck cancer. Radiother Oncol 94:30–35

Lassen P, Eriksen JG, Krogdahl A, Therkildsen MH, Ulhoi BP, Overgaard M, Specht L, Andersen E, Johansen J, Andersen LJ, Grau C, Overgaard J (2011) The influence of HPV-associated p16-expression on accelerated fractionated radiotherapy in head and neck cancer: evaluation of the randomised DAHANCA 6&7 trial. Radiother Oncol 100:49–55

Lassen P, Overgaard J, Eriksen JG (2013) Expression of EGFR and HPV-associated p16 in oropharyngeal carcinoma: correlation and influence on prognosis after radiotherapy in the randomized DAHANCA 5 and 7 trials. Radiother Oncol 108:489–494

Lau HY, Brar S, Klimowicz AC, Petrillo SK, Hao D, Brockton NT, Kong CS, Lees-Miller SP, Magliocco AM (2011) Prognostic significance of p16 in locally advanced squamous cell carcinoma of the head and neck treated with concurrent cisplatin and radiotherapy. Head Neck 33:251–256

Lewis JS (2012) p16 immunohistochemistry as a standalone test for risk stratification in oropharyngeal squamous cell carcinoma. Head Neck Pathol 6(Suppl 1):S75–S82

Licitra L, Perrone F, Bossi P, Suardi S, Mariani L, Artusi R, Oggionni M, Rossini C, Cantu G, Squadrelli M, Quattrone P, Locati LD, Bergamini C, Olmi P, Pierotti MA, Pilotti S (2006) High-risk human papillomavirus affects prognosis in patients with surgically treated oropharyngeal squamous cell carcinoma. J Clin Oncol 24:5630–5636

Lindel K, Beer KT, Laissue J, Greiner RH, Aebersold DM (2001) Human papillomavirus positive squamous cell carcinoma of the oropharynx: a radiosensitive subgroup of head and neck carcinoma. Cancer 92:805–813

Lingen MW, Xiao W, Schmitt A, Jiang B, Pickard R, Kreinbrink P, Perez-Ordonez B, Jordan RC, Gillison ML (2013) Low etiologic fraction for high-risk human papillomavirus in oral cavity squamous cell carcinomas. Oral Oncol 49:1–8

Marur S, D'Souza G, Westra WH, Forastiere AA (2010) HPV-associated head and neck cancer: a virus-related cancer epidemic. Lancet Oncol 11:781–789

Mehanna H, Beech T, Nicholson T, El-Hariry I, McConkey C, Paleri V, Roberts S (2013) Prevalence of human papillomavirus in oropharyngeal and nonoropharyngeal head and neck cancer-systematic review and meta-analysis of trends by time and region. Head Neck 35:747–755

Mellin H, Friesland S, Lewensohn R, Dalianis T, Munck-Wikland E (2000) Human papillomavirus (HPV) DNA in tonsillar cancer: clinical correlates, risk of relapse, and survival. Int J Cancer 89:300–304

Mellin DH, Lindquist D, Bjornestal L, Ohlsson A, Dalianis T, Munck-Wikland E, Elmberger G (2005) P16(INK4a) correlates to human papillomavirus presence, response to radiotherapy and clinical outcome in tonsillar carcinoma. Anticancer Res 25:4375–4383

Mortensen LS, Johansen J, Kallehauge J, Primdahl H, Busk M, Lassen P, Alsner J, Sorensen BS, Toustrup K, Jakobsen S, Petersen J, Petersen H, Theil J, Nordsmark M, Overgaard J (2012) FAZA PET/CT hypoxia imaging in patients with squamous cell carcinoma of the head and neck treated with radiotherapy: results from the DAHANCA 24 trial. Radiother Oncol 105:14–20

Nevins JR (2001) The Rb/E2F pathway and cancer. Hum Mol Genet 10(7):699–703

O'Sullivan B, Huang SH, Perez-Ordonez B, Massey C, Siu LL, Weinreb I, Hope A, Kim J, Bayley AJ, Cummings B, Ringash J, Dawson LA, Cho BC, Chen E, Irish J, Gilbert RW, Hui A, Liu FF, Zhao H, Waldron JN, Xu W (2012) Outcomes of HPV-related oropharyngeal cancer patients treated by radiotherapy alone using altered fractionation. Radiother Oncol 103:49–56

O'Sullivan B, Huang SH, Siu LL, Waldron J, Zhao H, Perez-Ordonez B, Weinreb I, Kim J, Ringash J, Bayley A, Dawson LA, Hope A, Cho J, Irish J, Gilbert R, Gullane P, Hui A, Liu FF, Chen E, Xu W (2013) Deintensification candidate subgroups in human papillomavirus-related oropharyngeal cancer according to minimal risk of distant metastasis. J Clin Oncol 31:543–550

Overgaard J (2011) Hypoxic modification of radiotherapy in squamous cell carcinoma of the head and neck—a systematic review and meta-analysis. Radiother Oncol 100:22–32

Overgaard J, Hansen HS, Overgaard M, Bastholt L, Berthelsen A, Specht L, Lindelov B, Jorgensen K (1998) A randomized double-blind phase III study of nimorazole as a hypoxic radiosensitizer of primary radiotherapy in supraglottic larynx and pharynx carcinoma. Results of the Danish Head and Neck Cancer Study (DAHANCA) Protocol 5-85. Radiother Oncol 46:135–146

Overgaard J, Hansen HS, Specht L, Overgaard M, Grau C, Andersen E, Bentzen J, Bastholt L, Hansen O, Johansen J, Andersen L, Evensen JF (2003) Five compared with six fractions per week of conventional radiotherapy of squamous-cell carcinoma of head and neck: DAHANCA 6 and 7 randomised controlled trial. Lancet 362:933–940

Pajares B, Trigo JM, Toledo MD, Alvarez M, Gonzalez-Hermoso C, Rueda A, Medina JA, Luque V, Jerez JM, Alba E (2013) Differential outcome of concurrent radiotherapy plus epidermal growth factor receptor inhibitors versus radiotherapy plus cisplatin in patients with human papillomavirus-related head and neck cancer. BMC Cancer 13:26

Pignon JP, Le MA, Maillard E, Bourhis J (2009) Meta-analysis of chemotherapy in head and neck cancer (MACH-NC): an update on 93 randomised trials and 17,346 patients. Radiother Oncol 92:4–14

Ragin CC, Taioli E (2007) Survival of squamous cell carcinoma of the head and neck in relation to human papillomavirus infection: review and meta-analysis. Int J Cancer 121:1813–1820

Rieckmann T, Tribius S, Grob TJ, Meyer F, Busch CJ, Petersen C, Dikomey E, and Kriegs M (2013) HNSCC cell lines positive for HPV and p16 possess higher cellular radiosensitivity due to an impaired DSB repair capacity. Radiother Oncol S0167–S8140

Rischin D, Young RJ, Fisher R, Fox SB, Le QT, Peters LJ, Solomon B, Choi J, O'Sullivan B, Kenny LM, McArthur GA (2010a) Prognostic significance of p16INK4A and human papillomavirus in patients with oropharyngeal cancer treated on TROG 02.02 phase III trial. J Clin Oncol 28:4142–4148

Rischin D, Peters LJ, O'Sullivan B, Giralt J, Fisher R, Yuen K, Trotti A, Bernier J, Bourhis J, Ringash J, Henke M, Kenny L (2010b) Tirapazamine, cisplatin, and radiation versus cisplatin and radiation for advanced squamous cell carcinoma of the head and neck (TROG 02.02, HeadSTART): a phase III trial of the Trans-Tasman Radiation Oncology Group. J Clin Oncol 28:2989–2995

Settle K, Posner MR, Schumaker LM, Tan M, Suntharalingam M, Goloubeva O, Strome SE, Haddad RI, Patel SS, Cambell EV III, Sarlis N, Lorch J, Cullen KJ (2009) Racial survival disparity in head and neck cancer results from low prevalence of human papillomavirus infection in black oropharyngeal cancer patients. Cancer Prev Res 2:776–781

Shi W, Kato H, Perez-Ordonez B, Pintilie M, Huang S, Hui A, O'Sullivan B, Waldron J, Cummings B, Kim J, Ringash J, Dawson LA, Gullane P, Siu L, Gillison M, Liu FF (2009) Comparative prognostic value of HPV16 E6 mRNA compared with in situ hybridization for human oropharyngeal squamous carcinoma. J Clin Oncol 27:6213–6221

Slebos RJ, Yi Y, Ely K, Carter J, Evjen A, Zhang X, Shyr Y, Murphy BA, Cmelak AJ, Burkey BB, Netterville J, Levy S, Yarbrough WG, Chung CH (2006) Gene expression differences associated with human papillomavirus status in head and neck squamous cell carcinoma. Clin Cancer Res 12:701–709

Smeets SJ, Braakhuis BJ, Abbas S, Snijders PJ, Ylstra B, van de Wiel MA, Meijer GA, Leemans CR, Brakenhoff RH (2006) Genome-wide DNA copy number alterations in head and neck squamous cell carcinomas with or without oncogene-expressing human papillomavirus. Oncogene 25:2558–2564

Smeets SJ, Hesselink AT, Speel EJ, Haesevoets A, Snijders PJ, Pawlita M, Meijer CJ, Braakhuis BJ, Leemans CR, Brakenhoff RH (2007) A novel algorithm for reliable detection of human papillomavirus in paraffin embedded head and neck cancer specimen. Int J Cancer 121:2465–2472

Smith EM, Ritchie JM, Summersgill KF, Klussmann JP, Lee JH, Wang D, Haugen TH, Turek LP (2004) Age, sexual behavior and human papillomavirus infection in oral cavity and oropharyngeal cancers. Int J Cancer 2004(108):766–772

Sorensen BS, Busk M, Olthof N, Speel EJ, Horsman MR, Alsner J, Overgaard J (2013) Radiosensitivity and effect of hypoxia in HPV positive head and neck cancer cells. Radiother Oncol S0167–S8140

Stransky N, Egloff AM, Tward AD, Kostic AD, Cibulskis K, Sivachenko A, Kryukov GV, Shefler E, Stojanov P, Carter S, Voet D, Auclair D, Berger MF, Guiducci C, Onofrio RC, Parkin M, Romkes M, Weissfeld JL, Seethala RR, Wang L, Rangel-Escareño C, Fernandez-Lopez JC, Hidalgo-Miranda A, Melendez-Zajgla J, Ardlie K, Gabriel BS, Meyerson M, Lander ES, Getz G, Grandis JR (2011) The mutational landscape of head and neck squamous cell carcinoma. Science 333:1157–1160

Sudhoff HH, Schwarze HP, Winder D, Steinstraesser L, Görner M, Stanley M, Goon PKC (2011) Evidence for a causal association for HPV in head and neck cancers. Eur Arch Otorhinolaryngol 268:1541–1547

Topalian SL, Hodi FS, Brahmer JR, Gettinger SN, Smith DC, McDermott DF, Powderly JD, Carvajal RD, Sosman JA, Atkins MB, Leming PD, Spigel DR, Antonia SJ, Horn L, Drake CG, Pardoll DM, Chen L, Sharfman WH, Anders RA, Taube JM, McMiller TL, Xu H, Korman AJ, Jure-Kunkel M, Agrawal S, McDonald D, Kollia GD, Gupta A, Wigginton JM, Sznol M (2012) Safety, activity, and immune correlates of anti-PD-1 antibody in cancer. N Engl J Med 366:2443–2454

Toustrup K, Sorensen BS, Lassen P, Wiuf C, Alsner J, Overgaard J (2012) Gene expression classifier predicts for hypoxic modification of radiotherapy with nimorazole in squamous cell carcinomas of the head and neck. Radiother Oncol 102:122–129

Wansom D, Light E, Worden F, Prince M, Urba S, Chepeha DB, Cordell K, Eisbruch A, Taylor J, D'Silva N, Moyer J, Bradford CR, Kurnit D, Kumar B, Carey TE, Wolf GT (2010) Correlation of cellular immunity with human papillomavirus 16 status and outcome in patients with advanced oropharyngeal cancer. Arch Otolaryngol Head Neck Surg 136:1267–1273

Weinberger PM, Yu Z, Haffty BG, Kowalski D, Harigopal M, Brandsma J, Sasaki C, Joe J, Camp RL, Rimm DL, Psyrri A (2006) Molecular classification identifies a subset of human papillomavirus–associated oropharyngeal cancers with favorable prognosis. J Clin Oncol 24:736–747

Westra WH (2012) The morphologic profile of HPV-related head and neck squamous carcinoma: implications for diagnosis, prognosis, and clinical management. Head Neck Pathol 6(Suppl 1): S48–S54

Worden FP, Kumar B, Lee JS, Wolf GT, Cordell KG, Taylor JM, Urba SG, Eisbruch A, Teknos TN, Chepeha DB, Prince ME, Tsien CI, D'Silva NJ, Yang K, Kurnit DM, Mason HL, Miller TH, Wallace NE, Bradford CR, Carey TE (2008) Chemoselection as a strategy for organ preservation in advanced oropharynx cancer: response and survival positively associated with HPV16 copy number. J Clin Oncol 26:3138–3146

Zur Hausen H (1994) Molecular pathogenesis of cancer of the cervix and its causation by specific human papillomavirus types. Curr top microbiol immunol 186:131–156

Zur Hausen H (2002) Papillomaviruses and cancer: from basic studies to clinical application. Nature Rev Cancer 2:342–350

FDG and Beyond

Dirk De Ruysscher, Karin Haustermans and Daniela Thorwarth

Abstract

Although many PET tracers are in use, FDG still is the most widely used in clinical oncology practice. FDG therefore deserves an in-depth discussion, which is even more interesting because of the huge increase in the molecular biology of glucose metabolism. Obviously, other tracers are of increasing importance as well, and these will be discussed in short.

Keyword

Molecular imaging · Target volume · PET · FDG · Tracer · Hypoxia

Although many PET tracers are in use, FDG still is the most widely used in clinical oncology practice. FDG therefore deserves an in-depth discussion, which is even more interesting because of the huge increase in the molecular biology of glucose metabolism. Obviously, other tracers are of increasing importance as well, and these will be discussed in short.

D. De Ruysscher (✉) · K. Haustermans
Radiation Oncology, University Hospitals Leuven/KU Leuven, Louvain, Belgium
e-mail: dirk.deruysscher@maastro.nl

K. Haustermans
e-mail: karin.haustermans@uzleuven.be

D. Thorwarth
Section for Biomedical Physics, University Hospital for Radiation Oncology Tübingen, Tübingen, Germany
e-mail: daniela.thorwarth@med.uni-tuebingen.de

D. De Ruysscher
Maastricht University Medical Center, GROW, Maastro clinic, Louvain, Belgium

© Springer-Verlag Berlin Heidelberg 2016
M. Baumann et al. (eds.), *Molecular Radio-Oncology*, Recent Results
in Cancer Research 198, DOI 10.1007/978-3-662-49651-0_8

1 FDG

In order to understand thoroughly the biological meaning of FDG uptake, it is necessary to have some insight into the way glucose is taken up by cells and how this is regulated.

1.1 Uptake of Deoxyglucose

2-Deoxy-2[^{18}F]fluoro-D-glucose or FDG is still the working horse for clinical PET imaging in oncology. It exploits the preferential utilisation of aerobic glycolysis by cancer cells. Like regular D-glucose, FDG enters the cell via the glucose transporters GLUT1 and GLUT3, which are ATP-independent (Bensinger and Christofk 2012). FDG is, again like glucose, phosphorylated by hexokinase to FDG-6-phosphate. While glucose-6-phosphate is converted to fructose-6-phosphate by an isomerisation process and thus comes into the glycolysis pathway, or is oxidised to 6-phosphonogluconolactone to come into the pentose phosphate pathway, FDG-6-phosphate is not metabolised. This is due to the lack of an oxygen atom at the C-2 position of the molecule. FDG-6-phosphate is unable to diffuse out of the cell, and the process of dephosphorylation is very slow. FDG-6-phosphate is thus trapped in the cell at a rate that is proportional to the glucose consumption. FDG uptake gives therefore information about the uptake of glucose by ATP-independent transporters, i.e. specific GLUTs, and hexokinase activity.

Many common cancers show a high FDG uptake, including lung, breast and colorectal carcinoma, but also melanoma and many lymphomas (Scheibler et al. 2012). However, some cancers are not uniformly FDG-avid on PET scans such as hepatocellular carcinoma and pancreatic and prostate cancer. Reasons for the low FDG uptake visualisation on PET scans include alternative energy sources for glucose such as fatty acids, poor perfusion of the tumour, low density of tumour cells or a high background signal, e.g. by bladder filing. Some malignancies such as well-differentiated hepatocellular carcinoma exhibit such high-level glucose-6-phosphatase that FDG-6-phosphate is, contrary to the situation in most cancer cells, dephosphorylated (Torizuka et al. 1995). FDG subsequently can leave the cell. Some cancer cells are dependent on ATP-dependent glucose uptake (Bettendorff et al. 2002). These receptors are not a substrate for deoxyglucose and are thus not visualised by FDG.

1.2 Transcriptional Regulation of Glucose Uptake

Glucose uptake is regulated via a complex and incompletely understood mechanism. The hypoxia-inducible factor 1 (HIF1) regulates the expression of glucose transporters and of most of the glycolytic enzymes (Semenza 2012). HIF1 upregulates glucose uptake and increases the expression of pyruvate dehydrogenase kinases (PDKs) that phosphorylate and inactivate the mitochondrial pyruvate dehydrogenase complex. This enzyme controls the entry of pyruvate into the tri-carboxylic acid (TCA) cycle. In normal cells under normal oxygen concentrations, HIF1-α is constantly degraded, but in hypoxic conditions it is stabilised. Stabilised HIF1 increases the influx of glucose and stimulates glycolysis, but also decreases the pyruvate flux into the TCA cycle. Oxygen consumption is reduced and ATP production diminishes from 36 mol ATP per mol glucose to only 2 mol ATP per mol glucose in case of anaerobic glycolysis. However, HIF1 stabilisation occurs not only in hypoxia, but is also very common in many cancers in the presence of oxygen. It may be caused by enhanced transcription downstream of the PI3K/AKT/mTOR pathway. In this scenario of aerobic glycolysis (Warburg effect), 4 mol ATP is made per mol glucose. Both anaerobic glycolysis and aerobic gly-colysis thus lead to increased FDG uptake.

The MYC oncogene upregulates many glucose transporters, glycolytic enzymes, PDK1 and lactate dehydrogenase A (Osthus et al. 2000; Shim et al. 1997; Dang et al. 2008). MYC thus enhances the Warburg effect by increasing glycolysis while at the same time decreasing the entry of pyruvate into the TCA cycle. At the same time, MYC activates the transcription of glutamine transporters and glutaminase-1, leading to a higher conversion of glutamine to glutamate (Gao et al. 2009), an important carbogen and nitrogen source, by repression of miRNA-23a/b expression (Gao et al. 2009).

The well-known tumour suppressor p53 suppresses glycolysis regulating fructose-2,6-bisphosphatase (Bensaad et al. 2006). At the same time, p53 promotes the oxidative phosphorylation by increased synthesis of cytochrome c oxidase-2 (Matoba et al. 2006). The loss of p53 expression in tumour cells will thus lead into increased glucose uptake and decreased oxidative phosphorylation.

In conclusion, FDG uptake is a reflection of the tightly regulated uptake of glucose and the Warburg effect. These complex mechanisms explain why FDG uptake is related to cell viability (Dooms et al. 2009), hypoxia (van Baardwijk et al. 2007) and cell density, but also to MYC amplification, p53 mutation, activation of PI3K/AKT/mTOR and many others. It therefore does not come as a surprise that FDG uptake is by no means specific for a given biological characteristic, but is related to many unfavourable features. FDG thus remains the most frequently used PET tracer in oncology.

1.3   Use of FDG in Radiation Oncology

As FDG has been shown to be taken up by the viable parts of most tumours, it is widely used for radiotherapy (RT) staging, therapy decision-making and treatment planning, but also treatment alteration, response monitoring and follow-up assessment (MacManus et al. 2009; Arens et al. 2011; Mak et al. 2011; Das and Ten Haken 2011; Bentzen and Grégoire 2011; Wahl et al. 2011; Nestle et al. 2009). Unfortunately, in some tumours FDG cannot be used in a reliable manner as its uptake is not visible due to FDG accumulation in surrounding normal tissues such as brain, stomach or heart or excreted FDG in the urine.

FDG PET has been shown to have a high impact on the diagnosis and staging of a variety of different cancers, such as lung, head and neck and colorectal cancer, melanoma, lymphoma, breast and gynaecological cancers as well as oesophageal tumours (Gambhir et al. 2001). Combined FDG PET/CT has been shown to perform superior-to-stand-alone RT planning CT in a number of different cancer sites such as lung, head and neck, or colorectal or gynaecological tumours (Delbeke and Martin 2004; Troost et al. 2010; De Ruysscher and Kirsch 2010; Lambrecht and Haustermans 2010; Haie-Meder et al. 2010).

In non-small cell lung cancer (NSCLC), FDG PET/CT is commonly used for staging, RT target volume definition and treatment planning. In prospective trials where FDG PET was used for tumour staging, about 20 % of the patients considered for curative RT were excluded from radical RT because of advanced disease diagnosed during FDG PET (Mac Manus and Hicks 2012). Incorporation of FDG PET into patient selection and RT treatment planning has led to significant improvements for patients with NSCLC (Mac Manus 2010). The use of FDG for RT planning allows better target volume definition, reduced inter-observer variability and selective irradiation of involved mediastinal lymph nodes (De Ruysscher et al. 2012; MacManus et al. 2009). Studies that compared PET-based target volume delineation to only CT-based contouring of the gross target volume (GTV) reported significant differences (Mac Manus and Hicks 2012). A recent clinical study reported on frequent changes in the management of patients with NSCLC due to FDG PET/CT findings and excellent association of FDG PET with overall survival (Mac Manus et al. 2013).

Also head and neck cancer (HNC) has been extensively studied with FDG PET/CT. Higher precision and better reproducibility have been observed when using FDG PET for the GTV definition (Grégoire et al. 2012; Arens et al. 2011; Mak et al. 2011; Gornik and Weber 2011; Nestle et al. 2009). Predictive value of FDG uptake before the start of RT has been reported recently (Picchio et al. 2013; Schinagl et al. 2011). Methodological approaches for the direct integration of PET information into RT planning are still under investigation (Picchio et al. 2013; Schinagl et al. 2011).

In the management of cervical cancer, FDG PET has been shown to be more sensitive than CT in detecting lymph node metastases (Grigsby 2009). Increased FDG uptake in para-aortic lymph nodes has been associated with lower control probabilities. Similarly, positive uptake in the primary tumour after the end of therapy was correlated with less favourable outcome (Grigsby 2009).

FDG is increasingly used for improved target volume delineation. A variety of different methodological approaches for manual, semi-automatic or automatic PET-based GTV contouring have been proposed and extensively studied in the last years (Shepherd et al. 2012; Erdi et al. 1997; Schaefer et al. 2008; Geets et al. 2007). In addition to large differences in complexity and implementation, validation of PET-based delineation strategies is scarce. Furthermore, different physical and biological factors as well as patient management and examination protocols may have a major impact on PET image characteristics such as spatial resolution, signal-to-noise ratio and tracer quantification. As a consequence, those factors will also affect target volume delineation (Schinagl et al. 2013). Several studies that compared automated PET-based contouring to the GTVs delineated by trained radiation oncology specialists reported the superiority of manually delineated volumes (Schinagl et al. 2013; Bayne et al. 2010).

Data published so far on studies investigating the potential of FDG PET/CT in RT suggest two possibilities for the future use of FDG PET in RT: (i) PET image data are predictors but can only be used for patient selection or (ii) PET signal information can in addition be used to alter or intensify RT individually (Grégoire et al. 2012). The latter approach is called dose painting (DP) and aims at prescribing higher doses to volumes showing positive PET tracer uptake (Thorwarth et al. 2010). The idea of DP has been extensively studied in theoretical studies investigating the technical feasibility and the dosimetric effect of such treatment adaptations. Overall, two different DP strategies have been proposed so far: (i) homogeneously escalated dose level to a GTV_{PET} or (ii) prescription of locally varying increased doses according to the signal of each single PET voxel. To date, only a few studies were published that realised PET-based dose escalation in HNC or NSCLC (Madani et al. 2011; Berwouts et al. 2013; Van Elmpt et al. 2012).

In addition, a number of different studies have shown the value of FDG PET/CT for early response monitoring of (chemo-)radiotherapy in several tumour sites (Usmanij et al. 2013; Cuenca et al. 2013; Van Elmpt et al. 2012; Hatt et al. 2013). A recent study in oesophageal cancer investigated the potential of early response assessment via FDG PET/CT after 2 weeks of radiochemotherapy (20Gy plus 2 cycles of chemotherapy). The authors concluded that the metabolic response defined as 1-SUV2/SUV1 showed a great prognostic value in n = 72 oesophageal cancer patients (Cuenca et al. 2013). Another recently published study reported similar results for a study aiming at response assessment with FDG PET/CT in n = 28 NSCLC patients. In this study, early metabolic changes were measured using the difference in the total lesion glycolysis (TLG) between the pre-treatment FDG PET scan and the second scan at the end of the second week of therapy. Here, changes in TLG during the first two weeks of therapy were reported to be prognostic for response to concomitant radiochemotherapy in NSCLC (Usmanij et al. 2013). Furthermore, pre-treatment TLG was observed to be correlated with progression-free survival (PFS) in this patient group (Usmanij et al. 2013). A similar study published by Van Elmpt et al. (2012) investigated response assessment in n = 34 NSCLC patients using changes in mean SUV in the target volume comparing pre-treatment FDG PET/CT scans to scans acquired after two weeks of radiochemotherapy. This study concludes that a decrease in FDG uptake in the primary tumour correlates with higher long-term overall survival, whereas changes in tumour volume defined on CT did not show a correlation with overall survival (Van Elmpt et al. 2012). Also for rectal cancer, the potential of early response prediction based on sequential FDG PET was shown in a clinical study (Hatt et al. 2013).

As a consequence, FDG PET/CT might in the future be a very efficient tool for early response assessment and eventually also for subsequent decisions on therapy alterations and adaptations.

In 2000, initially guidelines for the evaluation of response to treatment in solid tumours (RECIST) had been published (Therasse et al. 2000, 2006), which have been revised later (RECIST 1.1) (Eisenhauer et al. 2009). Those RECIST criteria were recommended to be used for the measurement and extrapolation of response to treatment in RT. Wahl et al. (Wahl et al. 2009) modified those criteria for dedicated use of FDG PET for response measurements and follow-up examinations (PET response criteria in solid tumours, PERCIST 1.0).

2   Other Tracers, Excluding Hypoxia

The uptake of ^{18}F-fluorothymidine (^{18}F-FLT), a marker of DNA synthesis, correlates with tumour proliferation (Apisarnthanarax et al. 2006; Buck et al. 2003; Muzi et al. 2005; Wagner et al. 2003; Yamamoto et al. 2007; Yap et al. 2006). FLT can detect changes in proliferation during and after irradiation in colorectal tumours and breast cancer cell lines (Pan et al. 2008; Roels et al. 2008; Wieder et al. 2007). FLT PET enables to image proliferation during chemo-radiotherapy (Everitt et al. 2009). FLT PET has recently been shown to allow for early prediction of therapy response in HNC (Hoeben et al. 2013).

Amino acid tracers may have the advantage over FDG in that they more specifically accumulate in viable cancer cells (Kubota et al. 1995). However, clinical data remain scarce (Grosu and Weber 2010). Amino acid PET is to date mostly used in brain tumours, as in the brain amino acids to not present with physiologic uptake as, for example, FDG does. 11C-Methionine (MET) PET is currently the most popular amino acid tracer used in PET imaging of brain tumours (Glaudemans et al. 2013). It provides a high detection rate and allows for accurate lesion delineation for RT treatment planning, especially in glioblastoma but also in other tumours such as metastatic brain tumours. A recent study showed that the usage of MET PET for the definition of target volumes planned for stereotactic irradiation with intensity-modulated RT (IMRT) may contain additional information compared to MRI, which remains the gold standard for stereotactic irradiations in the brain (Miwa et al. 2012). But also other amino acid PET tracers, such as O-(2-^{18}F-fluoroethyl)-L-tyrosine (FET) PET may be very effective for RT treatment planning and also for the assessment of response to treatment. Galldiks et al. could show the added value of FET PET examinations in comparison with contrast-enhanced MRI data in glioblastoma (Galldiks et al. 2012). This study concluded that in contrast to volumes defined from gadolinium MRI, changes in FET PET may be a valuable parameter to measure treatment response in glioblastoma (Galldiks et al. 2012).

Choline PET/CT, labelled with either ^{11}C or ^{18}F, is mainly used for imaging of prostate cancer (Picchio et al. 2010). Nevertheless, for primary prostate cancer, the additional value of choline PET/CT to MRI has been shown to be very limited for the localisation of intraprostatic especially when multiparametric MRI is used (Van den Bergh et al. 2012, 2013). In contrast, for recurrent prostate cancer that has already been treated primarily with RT and present with suspicion for relapse

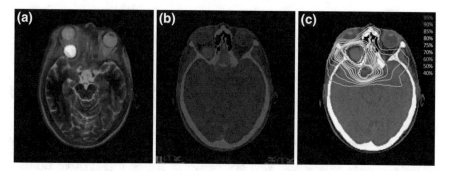

Fig. 1 [68 Ga]-DOTATATE PET/MR imaging for accurate RT target volume delineation and treatment planning in meningioma. **a** Hybrid PET/MR imaging using [68 Ga]-DOTATATE. Small additional lesion close to the pituitary gland is only visible in the DOTATATE PET data. **b** Fusion of DOTATATE PET to the planning CT. **c** Planning CT with gross target volume (GTV) in red consisting of the two lesions visible in the PET/MR data in (**a**), planning target volume (PTV) in yellow defined as GTV plus a 2-mm expansion in all three directions. In addition, the clinical IMRT plan is shown represented by different isodose lines (see legend in the figure) highly conformal to the PET-based target volume. For treatment planning, the treatment planning system Hyperion (Eberhard-Karls University Tübingen, Germany) was used

during follow-up, the detection rate of choline PET is very high and has been reported to be proportional to trigger PSA (prostate-specific antigen) (Chondrogiannis et al. 2013). As a consequence, choline PET may have an important impact on the therapeutic strategy in patients with recurrent prostate cancer and can help to determine appropriate treatment (Soyka et al. 2012).

68Ga-DOTATOC or 68Ga-DOTATATE PET/CT is widely used for imaging of meningioma in order to accurately define target volumes for RT treatment (Thorwarth et al. 2011; Graf et al. 2013; Combs et al. 2013). Meningiomas express the somatostatin receptor subtype 2 (SSTR2) (Reubi et al. 1986); therefore, the 86Ga-labelled somatostatin receptor ligands DOTATOC and DOTATATE (Velikyan et al. 2012) can be used as tracers for the visualisation of the geometric extension of meningiomas with PET (Khan et al. 2009; Miederer et al. 2009; Henze et al. 2005). Several studies could show that DOTATOC PET/CT imaging is of additional value compared to MRI for RT target volume definition (Thorwarth et al. 2011; Graf et al. 2013; Combs et al. 2013) (Fig. 1).

3   Conclusions

FDG PET integration in RT is now standard practice and has improved patient care substantially. FDG will most likely remain the working horse in the near future in oncology, but new more specific tracers are emerging, some of which have been successfully introduced in daily clinical practice.

Conflict of Interest None to declare.

References

Apisarnthanarax S, Alauddin MM, Mourtada F et al (2006) Early detection of chemoradioresponse in esophageal carcinoma by 3'-deoxy-3'-3H-fluorothymidine using preclinical tumor models. Clin Cancer Res 12:4590–4597

Arens AI, Troost EG, Schinagl D, Kaanders JH, Oyen WJ (2011) FDG-PET/CT in radiation treatment planning of head and neck squamous cell carcinoma. Q J Nucl Med Mol Imaging 55 (5):521–528

Bayne M, Hicks RJ, Everitt S et al (2010) Reproducibility of "intelligent" contouring of gross tumor volume in non-small-cell lung cancer on PET/CT images using a standardized visual method. Int J Radiat Oncol Biol Phys 77(4):1151–1157

Bensaad K, Tsuruta A, Selak MA, Vidal MN, Nakano K, Bartrons R et al (2006) TIGAR, a p53-inducible regulator of glycolysis and apoptosis. Cell 126:107–120

Bensinger SJ, Christofk HR (2012) New aspects of the Warburg effect in cancer cell biology. Semin Cell Dev Biol 23(4):352–361

Bentzen SM, Grégoire V (2011) Molecular imaging-based dose painting: a novel paradigm for radiation therapy prescription. Semin Radiat Oncol 21(2):101–110

Berwouts D, Olteanu LA, Duprez F et al (2013) Three-phase adaptive dose-painting-by-numbers for head-and-neck cancer: initial results of the phase I clinical trial. Radiother Oncol 107 (3):310–316

Bettendorff L, Lakaye B, Margineanu I, Grisar T, Wins P (2002) ATP-driven, Na$^{(+)}$-independent inward Cl$^-$ pumping in neuroblastoma cells. J Neurochem 81(4):792–801

Buck AK, Halter G, Schirrmeister H et al (2003) Imaging proliferation in lung tumors with PET: ^{18}F-FLT versus ^{18}F-FDG. J Nucl Med 44:1426–1431

Chondrogiannis S, Marzola MC, Perretti A et al (2013) Role of ^{18}F-choline PET/CT in suspicion of relapse following definitive radiotherapy for prostate cancer. Eur J Nucl Med Mol Imaging 40(9):1356–1364

Combs SE, Welzel T, Habermehl D et al (2013) Prospective evaluation of early treatment outcome in patients with meningiomas treated with particle therapy based on target volume definition with MRI and 68 Ga-DOTATOC. Acta Oncol 52(3):514–520

Cuenca X, Hennequin C, Hindié E et al (2013) Evaluation of early response to concomitant chemoradiotherapy by interim ^{18}F-FDG PET/CT imaging in patients with locally advanced oesophageal carcinomas. Eur J Nucl Med Mol Imaging 40(4):477–485

Dang CV, Kim JW, Gao P, Yustein J (2008) The interplay between MYC and HIF in cancer. Nat Rev Cancer 8:51–56

Das SK, Ten Haken RK (2011) Functional and molecular image guidance in radiotherapy treatment planning optimization. Semin Radiat Oncol 21(2):111–118

De Ruysscher D, Kirsch CM (2010) PET scans in radiotherapy planning of lung cancer. Radiother Oncol 96(3):335–338

De Ruysscher D, Nestle U, Jeraj R, Macmanus M (2012) PET scans in radiotherapy planning of lung cancer. Lung Cancer 75(2):141–145

Delbeke D, Martin WH (2004) Metabolic imaging with FDG: a primer. Cancer J 10:201–213

Dooms C, van Baardwijk A, Verbeken E, van Suylen RJ, Stroobants S, De Ruysscher D, Vansteenkiste J (2009) Association between ^{18}F-fluoro-2-deoxy-D-glucose uptake values and tumor vitality: prognostic value of positron emission tomography in early-stage non-small cell lung cancer. J Thorac Oncol 4(7):822–828

Eisenhauer EA, Therasse P, Bogaerts J et al (2009) New response evaluation criteria in solid tumors: revised RECIST guideline (version 1.1). Eur J Cancer 45:228–247

Erdi YE, Mawlawi O, Larson SM et al (1997) Segmentation of lung lesion volume by adaptive positron emission tomography image thresholding. Cancer 80:2505–2509

Everitt S, Hicks RJ, Ball D et al (2009) Imaging cellular proliferation during chemo-radiotherapy: a pilot study of serial ^{18}F-FLT positron emission tomography/computed tomography imaging for non-small-cell lung cancer. Int J Radiat Oncol Biol Phys 75:1098–1104

Galldiks N, Langen KJ, Holy K et al (2012) Assessment of treatment response in patients with glioblastoma using O-(2-^{18}F-fluoroethyl)-L-tyrosine PET in comparison to MRI. J Nucl Med 53(7):1048–1057

Gambhir SS, Czernin J, Schwimmer J, Silverman DH, Coleman RE, Phelps ME (2001) A tabulated summary of the FDG literature. J Nucl Med 42(5 Suppl):1S–93S

Gao P, Tchernyshyov I, Chang TC, Lee YS, Kita K, Ochi T et al (2009a) c-Myc suppression of miR-23a/b enhances mitochondrial glutaminase expression and glutamine metabolism. Nature 458:762–765

Gao P, Tchernyshyov I, Chang TC, Lee YS, Kita K, Ochi T et al (2009b) c-Myc suppression of miR-23a/b enhances mitochondrial glutaminase expression and glutamine metabolism. Nature 458:762–765

Geets X, Lee JA, Bol A, Lonneux M, Grégoire V (2007) A gradient-based method for segmenting FDG-PET images: methodology and validation. Eur J Nucl Med Mol Imaging 34:1427–1438

Glaudemans AW, Enting RH, Heesters MA et al (2013) Value of 11C-methionine PET in imaging of brain tumours and metastases. Eur J Nucl Med Mol Imaging 40(4):615–635

Gornik G, Weber W (2011) New tracers beyond FDG in head and neck oncology. Q J Nucl Med Mol Imaging 55(5):529–540

Graf R, Nyuyki F, Steffen IG et al (2013) Contribution of 68 Ga-DOTATOC PET/CT to target volume delineation of skull base meningiomas treated with stereotactic radiation therapy. Int J Radiat Oncol Biol Phys 85(1):68–73

Grégoire V, Jeraj R, Lee JA, O'Sullivan B (2012) Radiotherapy for head and neck tumours in 2012 and beyond: conformal, tailored, and adaptive? Lancet Oncol 13(7):e292–e300

Grigsby PW (2009) PET/CT imaging to guide cervical cancer therapy. Futures Oncol 5:953–958

Grosu A-L, Weber W (2010) PET for radiation treatment planning of brain tumours. Radiother Oncol 96(3):325–327

Haie-Meder C, Mazeron R, Magné N (2010) Clinical evidence on PET–CT for radiation therapy planning in cervix and endometrial cancer. Radiother Oncol 96(3):351–355

Hatt M, van Stiphout R, le Pogam A, Lammering G, Visvikis D, Lambin P (2013) Early prediction of pathological response in locally advanced rectal cancer based on sequential ^{18}F-FDG PET. Acta Oncol 52(3):619–626

Henze M, Dimitrakopoulou-Strauss A, Milker-Zable S et al (2005) Characterization of ^{68}Ga-DOTA-D-Phe1-Tyr3-octreoide kinetics in patients with meningiomas. J Nucl Med 46(5):763–769

Hoeben BA, Troost EG, Span PN et al (2013) ^{18}F-FLT PET during radiotherapy or chemoradiotherapy in head and neck squamous cell carcinoma is an early predictor of outcome. J Nucl Med 54(4):532–540

Khan MU, Khan S, El-Refaie S et al (2009) Clinical indications for Gallium-68 positron emission tomography imaging. Eur J Surg Oncol 35:561–567

Kubota R, Kubota K, Yamada S et al (1995) Methionine uptake by tumor tissue: a microautoradiographic comparison with FDG. J Nucl Med 36:484–492

Lambrecht M, Haustermans K (2010) Clinical evidence on PET-CT for radiation therapy planning in gastro-intestinal tumors. Radiother Oncol 96(3):339–346

Mac Manus MP (2010) Use of PET/CT for staging and radiation therapy planning in patients with non-small cell lung cancer. Q J Nucl Med Mol Imaging 54(5):510–520

Mac Manus MP, Hicks RJ (2012) The role of positron emission tomography/computed tomography in radiotherapy planning for patients with lung cancer. Semin Nucl Med 42(5):308–319

Mac Manus MP, Everitt S, Bayne M et al (2013) The use of fused PET/CT images for patient selection and radical radiotherapy target volume definition in patients with non-small cell lung cancer: results of a prospective study with mature survival data. Radiother Oncol 106(3):292–298

MacManus M, Nestle U, Rosenzweig KE et al (2009) Use of PET and PET/CT for radiation therapy planning: IAEA expert report 2006–2007. Radiother Oncol 91(1):85–94

Madani I, Duprez F, Boterberg T et al (2011) Maximum tolerated dose in a phase I trial on adaptive dose painting by numbers for head and neck cancer. Radiother Oncol 101(3):351–355

Mak D, Corry J, Lau E, Rischin D, Hicks RJ (2011) Role of FDG-PET/CT in staging and follow-up of head and neck squamous cell carcinoma. Q J Nucl Med Mol Imaging 55(5):487–499

Matoba S, Kang JG, Patino WD, Wragg A, Boehm M, Gavrilova O et al (2006) p53 regulates mitochondrial respiration. Science 312:1650–1653

Miederer M, Seidl S, Buck A et al (2009) Correlation of immunohistopathological expression of somatostatin receptor 2 with standardized uptake values in ^{68}Ga-DOTATOC-PET/CT. Eur J Nucl Med Mol Imaging 36(1):48–52

Miwa K, Matsuo M, Shinoda J et al (2012) Clinical value of [^{11}C]methionine OET for stereotactic radiation therapy with intensity modulated radiation therapy to metastatic brain tumors. Int J Radiat Oncol Biol Phys 84(5):1139–1144

Muzi M, Vesselle H, Grierson JR et al (2005) Kinetic analysis of 3'-deoxy-3'-fluorothymidine PET studies: validation studies in patients with lung cancer. J Nucl Med 46:274–282

Nestle U, Weber W, Hentschel M, Grosu A-L (2009) Biological imaging in radiotherapy: role of positron emission tomography. Phys Med Biol 54:R1–R25

Osthus RC, Shim H, Kim S, Li Q, Reddy R, Mukherjee M et al (2000) Deregulation of glucose transporter 1 and glycolytic gene expression by c-MycJ. Biol Chem 275:21797–21800

Pan MH, Huang SC, Liao YP et al (2008) FLT-PET imaging of radiation responses in murine tumors. Mol Imaging Biol 10:325–334

Picchio M, Giovannini E, Grivellaro C et al (2010) Clinical evidence on PET/CT for radiation therapy planning in prostate cancer. Radiother Oncol 96(3):347–350

Picchio M, Kirienko M, Mapelli P et al (2013) Predictive value of ^{18}F-FDG PET/CT for the outcome of ^{18}F-FDG PET-guided radiotherapy in patients with head and neck cancer. Eur J Nucl Med Mol Imaging (epub)

Reubi JC, Maurer R, Klijn JG et al (1986) High incidence of somatostatin receptors in human meningiomas: biochemical characterization. J Clin Endocrinol Metab 63(2):433–438

Roels S, Slagmolen P, Nuyts J et al (2008) Biological image-guided radiotherapy in rectal cancer: is there a role for FMISO or FLT, next to FDG? Acta Oncol 47:1237–1248

Schaefer A, Kremp S, Hellwig D, Rübe C (2008) Kirsch Cm, Nestle U. A contrast-oriented algorithm for FDG-PET-based delineation of tumour volumes for the radiotherapy of lung cancer: derivation from phantom measurements and validation in patient data. Eur J Nucl Med Mol Imaging 35:1989–1999

Scheibler F, Zumbé P, Janssen I, Viebahn M, Schröer-Günther M, Grosselfinger R, Hausner E, Sauerland S, Lange S (2012) Randomized controlled trials on PET: a systematic review of topics, design, and quality. J Nucl Med 53(7):1016–1025

Schinagl DA, Span PN, Oyen WJ, Kaanders JH (2011) Can FDG PET predict radiation treatment outcome in head and neck cancer patients? Results of a prospective study. Eur J Nucl Med Mol Imaging 38:1449–1458

Schinagl DA, Span PN, van den Hoogen FJ et al (2013) Pathology-based validation of FDG PET segmentation tools for volume assessment of lymph node metastases from head and neck cancer. Eur J Nucl Med Mol Imaging (epub)

Semenza GL (2012) Hypoxia-inducible factors in physiology and medicine. Cell 148(3):399–408

Shepherd T, Teras M, Beichel R et al (2012) Comparative study with new accuracy metrics for target volume contouring in PET image guided radiation therapy. IEEE Trans Med Imaging (epub)

Shim H, Dolde C, Lewis BC, Wu CS, Dang G, Jungmann RA et al (1997) c-Myc transactivation of LDH-A: implications for tumor metabolism and growth. Proc Natl Acad Sci USA 94:6658–6663

Soyka JD, Muster MA, Schmid DT et al (2012) Clinical impact of ^{18}F-choline PET/CT in patients with recurrent prostate cancer. Eur J Nucl Med Mol Imaging 39(6):936–943

Therasse P, Arbuck SG, Eisenhauer EA et al (2000) New guidelines to evaluate the response to treatment of solid tumors. European Organization for Research and Treatment of Cancer, National Institute of the United States, National Cancer Institute of Canada. J Natl Cancer Inst 92:205–216

Therasse P, Eisenhauer EA, Verweij J (2006) RECIST revisited: a review of validation studies on tumor assessment. Eur J Cancer 42:1031–1039

Thorwarth D, Geets X, Paiusco M (2010) Physical radiotherapy treatment planning based on functional PET/CT data. Radiother Oncol 96(3):317–324

Thorwarth D, Henke G, Müller AC et al (2011) Simultaneous 68 Ga-DOTATOC-PET/MRI for IMRT treatment planning for meningioma: first experience. Int J Radiat Oncol Biol Phys 81 (1):277–283

Torizuka T, Tamaki N, Inokuma T, Magata Y, Sasayama S, Yonekura Y, Tanaka A, Yamaoka Y, Yamamoto K, Konishi J (1995) In vivo assessment of glucose metabolism in hepatocellular carcinoma with FDG-PET. J Nucl Med 36(10):1811–1817

Troost EGC, Schinagl DAX, Bussink J et al (2010) Clinical evidence on PET–CT for radiation therapy planning in head and neck tumours. Radiother Oncol 96(3):328–334

Usmanij EA, Geus-Oei F, Troost EG et al (2013) ^{18}F-FDG PET early response evaluation of locally advanced non-small cell lung cancer treated with concomitant radiochemotherapy. J Nucl Med 54(9):1528–1534

van Baardwijk A, Dooms C, van Suylen RJ, Verbeken E, Hochstenbag M, Dehing-Oberije C, Rupa D, Pastorekova S, Stroobants S, Buell U, Lambin P, Vansteenkiste J, De Ruysscher D (2007) The maximum uptake of (18)F-deoxyglucose on positron emission tomography scan correlates with survival, hypoxia inducible factor-1alpha and GLUT-1 in non-small cell lung cancer. Eur J Cancer 43(9):1392–1398

Van den Bergh L, Koole M, Isebaert S et al (2012) Is there an additional value of ^{11}C-Choline PET-CT to T2-weighted MRI images in the localization of intraprostatic tumor nodules? Int J Radiat Oncol Biol Phys 83(5):1486–1492

Van den Bergh L, Isebaert S, Koole M et al (2013) Does 11C-Choline PET-CT contribute to multiparametric MRI for prostate cancer localization? Strahlenther Oncol (epub)

van Elmpt W, De Ruysscher D, van der Salm A et al (2012a) The PET-boost randomised phase II dose-escalation trial in non-small cell lung cancer. Radiother Oncol 104(1):67–71

Van Elmpt W, Ollers M, Dingemans AM, Lambin P, De Ruysscher D (2012b) Response assessment using ^{18}F-FDG PET early in the course of radiotherapy correlates with survival in advanced-stage non-small cell lung cancer. J Nucl Med 53(10):1514–1520

Velikyan I, Xu H, Nair M, Hall H (2012) Robust labelling and comparative preclinical characterization of DOTA-TOC and DOTA-TATE. Nucl Med Biol 39(5):68–73

Wagner M, Seitz U, Buck A et al (2003) 3'-[^{18}F]fluoro-3'-deoxythymidine ([^{18}F]-FLT) as positron emission tomography tracer for imaging proliferation in a murine B-Cell lymphoma model and in the human disease. Cancer Res 63:2681–2687

Wahl RL, Jacene H, Kasamon Y, Lodge MA (2009) From RECIST to PERCIST: evolving considerations for PET response criteria in solid tumors. J Nucl Med 50(Suppl 1):122S–150S

Wahl RL, Herman JM, Ford E (2011) The promise and pitfalls of positron emission tomography and single-photon emission computed tomography molecular imaging-guided radiation therapy. Semin Radiat Oncol 21(2):88–100

Wieder HA, Geinitz H, Rosenberg R et al (2007) PET imaging with [^{18}F]3'-deoxy-3'-fluorothymidine for prediction of response to neoadjuvant treatment in patients with rectal cancer. Eur J Nucl Med Mol Imaging 34:878–883

Yamamoto Y, Nishiyama Y, Ishikawa S et al (2007) Correlation of ^{18}F-FLT and ^{18}F-FDG uptake on PET with Ki-67 immunohistochemistry in non-small cell lung cancer. Eur J Nucl Med Mol Imaging 34:1610–1616

Yap CS, Czernin J, Fishbein MC et al (2006) Evaluation of thoracic tumors with ^{18}F-fluorothymidine and ^{18}F-fluorodeoxyglucose-positron emission tomography. Chest 129:393–401

On the Reliability of Automatic Volume Delineation in Low-Contrast [18F]FMISO-PET Imaging

Robert Haase, Michael Andreeff and Nasreddin Abolmaali

Abstract

Hypoxia is a marker of poor prognosis in malignant tumors independent from the selected therapeutic method and the therapy should be intensified in such tumors. Hypoxia imaging with positron emission tomography (PET) is limited by low contrast to noise ratios with every available tracer. In radiation oncology appropriate delineation is required to allow therapy and intensification. While manual segmentation results are highly dependent from experience and observers condition (high inter- and intra observer variability), threshold- and gradient-based algorithms for automatic segmentation frequently fail in low contrast data sets. Likewise, calibration of these algorithms using phantoms is not useful. Complex computational models such as swarm intelligence-based algorithms are promising tools for optimized segmentation results and allow observer independent interpretation of multimodal and multidimensional imaging data.

R. Haase · N. Abolmaali
OncoRay, National Center for Radiation Research in Oncology, Medical Faculty Carl Gustav Carus, TU Dresden, Fetscherstraße 74, 01307 Dresden, Germany

M. Andreeff
Clinic and Policlinic for Nuclear Medicine, University Hospital Carl Gustav Carus, TU Dresden, Fetscherstraße 74, 01307 Dresden, Germany

N. Abolmaali
Institute and Policlinic of Diagnostic Radiology, University Hospital Carl Gustav Carus, TU Dresden, Fetscherstraße 74, 01307 Dresden, Germany

N. Abolmaali (✉)
Clinic for Radiology, Akademisches Lehrkrankenhaus Dresden-Friedrichstadt, Friedrichstraße 41, 01067 Dresden, Germany
e-mail: Abolmaali-Na@khdf.de

© Springer-Verlag Berlin Heidelberg 2016
M. Baumann et al. (eds.), *Molecular Radio-Oncology*, Recent Results
in Cancer Research 198, DOI 10.1007/978-3-662-49651-0_9

Keywords
Tumor microenvironment · Hypoxia imaging · FMISO-PET · Ant colony
optimization algorithm · Swarm intelligence · Image analysis

1   Introduction

In diagnostic imaging for oncology, non-invasive detection and localization of
biological properties in vivo like hypoxia of solid tumours is of increasing interest
and based on several publications (Lee et al. 2008; Thorwarth and Alber 2010; Choi
et al. 2010), numerous studies are ongoing to achieve a rational clinical application.
Early work demonstrating the use of the tracer [^{18}F]-fluoromisonidazole (FMISO)
in positron emission tomography (PET) showed the capability of assessing hypoxia
in vivo (Rasey et al. 1996). While FMISO-PET imaging remains promising (Le
et al. 2010; Abolmaali et al. 2009), controversies about imaging accuracy and
reproducibility are discussed (Nehmeh et al. 2008; Mortensen et al. 2010; Yasuda
et al. 2013; Okamoto et al. 2013). Hypoxia imaging visualizes changes in the
tumour microenvironment during therapy (Lee et al. 2009), and resulting
imaging-derived parameters appear to be promising prognostic factors for the
evaluation of therapy response (Rajendran et al. 2006; Eschmann et al. 2005;
Hugonnet et al. 2011; Zips et al. 2012). On the other hand, it was also reported that

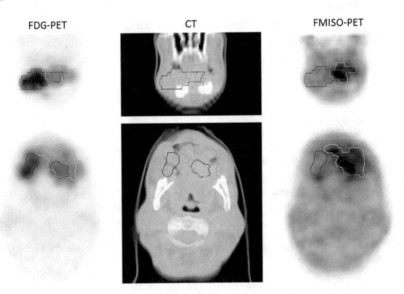

Fig. 1 Using FMISO-PET, a new perspective on tumour biology could be added to the
established imaging modalities. In this patient, a tumour at the base of the mouth contains two
subvolumes comprising differences in biological properties: the right lateral part delineated in *red*
accumulates FDG more than the part on the left side. The region of increased FMISO uptake
outlined in *green* appears reverse

neither the presence nor the absence of increased FMISO uptake after four weeks of chemoradiotherapy may correlate with therapy outcome (Lee et al. 2009). Neverthe-less, a major aim of hypoxia imaging is to inform the clinician on the presence of hypoxia and to support him in making therapeutic decisions. By adding a reliable method for hypoxia detection to the imaging procedure, the clinician could get another perspective to tumour biology as emphasized in Fig. 1. Tumour hypoxia may indicate decreased response independent from chosen therapy (Höckel et al. 1993) and indi-vidualizing therapy after analysis of biological imaging data may improve therapeu-tical success. Upcoming approaches in the field of radiotherapy, such as intensity-modulated radiotherapy (IMRT) and image-guided radiotherapy (IGRT), allow for the inclusion of biological aspects such as hypoxia into RT planning, but none of the proposed strategies (Thorwarth and Alber 2010; Lee et al. 2008; Madani et al. 2007) has reached wide acceptance in clinical practice yet. Other hypoxia tracers such as [^{18}F]-EF5 and [^{18}F]-FAZA have also been investigated (Komar et al. 2008; Beck et al. 2007; Souvatzoglou et al. 2007). But tracer uptake within the tumour is not higher using these tracers compared to FMISO (Souvatzoglou et al. 2007; Dubois et al. 2009; Grönroos and Minn 2007). Furthermore, image contrast is just at the same order of magnitude using FMISO. On the contrary, [18F]-fluorodeoxyglucose (FDG) PET delivers images containing significantly higher standard uptake values (SUV) within the tumour volume and lower SUVs in normal tissues. Accordingly, FDG PET images show an image contrast about one order of magnitude higher than when using FMISO (Abolmaali et al. 2011). Improvements of FMISO-PET image quality may be obtained by the following: 1) using new scanner technology such as improved detectors (Yasuda et al. 2013), 2) introduction of signal improving algorithms (Hofheinz et al. 2011), 3) developing imaging protocols producing data sets with the best achievable contrast (Abolmaali et al. 2011) and 4) methods for partial volume correction (Hof-heinz et al. 2012). However, reliable target volume delineation is a prerequisite. Thus, it is worthwhile developing approaches for accurate delineation of hypoxic volumes in low-contrast FMISO-PET images. This article summarizes the abilities of standard threshold-based segmentation approaches in this field and the given limitations. Alternatives utilizing more complex algorithms are outlined.

2 Application of Conventional Threshold-Based Algorithms to FMISO-PET

In FMISO-PET image analysis, standardized thresholds were already applied to dif-ferentiate between normoxic and hypoxic tissues (Rajendran et al. 2006; Swanson et al. 2009). The possibility of rough differentiation between these tissues cannot be denied, since hypoxic tissues actually may show higher uptake than surrounding tissues. But the resulting delineation should be treated with caution. On the one hand, the methodology of applying thresholds to volume data is of limited accuracy because of the given spatial resolution of clinical PET scanners. A PET scanner may not be able to measure hypoxia-induced high-tracer uptake if necrosis and hypoxia are mixed inside the tumour volume (Swanson et al. 2009) or even worse a small amount of hypoxic cancerous stem cells survive in a necrotic environment. Pronounced perfusion in adjacent regions may have a similar effect on FMISO uptake in hypoxic regions (Cho et al. 2009). Currently, there is no reference standard for hypoxia quantification in vivo beside invasive pO2-measurements (Chapman et al. 2001) and the development of a non-invasive reference quantification is not foreseeable. Furthermore, correlation between FMISO-PET and pO2-measurements using Eppendorf electrodes was not observed in a clinical set-up, but FMISO-PET delivered lower hypoxia measurements compared to Eppendorf pO2 measurements (Mortensen et al. 2010). Therefore, the expected high false-negative rate of FMISO-PET in assessing hypoxia is difficult to measure in a clinical environment, where Eppendorf electrodes are not part of the examination routine.

Considering FMISO-PET images show higher uptake within hypoxic tumour volumes poses the question as to whether such a volume can be delineated correctly using a single predefined threshold. This aspect has been investigated for FDG PET imaging of peripheral lung lesions (Biehl et al. 2006), where the contrast between FDG avid lesions and normal lung parenchyma with very limited FDG uptake is high. The authors showed that even in this preferable situation, no single threshold applied to PET data is capable to delineate volumes accurately compared to reference delineations from computed tomography (CT). This conclusion is expected to be transferable to FMISO-PET since the same tomography technique is used and comparable biological mechanisms are generating the uptake. Nevertheless, results are expected to be even worse since FMISO-PET reveals significantly lower contrast between normal and hypoxic tissues. However, hypoxia measurements resulting from FMISO-PET imaging may allow predicting local progression free survival based on thresholding even though image quality is limited (Zips et al. 2012).

In general, there are three straight-forward ways for determining the threshold to segment PET data:

- The first is to assume a relative threshold depending on the mean activity measured in blood samples (Swanson et al. 2009; Thorwarth et al. 2005).
- Secondly, the threshold can be determined relative to the maximum activity inside tumour volume (Nehmeh et al. 2009).
- Thirdly, a threshold level can be applied that depends on the mean activity measured in a reference region of the PET data set (Eschmann et al. 2005; Abolmaali et al. 2011).

When determining an appropriate threshold and verifying it by manual visual observation, it depends not only on surrounding tissue, the pertinent organ and technological aspects, such as the chosen reconstruction algorithm. The chosen threshold and resulting final delineation depends also on the individual investigator and applied display window settings (Nestle et al. 2005). A similar effect of image characteristics to delineations was observed for automatic segmentation algorithms (Cheebsumon and van Velden 2011; Cheebsumon and Yaqub 2011). Furthermore, small changes on the threshold may in one case result in contour changes which are hard to see but in other cases may lead to dramatic volume differences. This fact, highlighted in Fig. 2, may be

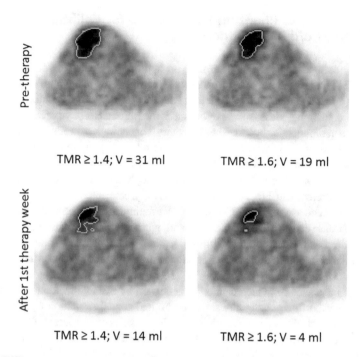

Fig. 2 Different target-to-muscle-ratio (TMR) thresholds applied on two FMISO-PET data sets acquired before therapy and after the first therapy week. The choice of the threshold appears decisive for volume delineation. Using a threshold of TMR $\geq$ 1.4 leads to the conclusion that the hypoxic volume halved during one week, the threshold TMR $\geq$ 1.6 suggests volume reduction by quartering. The observed differences are a result of the applied threshold, not entirely a result of biological properties

of importance when applying constant thresholds to repeated FMISO-PET imaging data to observe therapy progress. Varying thresholds may alternatively change the measured reproducibility of FMISO-PET. The work of Nehmeh et al. (2008) is often cited to underline limited reproducibility of FMISO-PET itself, but the authors found a strong correlation of activity distribution in patients scanned twice using FMISO-PET. The correlation decreased dramatically after applying a fixed background-dependent threshold to the data sets, as proposed by Rajendran and analysing the remaining voxels (Rajendran et al. 2006). One source of this aspect of limited reproducibility in FMISO-PET may be the threshold approach and not solely the imaging technique. Additionally the technique of using voxel-wise Pearson correlation coefficient seems to be inadequate to measure reproducibility of serial PET scans (Schwartz et al. 2011; Westgard 2008). The observations of Nehmeh et al. that FMISO-PET is of limited reproducibility was furthermore contradicted in a recent study applying similar analysis methods to a different patient cohort (Okamoto et al. 2013).

3 Limitations of Phantom Experiments for Calibration of Threshold-Based Algorithms

A widely accepted approach to determine an appropriate threshold for volume definition in PET imaging is the use of phantom experiments for calibrating segmentation algorithms (Nehmeh et al. 2009; Schaefer et al. 2008). Several groups utilized cylinder phantoms containing glass spheres for such measurements. Cylinder and spheres contained a radionuclide, but the mean activity concentration inside and outside the spheres differed. Varying activity levels were set up by using the same radionuclide but different solutions in spheres and cylinder to achieve constant activity ratios. Alternatively two different radionuclides in spheres and cylinder were placed. The radionuclides have different half-life, and thus, mean activity concentrations within sphere and cylinder will decrease differently with time. Resulting images show varying contrast with time (Haase et al. 2010). On the one hand, gathering images, when using the same radionuclide, is time-consuming requiring several phantom experiments. Using different nuclides is more efficient but introduces differing mean positron ranges in the imaging process. At the boundaries of the target objects, a gradient may appear in the dual radionuclide set-up, which cannot be generated by a single radionuclide. But this effect is expected to be negligible, since the limited spatial resolution of clinical PET scanners may not allow for measuring it. Using spheres with glass walls introduces another source of error in the process. There is no activity inside the glass walls, and therefore, the boundary between sphere and cylinder can be delineated more accurately than in patient data sets having no glass sphere around the target volume. This effect was surveyed earlier (Hofheinz et al. 2010; van den Hoff and Hofheinz 2013), and its importance for low-contrast PET was emphasized: thresholds determined in phantom experiments may not be appropriate if background activity is high in respect to the mean activity concentration in a target volume. Additionally the PET-detectable walls of the spheres, shown in Fig. 3, can lead to artefacts in the attenuation map used for correction of the PET signal. This fact leads to the idea of using wax spheres without

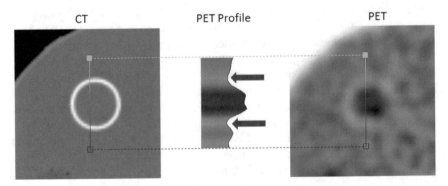

Fig. 3 In the CT data set of a phantom experiment, the glass walls of a target simulating sphere are clearly visible. However, if the ratio between target and background activity is low enough, in this case 1.5, the sphere also becomes visible in the corresponding PET image and the profile through the target volume (*red arrows*)

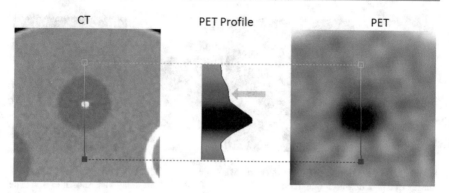

Fig. 4 When utilizing wax spheres as target volume simulation in a phantom experiment, the target volume may appear homogeneous in CT. But in the corresponding PET image, it is obvious that a subvolume of the sphere shows decreased signal intensity. The region is depicted in the profile through the target sphere with an *orange arrow*

inactive walls (Bazañez-Borgert et al. 2008). But creating wax spheres with homogenously distributed activity concentration is technically challenging (Haase et al. 2010). Resulting PET imaging data may show cold areas within the hot spheres as shown in Fig. 4. However, this kind of phantom experiments performed on a combined PET/CT scanner in principal offers the opportunity to calibrate and validate segmentation algorithms in general because of the CT-measurable volume of the spheres as reference measurement. But for a final evaluation of a determined threshold more sophisticated algorithms, the new methods should be validated by applying them to clinical data sets.

4 Image Contrast Limits Abilities of Established PET Segmentation Algorithms

Our investigations encouraged us to accept the hypothesis that there is no threshold-based algorithm which generates appropriate volume delineations for FMISO-PET. Major challenges of PET image segmentation, such as inhomogeneities and non-spherical target volumes, were reviewed before (Lee 2010). In addition, FMISO-PET segmentation is complicated by a low ratio of activity, i.e. the low contrast, between target volume and surrounding tissue. Threshold-based algorithms allow FDG PET data sets to be segmented more accurately. The edge between target and background is high due to high activity ratio between the tissues. But it must be stated that even when analysing FDG PET, estimation of the optimal threshold remains challenging. In non-small cell lung cancer (NSCLC), where the activity concentration in the surrounding lung tissue is low, the boundary of the target object can be segmented using a range of algorithms (Schaefer et al. 2008; Nehmeh et al. 2009; Hofheinz et al. 2012; Jentzen et al. 2007). But when analysing FMISO-PET data sets of the head and neck region, we found that the mean target-to-muscle-ratio (TMR) is often less than 2:1 (Abolmaali et al. 2011). The values of an amount of voxels inside the presumptive hypoxic subvolume may be equal or lower than grey

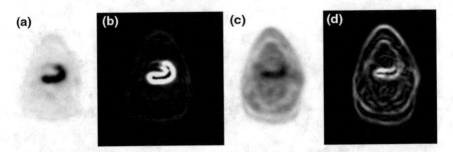

Fig. 5 Edge detection filter (Sobel operator) was applied to axial **a** FDG PET and **c** FMISO-PET images of a patient with hypopharyngeal cancer. Resulting gradient images are shown in **b**, **d**. The pixels in the filtered images **b** and **d** are white, if a high activity gradient is present in the surrounding pixels, and black, if the gradient is negligible. In the FMISO-PET image, several edges are visible and the edge of the target volume is not clearly differentiable

values of the surrounding tissue. The contrast is insufficient to differentiate tissue based directly on voxel values. This finding seems to be independent on the method; neither histogram-based algorithms nor methods calibrated by phantom measurements may deliver accurate delineations.

Gradient-based methods may also not be suitable to overcome these issues, because without high ratios between the structures to differentiate, there is no steep gradient which can be utilized as boundary between the volumes. To visualize the effect on gradient-based methods, two gradient images of an FDG and an FMISO-PET data set are shown in Fig. 5. It demonstrates that gradients between target and background in FMISO-PET are not distinguishable from gradients within or outside the target volume. Signal fluctuations between different tissues may be misinterpreted as boundary of a false-positive target volume.

5   Further Developments on Segmentation Algorithms for Low-Contrast PET Data

Nevertheless, there are several approaches published that may be able to deliver improved segmentation results when applied to low-contrast PET data such as FMISO-PET. Stated key aspects used multimodal information (Yu et al. 2009), spatial information (Montgomery et al. 2007) and intelligent algorithms (Haase et al. 2011; Hsu et al. 2008; Sharif et al. 2010). Methods like these may allow overcoming issues such as volume reproducibility in repeated FMISO-PET, explained in the first paragraph, as shown in Fig. 6.

All of these methods have still to be validated in detail for low-contrast FMISO-PET patient data. They are also connected by the fact that additional information to the value of voxels is utilized to find the solution to the segmentation problem. The measured uptake inside a single voxel alone does not allow its classification. This single activity value needs to be connected with data from other imaging modalities and/or with

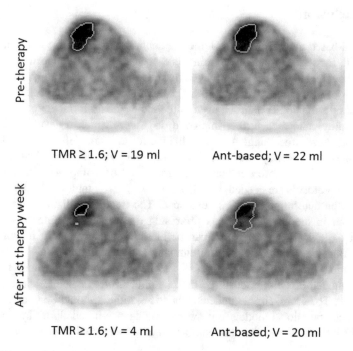

Fig. 6 When applying the ant-based segmentation algorithm proposed by our group (Haase et al. 2010), increased contour reproducibility and volume stability can be observed in repeated FMISO-PET compared to standard thresholds like TMR $\geq$ 1.6

voxels in its neighbourhood. In particular, in head and neck cancer, several different tissues are surrounding the periphery of the tumour compared to the central parts. Therefore, an approach is needed which is able to differentiate between the volumes having different properties in each imaging modality. For example, determining intersections between FMISO-PET indicated hypoxia and limited perfusion shown on dynamic contrast enhanced (DCE) magnetic resonance imaging (MRI) may deliver reliable information for interpreting the tumour microenvironment correctly (Cho et al. 2009). The combined analysis of FDG PET and CT data, currently becoming standard in clinical routine, offers advantages to tumour delineation (Nestle et al. 2009), and the number of automatic delineation approaches using the combination of FDG PET and CT is increasing. This trend may be the first step in introducing fully automatic, observer independent, multimodal segmentation approaches utilizing more than just two imaging modalities. First investigations in the field of multiparametric analysis of tumour microenvironment using different PET tracers, CT and MRI are promising (Kawai et al. 2011; Dirix et al. 2009). The research focus on FDG PET/CT fusion in the recent years ensures this approach to be a safe basis for combining several views of the same tumour and to deliver more perspectives than each modality could contribute alone.

6   Conclusions

Threshold-based algorithms for volume segmentation in PET were not found to be applicable for segmenting low-contrast data accurately. These algorithms may be able to show trends like decreasing hypoxic subvolume during therapy. But a single threshold for accurate delineation in one patient data set is not expected to deliver precise results in another data set, even of the same patient. If tracer uptake and thus image quality cannot be further improved, it is worthwhile to develop new algorithms for image processing. A new technique for accurate delineation of hypoxic subvolumes is urgently needed, especially for low-contrast data sets like FMISO-PET. To increase delineation accuracy, not only improved imaging techniques and protocols are needed, but also more intelligent, multimodal and complex segmentation algorithms must be developed. The trend of utilizing multimodality information in therapy planning is promising due to the dependencies between different biological aspects, which can be measured using modern imaging techniques. But the complexity of multimodal and multidimensional information interpretation may exceed human abilities, because comparing more than two imaging modalities with each three or four dimensions in image space is not a trivial task. Therefore, simple understandable algorithms should be combined with complex computational models, e.g. swarm intelligence-based algorithms, allowing for better interpretation of multimodal and multidimensional information.

Acknowledgments This work was supported by the ERDF European Regional Development Fund, project "Gemeinsames Zentrum für Strahlenforschung in der Onkologie", Contract Number 100066308.

References

Abolmaali N et al (2009) Imaging radiation biology for optimised radiation therapy. Int J. of Radiat. Biol. 85(9): 729–31. Available at: http://www.ncbi.nlm.nih.gov/pubmed/19728192 Accessed 22 Nov 2013

Abolmaali N et al (2011) Two or four hour [18F]FMISO-PET in HNSCC. When is the contrast best? Nuklearmedizin Nucl. Med. 50(1): 22–7. Available at: http://www.ncbi.nlm.nih.gov/pubmed/21165537 Accessed 22 Nov 2013

Bazañez-Borgert M et al (2008) Radioactive spheres without inactive wall for lesion simulation in PET. Zeitschrift für Medizinische Physik 18(1):37–42. Available at: http://linkinghub.elsevier.com/retrieve/pii/S0939388907000761 Accessed 22 Nov 2013

Beck R et al (2007) Pretreatment 18F-FAZA PET predicts success of hypoxia-directed radiochemotherapy using tirapazamine. J Nucl Med. 48(6): 973–80. Available at: http://www.ncbi.nlm.nih.gov/pubmed/17536108 Accessed 22 Nov 2013

Biehl KJ et al (2006) 18F-FDG PET definition of gross tumor volume for radiotherapy of non-small cell lung cancer: is a single standardized uptake value threshold approach appropriate? J. of Nucl. Med. 47(11): 1808–1182. Society of Nuclear Medicine. Available at: http://www.ncbi.nlm.nih.gov/pubmed/17079814

Chapman JD, Zanzonico P, Ling CC (2001) On measuring hypoxia in individual tumors with radiolabeled agents. J. of Nucl. Med. 42(11): 1653–1653. Society of Nuclear Medicine, Available at: http://www.ncbi.nlm.nih.gov/pubmed/11696634

Cheebsumon P, van Velden, FHP et al (2011) Effects of image characteristics on performance of tumor delineation methods: a test-retest assessment. J. of Nucl. Med. 52(10): 1550–1558. Society of Nuclear Medicine, Available at: http://www.ncbi.nlm.nih.gov/pubmed/21849398 Accessed 16 Nov 2013

Cheebsumon P, Yaqub M et al (2011) Impact of [18F]FDG PET imaging parameters on automatic tumour delineation: need for improved tumour delineation methodology. Eur. J. of Nucl. Med. and Mol. Imaging 38(12): 2136–2144. Available at: http://www.pubmedcentral.nih.gov/articlerender.fcgi?artid=3228515&tool=pmcentrez&rendertype=abstract Accessed 22 Nov 2013

Cho HJ et al (2009) Noninvasive multimodality imaging of the tumor microenvironment: registered dynamic magnetic resonance imaging and positron emission tomography studies of a preclinical tumor model of tumor hypoxia. Neoplasia 11(3):247–259

Choi W et al (2010) Planning study for available dose of hypoxic tumor volume using fluorine-18-labeled fluoromisonidazole positron emission tomography for treatment of the head and neck cancer. Radiother. and oncol.: J. of the Euro. Soc. for Ther. Radiol. and Oncol. 97(2): 176–182. Available at: http://www.ncbi.nlm.nih.gov/pubmed/20855118 Accessed 22 Nov 2013

Dirix P et al (2009) Dose painting in radiotherapy for head and neck squamous cell carcinoma: value of repeated functional imaging with (18)F-FDG PET, (18)F-fluoromisonidazole PET, diffusion-weighted MRI, and dynamic contrast-enhanced MRI. J. of Nucl. Med. 50(7): 1020–1027. Society of Nuclear Medicine, Available at: http://www.ncbi.nlm.nih.gov/pubmed/19525447 Accessed ember 22 Nov 2013

Dubois L et al (2009) [18F]EF3 is not superior to [18F]FMISO for PET-based hypoxia evaluation as measured in a rat rhabdomyosarcoma tumour model. Euro. J. of Nucl. Med. and Mol. Imaging 36(2): 209–218. Available at: http://www.ncbi.nlm.nih.gov/pubmed/18690432 Accessed 22 Nov 2013

Eschmann S-M et al (2005) Prognostic impact of hypoxia imaging with 18f-misonidazold pet in non-small cell lung cancer and head and neck cancer before radiotherapy. J Nucl Med 46 (2):253–260

Grönroos T, Minn H (2007) Imaging of tumour hypoxia using PET and 18F-labelled tracers: biology meets technology. Euro. J. of Nucl. Med. and Mol. Imaging 34(10): 1563–1565. Available at: http://www.ncbi.nlm.nih.gov/pubmed/17598110 Accessed 22 Nov 2013

Haase R et al (2010) A new segmentation approach for f-18-fluoromisonidazole positron emission tomography data based on ant colony optimization: considering reproducibility. In: Crossing the Borders with ABC, Automation, Biomedical Engineering and Computer Science, 55th IWK, TU Ilmenau, 505–510

Haase R et al (2011) Swarm intelligence for medical volume segmentation: the contribution of self-reproduction. In: Lecture notes on Computer Science 7006, on KI 2011: Advances in Artificial Intelligence, 111–121

Höckel M et al (1993) Intratumoral pO2 predicts survival in advanced cancer of the uterine cervix. Radiother. and Oncol. 26(1): 45–50. Available at: http://www.ncbi.nlm.nih.gov/pubmed/8438086

Hofheinz F et al (2010) Effects of cold sphere walls in PET phantom measurements on the volume reproducing threshold. Phys. in Med. and Biol 55(4): 1099–1113. Available at: http://www.ncbi.nlm.nih.gov/pubmed/20107246 Accessed 22 Nov 2013

Hofheinz F et al (2011) Suitability of bilateral filtering for edge-preserving noise reduction in PET. EJNMMI Res. 1(1): 23. Available at: http://www.pubmedcentral.nih.gov/articlerender.fcgi?artid=3250981&tool=pmcentrez&rendertype=abstract Accessed 22 Nov 2013

Hofheinz F et al (2012) Automatic volume delineation in oncological PET. Evaluation of a dedicated software tool and comparison with manual delineation in clinical data sets. Nuklearmedizin Nucl. Med. 51(1): 9–16. Available at: http://www.ncbi.nlm.nih.gov/pubmed/22027997 Accessed 22 Nov 2013

Hsu C-Y, Liu C-Y, Chen C-M (2008) Automatic segmentation of liver PET images. Comput. Med. Imaging and Graph.: The Off. J. of the Comput. Med. Imaging Soc. 32(7): 601–610. Available at: http://www.ncbi.nlm.nih.gov/pubmed/18722751 Accessed 22 Nov 2013

Hugonnet F et al (2011) Metastatic renal cell carcinoma: relationship between initial metastasis hypoxia, change after 1 month's sunitinib, and therapeutic response: an 18F-fluoromisonidazole PET/CT study. J. Nucl. Med. 52(7): 1048–1055. Available at: http://www.ncbi.nlm.nih.gov/pubmed/21680694 Accessed 22 Nov 2013

Jentzen W et al (2007) Segmentation of PET volumes by iterative image thresholding. J. of Nucl. Med.48(1): 108–114. Society of Nuclear Medicine, Available at: http://www.ncbi.nlm.nih.gov/pubmed/17204706

Kawai N et al (2011) Correlation of biological aggressiveness assessed by 11C-methionine PET and hypoxic burden assessed by 18F-fluoromisonidazole PET in newly diagnosed glioblastoma. Euro. J.of Nucl. Med. and Mol. Imaging 38(3): 441–450. Available at: http://www.ncbi.nlm.nih.gov/pubmed/21072512 Accessed 13 Nov 2013

Komar G et al (2008) 18F-EF5: a new PET tracer for imaging hypoxia in head and neck cancer. J. Nucl. Med. 49(12): 1944–1951. Available at: http://www.ncbi.nlm.nih.gov/pubmed/18997048 Accessed 22 Nov 2013

Le Q, Loo BW, Lee N (2010) Hypoxia imaging for image-guided radiotherapy In: Tamaki N, Kuge Y (eds) Molecular Imaging for Integrated Medical Therapy and Drug Development, 7–18. Available at: http://link.springer.com/10.1007/978-4-431-98074-2 Accessed 22 Nov 2013

Lee JA (2010) Segmentation of positron emission tomography images: some recommendations for target delineation in radiation oncology. Radioth. and Oncol. : J. of the Euro. Soc. for Ther. Radiol. and Oncol. 96(3): 302–307. Available at: http://www.ncbi.nlm.nih.gov/pubmed/20708286 Accessed 22 Nov 2013

Lee N et al (2009) Prospective trial incorporating pre-/mid-treatment [18 F]-misonidazole positron emisson tomography for head and neck cancer patients undergoing concurrent chemoradiotherapy. Int. J. Rad. Oncology Biol. Phys. 75(1):101–108

Lee NY. et al (2008) Fluorine-18-labeled fluoromisonidazole positron emission and computed tomography-guided intensity-modulated radiotherapy for head and neck cancer: a feasibility study. Int J. of Rad. Oncol. Biol. Phys. 70(1): 2–13. Available at: http://www.pubmedcentral.nih.gov/articlerender.fcgi?artid=2888477&tool=pmcentrez&rendertype=abstract Accessed 12 Nov 2013

Madani I et al (2007) Positron emission tomography-guided, focal-dose escalation using intensity-modulated radiotherapy for head and neck cancer. Int. J. of Rad. Oncol. Biol. Phys. 68(1): 126–135. Available at: http://www.ncbi.nlm.nih.gov/pubmed/17448871 Accessed 22 Nov 2013

Montgomery DWG, Amira A, Zaidi H (2007) Fully automated segmentation of oncological PET volumes using a combined multiscale and statistical model. Med. Phys. 34(2):722. Available at: http://link.aip.org/link/MPHYA6/v34/i2/p722/s1&Agg=doi Accessed 22 Nov 2013

Mortensen LS et al (2010) Identifying hypoxia in human tumors: A correlation study between 18F-FMISO-PET and the Eppendorf oxygen-sensitive electrode. Acta oncologica 49(7), Sweden, Stockholm, 934–40. Available at: http://www.ncbi.nlm.nih.gov/pubmed/20831480 Accessed 22 Nov 2013

Nehmeh SA et al (2008) Reproducibility of Intratumor Distribution of 18F-Fluoromisonidazole in Head and Neck Cancer. Int. J. of Rad. Oncol. Biol. Phys. 70(1): 235–242. Available at: http://linkinghub.elsevier.com/retrieve/pii/S0360301607038990 Accessed 20 Nov 2013

Nehmeh SA et al (2009) An iterative technique to segment PET lesions using a Monte Carlo based mathematical model. Med. Phy. 36(10): 4803–4809. Available at: http://link.aip.org/link/MPHYA6/v36/i10/p4803/s1&Agg=doi Accessed 22 Nov 2013

Nestle U et al (2009) Biological imaging in radiation therapy: role of positron emission tomography. Phys. in Med. and Biol. 54(1): 1–25. Available at: http://www.ncbi.nlm.nih.gov/pubmed/19060363 Accessed 22 Nov 2013

Nestle U et al (2005) Comparison of different methods for delineation of 18 f-fdg pet-positive tissue for target volume definition in radiotherapy of patients with non-small cell lung cancer. J Nucl Med 46(8):1342–1348

Okamoto S et al (2013) High reproducibility of tumor hypoxia evaluated by 18F-fluoromisonidazole PET for head and neck cancer. J. of Nucl. Med. 54(2): 201–207. Society of Nuclear Medicine, Available at: http://www.ncbi.nlm.nih.gov/pubmed/23321456 Accessed 22 Nov 2013

Rajendran JG et al (2006) Tumor hypoxia imaging with [F-18] fluoromisonidazole positron emission tomography in head and neck cancer. Clin. Cancer Res. 12(18): 5435–5441. Available at: http://www.ncbi.nlm.nih.gov/pubmed/17000677 Accessed 12 Nov 2013

Rasey JS et al (1996) Quantifying regional hypoxia in human tumors with positron emission tomography of [18F]fluoromisonidazole: a pretherapy study of 37 patients. Int. J. Radiat. Oncol. Biol. Phys. 36(2):417–428

Schaefer A et al (2008) A contrast-oriented algorithm for FDG-PET-based delineation of tumour volumes for the radiotherapy of lung cancer: derivation from phantom measurements and validation in patient data. Euro. J. of Nucl. Med. and Mol. Imaging 35(11):1989–1999. Available at: http://www.ncbi.nlm.nih.gov/pubmed/18661128 Accessed 22 Nov 2013

Schwartz J et al (2011) Repeatability of SUV measurements in serial PET. Med. Phy. 38(5): 2629–2638. Available at: http://link.aip.org/link/MPHYA6/v38/i5/p2629/s1&Agg=doi Accessed 22 Nov 2013

Sharif MS et al (2010) Artificial Neural Network-Based System for PET Volume Segmentation. Int. J. of Biomed. Imaging. Available at: http://www.pubmedcentral.nih.gov/articlerender.fcgi?artid=2948894&tool=pmcentrez&rendertype=abstract Accessed 22 Nov 2013

Souvatzoglou M et al (2007) Tumour hypoxia imaging with [18F]FAZA PET in head and neck cancer patients: a pilot study. Euro. J. of Nucl. Med. and Mol. Imaging 34(10): 1566–1675. Available at: http://www.ncbi.nlm.nih.gov/pubmed/17447061 Accessed 22 Nov 2013

Swanson KR et al (2009) Complementary but distinct roles for MRI and 18F-fluoromisonidazole PET in the assessment of human glioblastomas. J. of Nucl. Med. 50(1): 36–44. Society of Nuclear Medicine. Available at: http://www.ncbi.nlm.nih.gov/pubmed/19091885 Accessed 21 Nov 2013

Thorwarth D et al (2005) Kinetic analysis of dynamic 18F-fluoromisonidazole PET correlates with radiation treatment outcome in head-and-neck cancer. BMC cancer 5(152). Available at: http://www.pubmedcentral.nih.gov/articlerender.fcgi?artid=1325034&tool=pmcentrez&rendertype=abstract Accessed 22 Nov 2013

Thorwarth D, Alber M (2010) Implementation of hypoxia imaging into treatment planning and delivery. Radiother. and Oncol. 97(2): 172–175. Available at: http://www.ncbi.nlm.nih.gov/pubmed/20570382 Accessed 22 Nov 2013

Van den Hoff J. Hofheinz F (2013) Comments on comparative study with new accuracy metrics for target volume contouring in PET image guided radiation therapy. IEEE Trans. on Med. Imaging 32(6): 1146–1148. Available at: http://www.ncbi.nlm.nih.gov/pubmed/23247847

Westgard JO (2008) Use and interpretation of common statistical tests in method comparison studies. Clin. Chem. 54(3): 612. Available at: http://www.ncbi.nlm.nih.gov/pubmed/18310152 Accessed 22 Nov 2013

Yasuda K et al. (2013) [18F]fluoromisonidazole and a new PET system with semiconductor detectors and a depth of interaction system for intensity modulated radiation therapy for nasopharyngeal cancer. Int. J. of Rad. Oncol. Biol. Phys. 85(1): 142–147. Available at: http://www.ncbi.nlm.nih.gov/pubmed/22583608 Accessed 20 Nov 2013

Yu H et al (2009) Automated radiation targeting in head-and-neck cancer using region-based texture analysis of PET and CT images. Int. J. of Rad. Oncol. Biolo. Phy. 75(2): 618–25. Available at: http://www.ncbi.nlm.nih.gov/pubmed/19683403 Accessed 22 Nov 2013

Zips D et al (2012) Exploratory prospective trial of hypoxia-specific PET imaging during radiochemotherapy in patients with locally advanced head-and-neck cancer. Radiothe. and Oncol. : J. of the Euro. Soc. for Ther. Radiol. and Oncol. 105(1): 21–28. Available at: http://www.ncbi.nlm.nih.gov/pubmed/23022173 Accessed 18 Nov 2013

FMISO as a Biomarker for Clinical Radiation Oncology

Sebastian Zschaeck, Jörg Steinbach and Esther G.C. Troost

Abstract

Tumour hypoxia is a well-known negative prognostic marker in almost all solid tumours. [18F]Fluoromisonidazole (FMISO)-positron emission tomography (PET) is a non-invasive method to detect tumour hypoxia. Compared to other methods of hypoxia assessment it possesses some considerable advantages: It is non-invasive, it delivers spatial information on the hypoxia distribution within the entire tumour volume, and it can be repeated during the course of radio (chemo)therapy. This chapter briefly describes different methods of hypoxia

S. Zschaeck · E.G.C. Troost
OncoRay - National Center for Radiation Research in Oncology,
Medical Faculty and University Hospital Carl Gustav Carus,
Technische Universität Dresden and Helmholtz-Zentrum
Dresden-Rossendorf, Dresden, Germany

S. Zschaeck · E.G.C. Troost
German Cancer Consortium (DKTK), Dresden, Germany

S. Zschaeck (✉) · E.G.C. Troost
German Cancer Research Center (DKFZ), Heidelberg, Germany
e-mail: Sebastian.Zschaeck@uniklinikum-dresden.de

S. Zschaeck · E.G.C. Troost
Department of Radiation Oncology, Faculty of Medicine and University
Hospital Carl Gustav Carus, Technische Universität Dresden,
Fetscherstrasse 74, 01307 Dresden, Germany

J. Steinbach
Helmholtz-Zentrum Dresden-Rossendorf, Institute of Radiopharmaceutical
Cancer Research, Helmholtz-Zentrum Dresden-Rossendorf, Dresden, Germany

E.G.C. Troost
Helmholtz-Zentrum Dresden-Rossendorf, Institute of Radiooncology,
Helmholtz-Zentrum Dresden-Rossendorf, Dresden, Germany

© Springer-Verlag Berlin Heidelberg 2016
M. Baumann et al. (eds.), *Molecular Radio-Oncology*, Recent Results
in Cancer Research 198, DOI 10.1007/978-3-662-49651-0_10

evaluation and focuses on hypoxia PET imaging, with the most commonly used tracer being FMISO. The preclinical rationale and clinical studies to use FMISO-PET for patient stratification in radiation therapy are discussed as well as possible agents or radiation-dose modifications to overcome hypoxia.

Keywords

Hypoxia · FMISO · [18F]Fluoromisonidazole · PET · Positron emission tomography

1 Background on Tumour Cell Hypoxia

Tumour heterogeneity plays a pivotal role in several solid tumours regarding the outcome after surgery, radiotherapy and chemotherapy. Amongst the various tumour characteristics, tumour cell hypoxia is the most relevant in the field of radiation oncology. Hypoxia is generally differentiated into chronic, i.e. diffusion-limited hypoxia caused by rapid tumour growth with insufficient neo-vascularization and impaired oxygen supply, and acute hypoxia, i.e. acute decrease in perfusion due to functional impairment of the (neo-) vasculature. Tumour cell hypoxia is known to negatively affect patients' outcome irrespective of the chosen therapeutic approach (surgery, radiotherapy) as shown in a landmark study for cancer of the uterine cervix (Hockel et al. 1996). It is known to promote local tumour growth, lymph node involvement and distant metastases formation. In radiotherapy, the unfavourable therapeutic effect may be caused by hampering the formation of free radicals after photon irradiation, a prerequisite for the envisaged biological effect. This phenomenon can be expressed by the oxygen enhancement ratio (OER) that compares the biological efficacy of radiotherapy under oxic versus anoxic conditions.

Several strategies to improve outcome in patients presenting with hypoxic tumours have been developed and used in clinical studies. These include the following: hyperbaric oxygen breathing, carbogen breathing or the additional application of hypoxia sensitizers to the standard treatment (Jordan and Sonveaux 2012; Janssens et al. 2012). Furthermore, the nitroimidazole derivative nimorazole has been extensively studied in several Danish studies and is now routinely used for Danish head and neck squamous cell carcinoma (HNSCC) patients. Cytotoxic agents activated under hypoxic conditions include tirapazamine (Rischin et al. 2010) or the novel agent TH-302 (Borad et al. 2014). The benefit of hypoxia modification (by various means) in HNSCC even without stratification for the hypoxic status has been shown by a large meta-analysis by Overgaard, analysing 4805 patients treated within 32 randomized clinical trials (Overgaard 2011). With modern radiation techniques facilitating highly selective dose delivery, the concept of the biological target volume, introduced by Ling et al. (Ling et al. 2000) in 2000, has gained interest. For hypoxic tumours are radiation resistant, an increase in radiation dose, either to the whole tumour volume or selectively to the hypoxic subvolumes of the tumour only (dose painting), is aimed for. The latter approach can be either performed on a (manually or semi-manually) delineated subvolume or by prescribing individual doses to every voxel (dose painting by numbers) (Thorwarth et al. 2007). Obviously, it is important to assess the level of hypoxia both globally and on tumour subvolume level before and during (chemo)radiotherapy in order to facilitate these dose-painting techniques.

This chapter briefly addresses invasive measures to quantify hypoxia, but focuses on positron emission tomography (PET) of hypoxia-related markers as they may repeatedly image the entire tumour volume, and even more importantly, this technique is non-invasive.

2 Invasive Assessment of Tumour Cell Hypoxia

The classical gold standard for determination of the oxygen partial pressure has been the Eppendorf electrode. For its easy accessibility, the longest experience for pre-therapeutic Eppendorf electrode measurements exists in carcinomas of the uterine cervix (Hockel et al. 1996; Hoogsteen et al. 2009; Yaromina et al. 2006). This technique holds some important drawbacks: it has an invasive nature, is labour-intensive and cannot be used in all solid tumours for poor accessibility. Furthermore, Eppendorf electrode measurements only analyse small portions of the tumour and are unable to distinguish between vital hypoxic and anoxic necrotic tumour subvolumes.

Another attempt to measure tumour cell hypoxia is the immunohistochemical staining of histological samples that were obtained from the tumour or lymph node metastases. There are both exogenous markers, i.e. they need to be administered to the patient via an infusion or tablet, and endogenous markers, i.e. upregulated hypoxia-related markers. The most commonly used exogenous marker currently considered the reference standard is pimonidazole. Pimonidazole detects hypoxia below 10 mmHg (1.3 kPa) and has been used in preclinical and clinical studies (Hoogsteen et al. 2009; Yaromina et al. 2006). In the past, it required intravenous administration approximately 30–60 min before gathering the biopsy, but meanwhile an oral form exists and is FDA-approved. For logistic and financial reasons, endogenous markers of hypoxia have been pursued. These include hypoxia-inducible factor 1 alpha (HIF-1α), carbonic anhydrase-IX (CA-IX), vascular endothelial growth factor (VEGF) and the glucose transporters 1 and 3 (Glut-1 and Glut-3) (Troost et al. 2005; Ogawa et al. 2011; Goethals et al. 2006; Bussink et al. 2003). Noteworthy, the expression of these endogenous markers is influenced by a plethora of mechanisms and not exclusively driven by hypoxia. In accordance with Eppendorf electrode measurement, immunohistochemical staining of biopsies only represents a fraction of the entire tumour, is burdensome for the patients and is not ideal for repeated measurement of hypoxia.

Another attempt to quantify hypoxia is the use of serological blood biomarkers. Osteopontin is probably the best-established blood marker in the context of radiotherapy. In a HNSCC tumour cell line, hypoxia was found to upregulate osteopontin via a Ras-activated enhancer (Zhu et al. 2005). Plasma osteopontin correlated inversely with pO (Jordan and Sonveaux 2012) measured by Eppendorf electrodes in both HNSCC and NSCLC patient cohorts, and with worse clinical outcome in a variety of solid tumours (Le et al. 2003, 2006; Buijsen et al. 2014; Ostheimer et al. 2014). However, the factors influencing osteopontin levels and the additional value of combining several blood biomarkers (Osteopontin, VEGF and CA-IX) are subject of ongoing research (Ostheimer et al. 2014; Lukacova et al. 2005). A fourth strategy assessing tumour hypoxia is genetic analysis. Toustrup et al. (Toustrup et al. 2011) identified a hypoxia gene expression profile in vitro and validated the classifier in vivo in HNSCC xenograft models. In the latter model, they additionally checked whether tumour heterogeneity affected the gene profile, i.e. whether biopsies from mixed hypoxic and oxic areas yielded representative results compared to autoradiography with a hypoxia-related PET tracer. They found measurable upregulation of hypoxia genes even in tumour biopsies taken from mixed hypoxic and oxic subvolumes as identified with autoradiography PET imaging. Figure 1 gives an overview of established hypoxia detection methods.

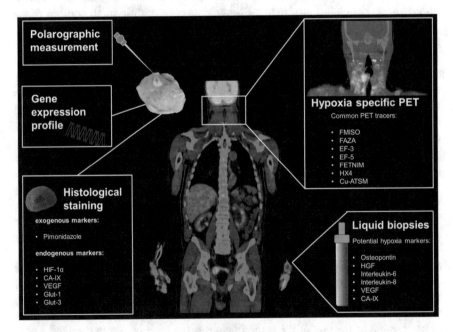

Fig. 1 Overview of different hypoxia detection methods

3 PET Imaging of Hypoxia and Relevance in (Radiation) Oncology

A non-invasive method for the detection and quantification of tumour cell hypoxia is PET imaging with hypoxia specific radiotracers, amongst which imidazole derivates are most commonly used. Imaging hypoxia via PET has several advantages for radiotherapy compared to the aforementioned methods: The entire tumour volume can be assessed at several time points prior to and during treatment, and it can be used for dose-redistribution based on biological tumour characteristics, e.g. hypoxia (Hendrickson et al. 2011). Notably, [^{18}F]Fluoro-deoxyglucose (FDG) may inherit some information on intratumoural hypoxia due to upregulation of Glut-1 by HIF-1α, but is aspecific and should, therefore, not be used for hypoxia imaging (Van Baardwijk et al. 2007).

Already in 1979, J.C. Chapman from the University of Alberta, Canada, recognized the importance of hypoxic sensitizers for radiation therapy and shortly thereafter he utilized ^{14}C-labelled misonidazole for the imaging of hypoxic areas in murine tumours (Chapman et al. 1981; Chapman 1979). He described the importance as future markers for hypoxic cells in tumours with potential clinical applicability (Garrecht and Chapman 1983). For diagnosis of ischaemia, Mathias et al. (1987) presented a first concept for radiotracers to be applied in nuclear medicine techniques based on hypoxic sensitizers.

Since then, [^{18}F]Fluoromisonidazole (FMISO) has become the hypoxia PET tracer most commonly used in a variety of solid tumours (Rajendran and Krohn 2015). Figure 2 shows the chemical structure of FMISO.

Additional imidazole tracers, including 5-[^{18}F]fluoro-5-deoxy-D-arabinofuranosyl-2-nitroimidazole (FAZA), [^{18}F]nitroimidazole-*N*-trifluoropropyl-acetamide (EF-3), [^{18}F]nitroimidazole-*N*-pentafluoropropyl-acetamide (EF-5), [^{18}F] fluoroerythronitroimidazole (FETNIM), or [^{18}F]fluoro-nitro-*H*-imidazol-methyl-*H*-triazol-propanol (HX4), have mainly been designed to improve the slow accumulation in comparison with FMISO within the tumour, and to enhance the signal-to-background ratio (SBR). Beside them, the SPECT or PET radiotracer 5-[$^{123/124}$I]iodo-5-deoxy-D-arabinofuranosyl-2-nitroimidazole (IAZA) is available (Reischl et al. 2007). Non-Imidazole tracers, e.g. [^{64}Cu]Cu-diacetyl-bis-*N*-methyl-thiosemicarbazone (Cu-ATSM) are less frequently used and may also reflect

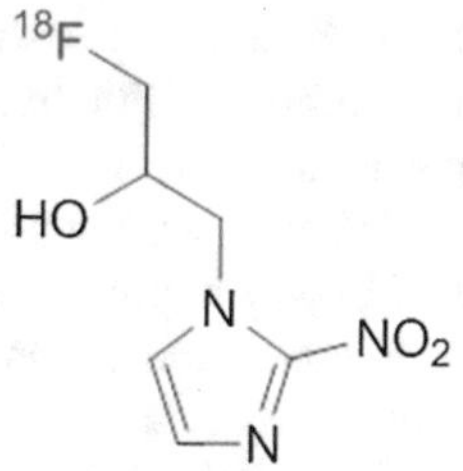

Fig. 2 Chemical structure of FMISO, the most important PET hypoxia marker

tumour perfusion rather than being a hypoxia-selective tracer (Movahedi et al. 2012). Due to the poor availability of ^{64}Cu a broad application is not visible. All these hypoxia specific tracers, except for Cu-ATSM, share the necessity of a relatively long interval between tracer injection and imaging and therefore are merely a surrogate of chronic instead of acute hypoxia. Off note, there are various additional imaging methods for the assessment of hypoxia, including blood oxygenation level-dependent (BOLD) magnetic resonance imaging (MRI) or optical spectroscopy, but discussion of these is beyond the scope of this chapter (Horsman et al. 2012; Chitneni et al. 2011).

4   Preclinical Validation Studies

Many in vivo studies focused on the correlation of different methods for hypoxia detection in order to move from invasive to non-invasive ones. One study compared FMISO uptake in rodent tumour xenograft models with robotic-guided multiple pO_2 measurement via electrodes and found a high non-concordance in some individual data pairs, possibly explained by partially necrotic, i.e. anoxic, subvolumes that do not take up the tracer (Chang et al. 2009). Numerous studies have shown a reasonably good correlation between hypoxic subvolumes as detected by pimonidazole immunohistochemistry and FMISO and FAZA uptake by autoradiography and/or microPET, under varying levels of oxygenation or artificially induced clamp hypoxia (Troost et al. 2008; Busk et al. 2008, 2009, 2013; Troost et al. 2006). Figure 3 depicts examples of pimonidazole-stained and FMISO-autoradiographed xenografts under different oxygen conditions.

In a study comparing the aforementioned hypoxia tracers FMISO, FAZA, HX4 and Cu-ATSM with pimonidazole and CA-IX immunohistochemistry in a head and neck xenograft tumour line, all except for Cu-ATSM showed similar distributions within the tumour (Carlin et al. 2014).

Comparing the different tracers per se, modelling as well as preclinical studies have suggested a superior SBR of FAZA compared to FMISO, however, data are conflicting (Busk et al. 2013; Busk et al. 2009). Peeters et al. (2015) recently compared FMISO, FAZA and HX4 in rats bearing syngeneic rhabdomyosarcoma R1 tumours. As expected and probably due to its high lipophilicity, the maximum SBR for FMISO was not reached until 6 h, as compared to 2 h for FAZA and 3 h for HX4. Remarkably, whereas all three tracers were able to monitor artificially induced hypoxia, only FMISO was able to successfully depict hypoxia-modifying treatment with nicotinamide and carbogen. Finally, the spatial reproducibility of FMISO in two consecutive scans obtained within a 48-h interval was best. The low conformity of FAZA shown in this study is somehow surprising for another study showed a good reproducibility of FAZA hypoxic volumes, even after fractionated radiotherapy (Busk et al. 2013). In other publications, FMISO and HX4 were both able to detect decreased levels of hypoxia after carbogen breathing (Troost et al. 2006; Dubois et al. 2011), and FAZA uptake decreased after pure oxygen breathing (Piert et al. 2005).

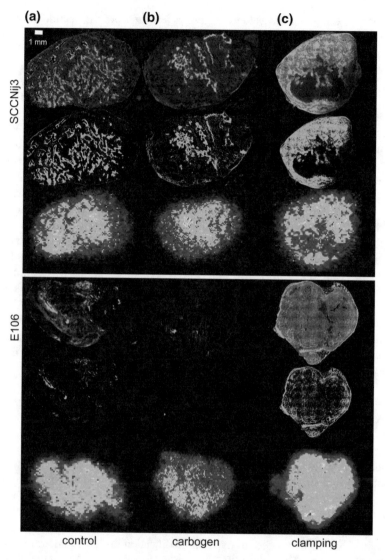

Fig. 3 Pseudo-coloured grey-value pimonidazole images (*top row*), images after segmentation of the pimonidazole signal (*middle row*), and FMISO autoradiography images (*bottom row*) of head and neck squamous cell carcinoma (SCCNij3) and glioblastoma (E106) xenograft tumour lines for control tumours, after carbogen breathing and clamping. Figure taken with kind permission from (Troost et al. 2006)

Data on Cu-ATSM are conflicting. Cu-ATSM has neither shown a good correlation with pimonidazole and CA-IX staining in solid tumour models, nor with FAZA uptake (Yuan et al. 2006; McCall et al. 2012). A correlation with FMISO uptake and oxygen probe measurement existed when applying an exceptional long time period between tracer injection and acquisition (O'Donoghue et al. 2005).

When investigating the value of hypoxia imaging, pre-therapeutic FAZA-PET was found to predict the therapeutic efficacy of adding nimorazole to radiotherapy in a preclinical sarcoma, but not in a glioma model (Bol et al. 2015). In rhabdomyosarcoma and NSCLC tumour models, Peeters et al. (2015) showed an association between the HX4-PET-derived hypoxic volume and tumour growth delay after treatment, and a benefit of the novel hypoxia specific cytotoxic agent TH-302 when combined with single-dose radiotherapy. In a recent study in HNSCC xenografts, Schütze et al. (2014) asserted the role of the FMISO-derived hypoxic volume and possible implications for subsequent dose escalation. Tumours with hypoxic volumes below the median had a significantly better local control rate after single-dose radiotherapy than those with hypoxic volumes above median. Interestingly, an increase of the single dose by another 10 Gy lead to similar increases of local control for both subgroups. Hence, tumour hypoxia as depicted by FMISO-PET is probably not barely a shift on the dose-effect curve for tumour control probability. If this had been the case, the same dose increase would have led to a much lower gain in tumour control in the hypoxic tumour subgroup. Rather, other effects most probably also play a role. The observations by Schütze et al. justify an attempt to moderately escalate the dose in hypoxic tumours to substantially increase the tumour control probability.

Taken together the preclinical data support the strong role of preclinical FMISO-PET-imaging as it correlates well with other established methods of hypoxia detection, it has a high reproducibility, and it reflects relevant therapy-induced changes.

5 Clinical Studies

After primary or (neo)adjuvant (chemo)radiotherapy, hypoxia in particular affects treatment outcome in tumours with unsatisfactory local control rates, e.g. glioblastomas, locally advanced NSCLC and locally advanced HNSCC (Mortensen et al. 2012; Rischin et al. 2006). In a recent review article, the prognostic value of PET-measured hypoxia, in particular FMISO-PET, for local tumour control has been highlighted (Rajendran and Krohn 2015). Moreover, a large meta-analysis underlined the positive effect of hypoxia modification on local tumour control and treatment outcome (Overgaard 2007). In order to select patients benefitting from treatment modification and to prevent those patients not benefitting from suffering undesired treatment-related side effects, methods to stratify patients are mandatory.

Stratification may be based on relatively simple parameters including tumour necrosis, on plasma markers, or a hypoxia gene set (Eustace et al. 2013). However, for aforementioned reasons, non-invasive imaging is of particular interest. Several recent studies have shown the prognostic value of hypoxia PET imaging regarding outcome after (chemo)radiotherapy in various solid tumours (Mortensen et al. 2012; Servagi-Vernat et al. 2014; Zips et al. 2012; Bollineni et al. 2014; Zegers et al. 2013). Zips et al. (2012) highlighted the prognostic value of FMISO-PET imaging obtained after one and two weeks of (chemo)radiotherapy in a cohort of 25 HNSCC patients.

Fig. 4 Example of 2 patients treated with cT3N2cM0 oropharyngeal cancer and FMISO-PET imaging. Patient **a** showed residual hypoxia and presented local recurrence 5 months after treatment. Patient **b** showed dissolution of hypoxia; this patient remained recurrence-free during follow-up

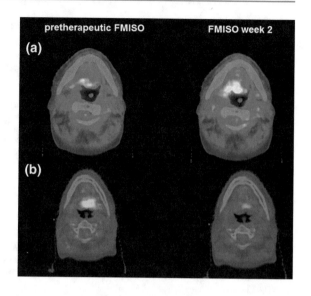

Conversely, FMISO-PET imaging obtained before treatment did not correlate with outcome. Figure 4 shows two patients of this study with sequential FMISO scans. In a small study cohort, Dirix et al. (2009) investigated FDG- and FMISO-PET, T1- and T2-weighted MRI, diffusion-weighted-(DWI-)MRI and dynamic contrast-enhanced (DCE-)MRI at various time points before and during primary radiotherapy in 15 HNSCC patients. Apart from the prognostic value of DWI- and DCE-MRI for locoregional recurrence, the prognostic value of FMISO-PET was underlined. A Danish study also found FAZA-PET imaging to stratify patients into groups according to loco-regional control (Mortensen et al. 2012). FMISO-PET imaging was part of a phase II clinical study on hypoxia-modification in patients with advanced HNSCC. In a substudy on 45 patients, FMISO-PET imaging prior to chemoradiotherapy was found to be a predictive marker selecting patients benefitting from the addition of tirapazamine (Rischin et al. 2006). In the cohort treated with chemoradiotherapy, 8 of 13 patients with tumour cell hypoxia as depicted by FMISO-PET experienced local relapse, whereas in the experimental arm, only 1 of 19 patients with hypoxia developed local recurrence.

Although older publications have shown conflicting results, recent studies have reported a good spatial reproducibility of repeated FMISO-PET-based hypoxic subvolumes obtained prior to initiation of (chemo)radiotherapy (Okamoto et al. 2013). Regarding reproducibility during treatment, Bittner et al. (2013) analysed the size, location and overlap of FMISO-PET positive subvolumes in 16 HNSCC patients. In patients with persistent hypoxia after 2 weeks of chemoradiotherapy, the FMISO-positive subvolumes mostly remained geographically stable. Summarizing these data, they prompt the scientific community to integrate hypoxia PET imaging into radiation treatment planning for hypoxia-directed dose escalation strategies.

At present, a German mono-institutional randomized phase II clinical trial investigates the clinical feasibility of FMISO-PET-based dose escalation in HNSCC (Welz et al. 2014). Patients in the standard arm undergo a conventional total dose of 70 Gy (chemo)radiotherapy, whereas in the experimental arm, patients receive 10 % dose escalation, i.e. 77 Gy, to the FMISO-PET-defined hypoxic subvolume. The planned interim analysis for the first 20 patients recruited into this study showed that dose escalation in this order of magnitude is well tolerated. Additionally, results of this study have thus far confirmed a prognostic model relating the dynamic FMISO-PET data to the individual tumour control probability established in an earlier study (Thorwarth et al. 2014).

References

Bittner M-I, Wiedenmann N, Bucher S, Hentschel M, Mix M, Weber WA et al (2013) Exploratory geographical analysis of hypoxic subvolumes using (18)F-MISO-PET imaging in patients with head and neck cancer in the course of primary chemoradiotherapy. Radiother Oncol 108 (3):511–516

Bol A, Labar D, Cao-Pham TT, Jordan B, Grégoire V et al (2015) Predictive value of (18)F-FAZA PET imaging for guiding the association of radiotherapy with nimorazole: a preclinical study. Radiother Oncol 114(2):189–194

Bollineni VR, Koole MJB, Pruim J, Brouwer CL, Wiegman EM, Groen HJM et al (2014) Dynamics of tumor hypoxia assessed by 18F-FAZA PET/CT in head and neck and lung cancer patients during chemoradiation: possible implications for radiotherapy treatment planning strategies. Radiother Oncol 113(2):198–203

Borad MJ, Reddy SG, Bahary N, Uronis HE, Sigal D, Cohn AL et al (2014) Randomized phase II trial of gemcitabine plus TH-302 versus gemcitabine in patients with advanced pancreatic cancer. J Clin Oncol

Buijsen J, van Stiphout RG, Menheere PPCA, Lammering G, Lambin P (2014) Blood biomarkers are helpful in the prediction of response to chemoradiation in rectal cancer: a prospective, hypothesis driven study on patients with locally advanced rectal cancer. Radiother Oncol 111 (2):237–242

Busk M, Horsman MR, Jakobsen S, Keiding S, van der Kogel AJ, Bussink J et al (2008) Imaging hypoxia in xenografted and murine tumors with 18F-fluoroazomycin arabinoside: a comparative study involving microPET, autoradiography, PO_2-polarography, and fluorescence microscopy. Int J Radiat Oncol Biol Phys 70(4):1202–1212

Busk M, Horsman MR, Jakobsen S, Hansen KV, Bussink J, van der Kogel A et al (2009) Can hypoxia-PET map hypoxic cell density heterogeneity accurately in an animal tumor model at a clinically obtainable image contrast? Radiother Oncol 92(3):429–436

Busk M, Mortensen LS, Nordsmark M, Overgaard J, Jakobsen S, Hansen KV et al (2013) PET hypoxia imaging with FAZA: reproducibility at baseline and during fractionated radiotherapy in tumour-bearing mice. Eur J Nucl Med Mol Imaging 40(2):186–197

Bussink J, Kaanders JHAM, van der Kogel AJ (2003) Tumor hypoxia at the micro-regional level: clinical relevance and predictive value of exogenous and endogenous hypoxic cell markers. Radiother Oncol 67(1):3–15

Carlin S, Zhang H, Reese M, Ramos NN, Chen Q, Ricketts S-A (2014) A comparison of the imaging characteristics and microregional distribution of 4 hypoxia PET tracers. J Nucl Med 55 (3):515–521

Chang J, Wen B, Kazanzides P, Zanzonico P, Finn RD, Fichtinger G et al (2009) A robotic system for 18F-FMISO PET-guided intratumoral pO_2 measurements. Med Phys 36(11):5301–5309

Chapman JD (1979) Hypoxic sensitizers–implications for radiation therapy. N Engl J Med 301 (26):1429–1432

Chapman JD, Franko AJ, Sharplin J (1981) A marker for hypoxic cells in tumours with potential clinical applicability. Br J Cancer 43(4):546–550

Chitneni SK, Palmer GM, Zalutsky MR, Dewhirst MW (2011) Molecular imaging of hypoxia. J Nucl Med 52(2):165–168

Dirix P, Vandecaveye V, De Keyzer F, Stroobants S, Hermans R, Nuyts S (2009) Dose painting in radiotherapy for head and neck squamous cell carcinoma: value of repeated functional imaging with (18)F-FDG PET, (18)F-fluoromisonidazole PET, diffusion-weighted MRI, and dynamic contrast-enhanced MRI. J Nucl Med 50(7):1020–1027

Dubois LJ, Lieuwes NG, Janssen MHM, Peeters WJM, Windhorst AD, Walsh JC et al (2011) Preclinical evaluation and validation of [18F]HX4, a promising hypoxia marker for PET imaging. Proc Natl Acad Sci USA 108(35):14620–14625

Eustace A, Irlam JJ, Taylor J, Denley H, Agrawal S, Choudhury A et al (2013) Necrosis predicts benefit from hypoxia-modifying therapy in patients with high risk bladder cancer enrolled in a phase III randomised trial. Radiother Oncol 108(1):40–47

Garrecht BM, Chapman JD (1983) The labelling of EMT-6 tumours in BALB/C mice with 14C-misonidazole. Br J Radiol 56(670):745–753

Goethals L, Debucquoy A, Perneel C, Geboes K, Ectors N, De Schutter H et al (2006) Hypoxia in human colorectal adenocarcinoma: comparison between extrinsic and potential intrinsic hypoxia markers. Int J Radiat Oncol Biol Phys 65(1):246–254

Hendrickson K, Phillips M, Smith W, Peterson L, Krohn K, Rajendran J (2011) Hypoxia imaging with [F-18] FMISO-PET in head and neck cancer: potential for guiding intensity modulated radiation therapy in overcoming hypoxia-induced treatment resistance. Radiother Oncol 101 (3):369–375

Hockel M, Schlenger K, Aral B, Mitze M, Schaffer U, Vaupel P (1996) Association between tumor hypoxia and malignant progression in advanced cancer of the uterine cervix. Cancer Res 56(19):4509–4515

Hoogsteen IJ, Lok J, Marres HAM, Takes RP, Rijken PFJW, van der Kogel AJ et al (2009) Hypoxia in larynx carcinomas assessed by pimonidazole binding and the value of CA-IX and vascularity as surrogate markers of hypoxia. Eur J Cancer 45(16):2906–2914

Horsman MR, Mortensen LS, Petersen JB, Busk M, Overgaard J (2012) Imaging hypoxia to improve radiotherapy outcome. Nat Rev Clin Oncol 9(12):674–687

Janssens GO, Rademakers SE, Terhaard CH, Doornaert PA, Bijl HP, van den Ende P et al (2012) Accelerated radiotherapy with carbogen and nicotinamide for laryngeal cancer: results of a phase III randomized trial. J Clin Oncol 30(15):1777–1783

Jordan BF, Sonveaux P (2012) Targeting tumor perfusion and oxygenation to improve the outcome of anticancer therapy. Front Pharmacol 3:94

Le Q-T, Sutphin PD, Raychaudhuri S, Yu SCT, Terris DJ, Lin HS et al (2003) Identification of osteopontin as a prognostic plasma marker for head and neck squamous cell carcinomas. Clin Cancer Res 9(1):59–67

Le Q-T, Chen E, Salim A, Cao H, Kong CS, Whyte R et al (2006) An evaluation of umor oxygenation and gene expression in patients with early stage non-small cell lung cancers. Clin Cancer Res 12(5):1507–1514

Ling CC, Humm J, Larson S, Amols H, Fuks Z, Leibel S et al (2000) Towards multidimensional radiotherapy (MD-CRT): biological imaging and biological conformality. Int J Radiat Oncol Biol Phys 47(3):551–560

Lukacova S, Khalil AA, Overgaard J, Alsner J, Horsman MR (2005) Relationship between radiobiological hypoxia in a C3H mouse mammary carcinoma and osteopontin levels in mouse serum. Int J Radiat Biol 81(12):937–944

Mathias CJ, Welch MJ, Kilbourn MR, Jerabek PA, Patrick TB, Raichle ME et al (1987) Radiolabeled hypoxic cell sensitizers: tracers for assessment of ischemia. Life Sci 41 (2):199–206

McCall KC, Humm JL, Bartlett R, Reese M, Carlin S (2012) Copper-64-diacetyl-bis(N(4)-methylthiosemicarbazone) pharmacokinetics in FaDu xenograft tumors and correlation with microscopic markers of hypoxia. Int J Radiat Oncol Biol Phys 84(3):e393–e399

Mortensen LS, Johansen J, Kallehauge J, Primdahl H, Busk M, Lassen P et al (2012) FAZA PET/CT hypoxia imaging in patients with squamous cell carcinoma of the head and neck treated with radiotherapy: results from the DAHANCA 24 trial. Radiother Oncol 105(1):14–20

Movahedi K, Schoonooghe S, Laoui D, Houbracken I, Waelput W, Breckpot K et al (2012) Nanobody-based targeting of the macrophage mannose receptor for effective in vivo imaging of tumor-associated macrophages. Cancer Res 72(16):4165–4177

O'Donoghue JA, Zanzonico P, Pugachev A, Wen B, Smith-Jones P, Cai S et al (2005) Assessment of regional tumor hypoxia using 18F-fluoromisonidazole and 64Cu(II)-diacetyl-bis (N4-methylthiosemicarbazone) positron emission tomography: Comparative study featuring microPET imaging, PO$_2$ probe measurement, autoradiography, and fluorescent microscopy in the R3327-AT and FaDu rat tumor models. Int J Radiat Oncol Biol Phys 61(5):1493–1502

Ogawa K, Chiba I, Morioka T, Shimoji H, Tamaki W, Takamatsu R et al (2011) Clinical significance of HIF-1alpha expression in patients with esophageal cancer treated with concurrent chemoradiotherapy. Anticancer Res 31(6):2351–2359

Okamoto S, Shiga T, Yasuda K, Ito YM, Magota K, Kasai K et al (2013) High reproducibility of tumor hypoxia evaluated by 18F-fluoromisonidazole PET for head and neck cancer. J Nucl Med 54(2):201–207

Ostheimer C, Bache M, Güttler A, Reese T, Vordermark D (2014a) Prognostic information of serial plasma osteopontin measurement in radiotherapy of non-small-cell lung cancer. BMC Cancer 14:858

Ostheimer C, Bache M, Güttler A, Kotzsch M, Vordermark D (2014b) A pilot study on potential plasma hypoxia markers in the radiotherapy of non-small cell lung cancer. Osteopontin, carbonic anhydrase IX and vascular endothelial growth factor. Strahlenther Onkol 190 (3):276–282

Overgaard J (2007) Hypoxic radiosensitization: adored and ignored. J Clin Oncol 25(26):4066–4074

Overgaard J (2011) Hypoxic modification of radiotherapy in squamous cell carcinoma of the head and neck—a systematic review and meta-analysis. Radiother Oncol 100(1):22–32

Peeters SGJA, Zegers CML, Lieuwes NG, van Elmpt W, Eriksson J, van Dongen GAMS et al (2015a) A comparative study of the hypoxia PET tracers [^{18}F]HX4, [^{18}F]FAZA, and [^{18}F] FMISO in a preclinical tumor model. Int J Radiat Oncol Biol Phys 91(2):351–359

Peeters SGJA, Zegers CML, Biemans R, Lieuwes NG, van Stiphout RGPM, Yaromina A et al (2015b) TH-302 in combination with radiotherapy enhances the therapeutic outcome and is associated with pretreatment [18F]HX4 hypoxia PET imaging. Clin Cancer Res

Piert M, Machulla H-J, Picchio M, Reischl G, Ziegler S, Kumar P et al (2005) Hypoxia-specific tumor imaging with 18F-fluoroazomycin arabinoside. J Nucl Med 46(1):106–113

Rajendran JG, Krohn KA (2015) F-18 fluoromisonidazole for imaging tumor hypoxia: imaging the microenvironment for personalized cancer therapy. Semin Nucl Med 45(2):151–162

Reischl G, Dorow DS, Cullinane C, Katsifis A, Roselt P, Binns D et al (2007) Imaging of tumor hypoxia with [124I]IAZA in comparison with [18F]FMISO and [18F]FAZA–first small animal PET results. J Pharm Pharm Sci 10(2):203–211

Rischin D, Hicks RJ, Fisher R, Binns D, Corry J, Porceddu S et al (2006) Prognostic significance of [18F]-misonidazole positron emission tomography-detected tumor hypoxia in patients with advanced head and neck cancer randomly assigned to chemoradiation with or without tirapazamine: a substudy of Trans-Tasman Radiation Oncology Group Study 98.02. J Clin Oncol 24(13):2098–2104

Rischin D, Peters LJ, O'Sullivan B, Giralt J, Fisher R, Yuen K et al (2010) Tirapazamine, cisplatin, and radiation versus cisplatin and radiation for advanced squamous cell carcinoma of the head and neck (TROG 02.02, HeadSTART): a phase III trial of the Trans-Tasman Radiation Oncology Group. J Clin Oncol 28(18):2989–2995

Schütze C, Bergmann R, Brüchner K, Mosch B, Yaromina A, Zips D et al (2014) Effect of [(18)F] FMISO stratified dose-escalation on local control in FaDu hSCC in nude mice. Radiother Oncol 111(1):81–87

Servagi-Vernat S, Differding S, Hanin F-X, Labar D, Bol A, Lee JA et al (2014) A prospective clinical study of ^{18}F-FAZA PET-CT hypoxia imaging in head and neck squamous cell carcinoma before and during radiation therapy. Eur J Nucl Med Mol Imaging 41(8):1544–1552

Thorwarth D, Eschmann S-M, Paulsen F, Alber M (2007) Hypoxia dose painting by numbers: a planning study. Int J Radiat Oncol Biol Phys 68(1):291–300

Thorwarth D, Monnich D, Wack L et al (2014) Validation of a hypoxia TCP model and dose painting in HNC: Planned interim analysis of a phase II trial. Radiother Oncol 111(Suppl 1):134

Toustrup K, Sørensen BS, Nordsmark M, Busk M, Wiuf C, Alsner J et al (2011) Development of a hypoxia gene expression classifier with predictive impact for hypoxic modification of radiotherapy in head and neck cancer. Cancer Res 71(17):5923–5931

Troost EGC, Bussink J, Kaanders JHAM, van Eerd J, Peters JPW, Rijken PFJW et al (2005) Comparison of different methods of CAIX quantification in relation to hypoxia in three human head and neck tumor lines. Radiother Oncol 76(2):194–199

Troost EGC, Laverman P, Kaanders JHAM, Philippens M, Lok J, Oyen WJG et al (2006) Imaging hypoxia after oxygenation-modification: comparing [18F]FMISO autoradiography with pimonidazole immunohistochemistry in human xenograft tumors. Radiother Oncol 80 (2):157–164

Troost EGC, Laverman P, Philippens MEP, Lok J, van der Kogel AJ, Oyen WJG et al (2008) Correlation of [18F]FMISO autoradiography and pimonidazole [corrected] immunohistochemistry in human head and neck carcinoma xenografts. Eur J Nucl Med Mol Imaging 35 (10):1803–1811

Van Baardwijk A, Dooms C, van Suylen RJ, Verbeken E, Hochstenbag M, Dehing-Oberije C et al (2007) The maximum uptake of (18)F-deoxyglucose on positron emission tomography scan correlates with survival, hypoxia inducible factor-1alpha and GLUT-1 in non-small cell lung cancer. Eur J Cancer 43(9):1392–1398

Welz S, Pfannenberg C, Reimold M et al (2014) Hypoxia dose-escalation with chemo-radiation in head and neck cancer: planned interim analysis of a randomized study. Radiother Oncol 111 (Suppl 1):155–156

Yaromina A, Zips D, Thames HD, Eicheler W, Krause M, Rosner A et al (2006) Pimonidazole labelling and response to fractionated irradiation of five human squamous cell carcinoma (hSCC) lines in nude mice: the need for a multivariate approach in biomarker studies. Radiother Oncol 81(2):122–129

Yuan H, Schroeder T, Bowsher JE, Hedlund LW, Wong T, Dewhirst MW (2006) Intertumoral differences in hypoxia selectivity of the PET imaging agent 64Cu(II)-diacetyl-bis (N4-methylthiosemicarbazone). J Nucl Med 47(6):989–998

Zegers CML, van Elmpt W, Wierts R, Reymen B, Sharifi H, Öllers MC et al (2013) Hypoxia imaging with [18F]HX4 PET in NSCLC patients: defining optimal imaging parameters. Radiother Oncol 109(1):58–64

Zhu Y, Denhardt DT, Cao H, Sutphin PD, Koong AC, Giaccia AJ et al (2005) Hypoxia upregulates osteopontin expression in NIH-3T3 cells via a Ras-activated enhancer. Oncogene 24(43):6555–6563

Zips D, Zöphel K, Abolmaali N, Perrin R, Abramyuk A, Haase R et al (2012) Exploratory prospective trial of hypoxia-specific PET imaging during radiochemotherapy in patients with locally advanced head-and-neck cancer. Radiother Oncol 105(1):21–28

Printed in the United States
By Bookmasters